Dear Reader,

When I started my gluten-free journey in 2010, I found it difficult to find recipes that were family friendly and easy to follow. Many of the recipes had expensive, hard-to-find ingredients and took a lot of time to cook, and honestly, my kids would not eat most of them.

So, I spent a lot of time in my kitchen testing different ingredients, trying to figure out how to modify our favorite meals to be gluten-free. Years later when I went dairy-free, I found it **easy to substitute** dairy-free alternatives in all of our favorite recipes. Eating gluten-free and dairy-free should not be very difficult or expensive, so I set out to fix that one recipe at a time. I have been able to modify classic recipes—like chocolate cake, so on your daughter's birthday, she can enjoy great-tasting cake just like the other kids. Another favorite is my gluten-free and dairy-free dinner rolls, so your dad, who was just recently diagnosed with celiac disease, can have his favorite rolls with Thanksgiving dinner too. I included a recipe for gluten-free and dairy-free fluffy pancakes, so now your **long-loved tradition** of making pancakes on Sunday morning can continue even though your partner is now gluten and dairy intolerant. You can also whip up gluten-free and dairy-free chocolate chip cookies, so your son can have cookies at the elementary school cookie party just like everyone else.

I could go on and on. These stories, and so many more just like them, are the reasons that I share my recipes in this cookbook with you. All of these **family favorites** can be easily made gluten-free and dairy-free. Baking and cooking are some of my love languages, and I love sharing what I make for my family. I hope that sharing my journey may help you with yours.

Happy baking and cooking,
Audrey Roberts

Welcome to the Everything® Series!

These handy, accessible books give you all you need to tackle a difficult project, gain a new hobby, comprehend a fascinating topic, prepare for an exam, or even brush up on something you learned back in school but have since forgotten.

You can choose to read an Everything® book from cover to cover or just pick out the information you want from our four useful boxes: Questions, Facts, Alerts, and Essentials. We give you everything you need to know on the subject, but throw in a lot of fun stuff along the way too.

question	fact
Answers to common questions.	Important snippets of information.

alert	essential
Urgent warnings.	Quick handy tips.

We now have more than 600 Everything® books in print, spanning such wide-ranging categories as cooking, health, parenting, personal finance, wedding planning, word puzzles, and so much more. When you're done reading them all, you can finally say you know Everything®!

PUBLISHER Karen Cooper

MANAGING EDITOR Lisa Laing

COPY CHIEF Casey Ebert

ASSOCIATE PRODUCTION EDITOR Jo-Anne Duhamel

ACQUISITIONS EDITOR Zander Hatch

SENIOR DEVELOPMENT EDITOR Laura Daly

EVERYTHING® SERIES COVER DESIGNER Erin Alexander

THE EVERYTHING®

GLUTEN-FREE & DAIRY-FREE COOKBOOK

AUDREY ROBERTS

of MamaKnowsGlutenFree.com

300 SIMPLE AND SATISFYING RECIPES WITHOUT GLUTEN OR DAIRY

ADAMS MEDIA

NEW YORK   LONDON   TORONTO   SYDNEY   NEW DELHI

"Every good and perfect gift is from above" (James 1:17).
To my loving husband and my wonderful children for all of their love and support.

adamsmedia

Adams Media
An Imprint of Simon & Schuster, Inc.
57 Littlefield Street
Avon, Massachusetts 02322

An Everything® Series Book.
Everything® and everything.com® are registered trademarks of Simon & Schuster, Inc.

First Adams Media trade paperback edition October 2019

ADAMS MEDIA and colophon are trademarks of Simon & Schuster.

For information about special discounts for bulk purchases, please contact Simon & Schuster Special Sales at 1-866-506-1949 or business@simonandschuster.com.

The Simon & Schuster Speakers Bureau can bring authors to your live event. For more information or to book an event contact the Simon & Schuster Speakers Bureau at 1-866-248-3049 or visit our website at www.simonspeakers.com.

Interior design by Colleen Cunningham
Photographs by Audrey Roberts

Manufactured in the United States of America

10 9 8 7 6

Library of Congress Cataloging-in-Publication Data
Names: Roberts, Audrey, author.
Title: The everything® gluten-free & dairy-free cookbook / Audrey Roberts of MamaKnowsGlutenFree.com.
Description: Avon, Massachusetts: Adams Media, 2019.
Series: Everything®.
Includes index.
Identifiers: LCCN 2019023007 (print) | LCCN 2019023008 (ebook) | ISBN 9781507211281 (pb) | ISBN 9781507211298 (ebook)
Subjects: LCSH: Gluten-free diet--Recipes. | Milk-free diet. | LCGFT: Cookbooks.
Classification: LCC RM237.86 .R586 2019 (print) | LCC RM237.86 (ebook) | DDC 641.3/09311--dc23
LC record available at https://lccn.loc.gov/2019023007
LC ebook record available at https://lccn.loc.gov/2019023008

ISBN 978-1-5072-1128-1
ISBN 978-1-5072-1129-8 (ebook)

Contents

4: POULTRY 83

5: BEEF AND PORK 115

12: DESSERTS   275

APPENDIX: WEEKLY MEAL PLANS   314

STANDARD US/METRIC MEASUREMENT CONVERSIONS   316

INDEX   317

Introduction

Gooey cinnamon roll cake, moist blueberry muffins, creamy casseroles, piping-hot deep-dish pizza, fluffy dinner rolls, classic party dips, and rich desserts—you might think you have to give up these foods because your doctor recommended a gluten- and dairy-free diet. But with *The Everything® Gluten-Free & Dairy-Free Cookbook*, you can still enjoy all these mouthwatering dishes and more!

If you've been diagnosed with celiac disease, a gluten intolerance, or dairy allergy or intolerance, changing your diet can be both life changing and lifesaving. You might have other health reasons besides those listed above to consider eliminating gluten or dairy from your diet as well.

With a gluten- and dairy-free diet, you may finally find relief from symptoms that have plagued you for years—all while still enjoying filling, flavorful dishes such as:

- Chocolate Cake Donuts
- Apple Cinnamon Quick Bread
- Southwest Tricolored Quinoa Salad
- Crunchy Coconut Chicken Bites
- Classic Shrimp Scampi
- Taco Soup
- Classic Vanilla Cake with Chocolate Buttercream

Instead of focusing on what you can't eat now, instead think about all the great foods you *can* eat, and celebrate the fact that you can still eat your favorite dishes—they'll just have slightly different ingredients in them. The three hundred recipes in this book will ensure that all your meals, snacks, and desserts are safe for you to eat and full of flavor. Best of all, the recipes use ingredients you can find at regular supermarkets, and you'll be able to make the dishes quickly and easily using step-by-step instructions.

Along with the tasty recipes, you'll also find other important information in this book for transitioning to a gluten- and dairy-free diet, such as how to avoid "hidden" gluten and dairy in foods you buy, and how to stock your pantry so you can make hundreds of mouthwatering dishes at a moment's notice. You'll learn tips on how to safely prepare gluten- and dairy-free foods without cross contamination, such as having separate toasters and labeling jars. To fully integrate your new diet into your daily life, you'll discover ideas on how to eat gluten- and dairy-free at work and while traveling.

While you can find some gluten- and dairy-free options at stores and restaurants nowadays, making dishes at home always yields tastier foods with flavors you can tailor to your and your family's personal preferences. Get ready to enjoy better health—start on your gluten-free and dairy-free lifestyle today!

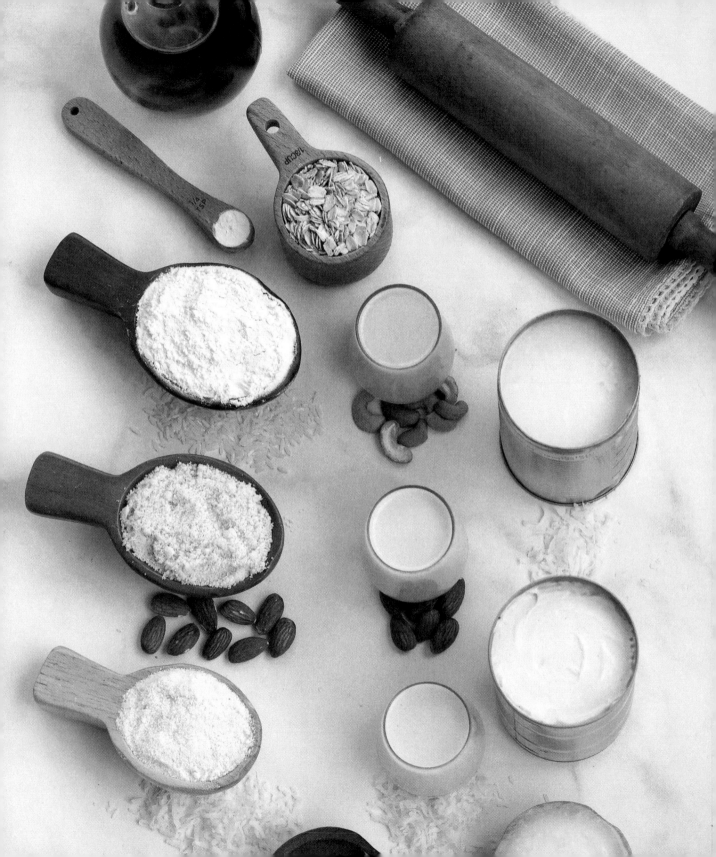

CHAPTER 1

Gluten-Free and Dairy-Free Living

Transitioning to a gluten- and dairy-free lifestyle doesn't have to be overwhelming or expensive. This chapter will explain exactly how consuming gluten and dairy could have been affecting the various systems in your body in an easy-to-understand way. Then you'll learn how to approach the change in your diet, from tips on product label reading to identifying which ingredients to reach for and which to stay away from. The tips in this chapter will help your switch to a gluten- and dairy-free diet be an easy transition.

Gluten-Free 101

Gluten is a naturally occurring protein found in several types of grains, such as wheat, barley, and rye. It is the substance that strengthens dough and gives bread its texture. By itself, gluten has the consistency of cornstarch and the stringy quality of chewing gum. It does not have a specific look, appearance, or color, so it can be hard to identify in foods.

Common Symptoms

If you are gluten intolerant or have celiac disease, eating gluten can cause adverse reactions and make you very sick. If people who have celiac disease eat gluten, the protein interferes with the absorption of nutrients by damaging parts of the small intestine called *villi*. Villi are small projections that line the small intestine and help your body absorb nutrients. When the villi are damaged, the small intestine is unable to properly absorb nutrients from the foods you eat. The inability to get nutrients from food is a serious issue that can lead to malnourishment and a whole host of other medical problems. Common symptoms of celiac disease are chronic diarrhea or constipation, bloating, gas, and anemia. In children, it can present as "failure to thrive" (when a child displays insufficient weight gain).

Another condition associated with gluten is non-celiac gluten sensitivity, also known as *gluten intolerance*. People with non-celiac gluten sensitivity do not test positive for celiac disease. However, they experience similar symptoms to people with celiac disease, and when gluten is removed from their diet, the symptoms resolve. The most frequently reported symptoms are abdominal pain, cramping, weight gain or loss, bloating, constipation, and diarrhea. These symptoms can be very disruptive to everyday life.

Diagnosing Gluten Issues

Because symptoms vary widely from person to person, diagnosing celiac disease or gluten sensitivities can unfortunately take a while. However, certain blood tests can diagnose celiac disease. Your doctor might also recommend an endoscopy to check the lining of the small intestine. (These tests require the patient to be eating gluten in order to be accurate.)

Another way to know if you should not eat gluten is to eliminate all gluten from your diet for at least a month to see if any of your symptoms disappear. That means *100 percent of all gluten* must be gone from your foods! Before you consider this option, talk to your doctor or your child's pediatrician. Following the gluten-free trial period, if you try eating gluten again and your symptoms return, then you have pretty good evidence that you should be gluten-free. Note that if you are being tested for celiac disease, you should not do an elimination diet until your doctor does the blood tests and possible endoscopy.

Treatments

There is no "cure" for celiac disease or gluten intolerance beyond following a gluten-free diet. The good news is that people with celiac disease and gluten intolerance will usually see significant symptom improvement once they completely remove gluten from their diets.

Which Foods Have Gluten?

One of the biggest challenges that people find early in the gluten-free journey is understanding how to identify which products contain gluten. Gluten is used in countless products for various reasons, such as a binder to hold ingredients together and to provide elasticity in dough. That's why you will find gluten in salad dressings, soy sauce, medications, spices, vitamins, candy, processed meats, sauces, gravy, and numerous other items most people do not even consider when thinking about gluten. It is critically important to read all labels and become educated on gluten-containing products and terms.

If it is not labeled, do not eat it. As a general rule, food allergen and gluten disclosure laws in the United States, Canada, and the EU provide that manufacturers must disclose the presence of wheat, barley, and rye (gluten) in their products. The tricky thing about labels is that some products are made with wheat-like soy sauce or with barley-like malt, and these will not be listed in bold print like wheat is in an ingredients list. So it is very important to know commonly used ingredients that are made out of gluten. You must be vigilant about reading and understanding labels, especially when eating processed foods. There are gluten-free certification standards where products that

meet a specific review can obtain certification as certified gluten-free. The guidelines require ongoing testing and inspection of all the ingredients, finished products, and manufacturing equipment.

There are several everyday foods and ingredients that contain gluten, and it is important to avoid them when meal planning.

These common food items that contain gluten are important to look out for:

- Breads, breading/coating mixes, and croutons
- Flour tortillas
- Most breakfast cereals
- Granola
- Pasta/noodles
- Baked goods: cakes, cookies, muffins
- Pre-prepared pie crusts, biscuits and rolls
- Crackers, pretzels, and some chips
- Soups
- Salad dressings
- Frozen meals
- Frozen waffles and pancakes
- Seasoning and sauce mixes
- Soy sauce
- Beer
- Whiskey
- Gin
- Vodka

These ingredients that contain gluten are important to look out for:

- All-purpose flour
- Semolina flour and durum flour
- Malt
- Malted barley
- Malted milk
- Malted syrup
- Wheat

- Rye
- Barley
- Spelt
- Millet
- Einkorn wheat
- KAMUT® Khorasan wheat
- Triticale
- Brewer's yeast
- Seitan (faux meat made from wheat)

This list is only a small portion of the most popular gluten-containing products. That's why you'll need to read every label to check before you purchase them. Many—but not all—companies list allergens in bold lettering on their labels. You'll also have to keep in mind that many gluten ingredients are not always listed as wheat (like soy sauce).

Dairy-Free 101

Dairy refers to foods and products made from the milk of cows, goats, and other mammals. It includes cheese, yogurt, cream, ice cream, butter, and a variety of other milk-derived products. It is a primary staple of the modern American diet, and dietary recommendations have touted the benefits of eating certain dairy products for many years. However, if you have an allergy or intolerance to dairy, consuming any of these can cause adverse reactions and make you very sick.

The two main proteins in cow's milk that can cause an allergic reaction are casein and whey. Casein is found in the solid portion of milk (the part that curdles), and whey is found in the liquid portion of milk that remains after the milk curdles.

Common Symptoms

Allergic reaction and lactose intolerance are the two most common issues people face with consuming dairy. The most frequently reported symptoms resulting from milk allergic reactions are upset stomach, the presence of hives, and vomiting. However, a potentially life-threatening reaction, anaphylaxis, may also occur, impairing breathing and causing the person to go into shock. Needless to say, a dairy allergy is a condition that requires attention to detail when it comes to diet.

The most frequently reported symptoms resulting from lactose intolerance are diarrhea, gas, bloating, and abdominal cramps. People who are lactose intolerant cannot digest the sugar in dairy, because they have a deficiency of an enzyme produced in the cells of the lining of the small intestine. This enzyme is called *lactase*. Although not life-threatening, lactose intolerance can really affect your quality of life.

There are also other symptoms of lactose intolerance that are often not discussed, such as migraine, stuffy nose, and eczema.

Diagnosing Dairy Issues

Doctors use diagnostic tests for screening for dairy allergies. The most commonly used tests are a skin-prick test and a blood test. Both of these tests look for immunoglobulin E (IgE) antibodies that are detectable when your body is exposed to a substance that causes a sensitive reaction and produces antibodies. These antibodies trigger the release of chemicals that produce the symptoms.

One way to know if you should not ingest dairy because you have lactose intolerance is to eliminate it from your diet for a month and see if your symptoms disappear. Before you consider this option, talk to your doctor or your child's pediatrician. That means *100 percent of all dairy and dairy-related products* must be gone from your foods! Following the dairy-free trial period, if you try eating dairy again and your symptoms return, then you have pretty good evidence that you should be dairy-free.

Treatment

Just like celiac disease and gluten intolerance, there is no cure for dairy allergies or lactose intolerance. People with these conditions must avoid consuming dairy by following a dairy-free diet every day.

How Do You Know What Foods Have Dairy?

Identifying which foods are safe to eat for a person with a dairy allergy or lactose intolerance requires attention to detail. Some foods may be labeled "lactose-free" but still contain allergy-related milk proteins. You may find dairy proteins in places you wouldn't expect them, such as candy, salad dressings, medications, hot dogs, vitamins, processed meats, sauces, and gravy. Once again, it is critically important to read labels and become educated on dairy-containing products and terms.

The Food Allergen Labeling and Consumer Protection Act requires that the top eight allergens be listed on food labels sold in the United States. However, the names for dairy-containing ingredients are sometimes not obvious, meaning, for example, they do not include the word *milk* but do contain dairy. Many food manufacturers now provide quality assurance of dairy-free and third-party testing as evidence. One stamp that you can look for on a product is "certified vegan by Vegan Action." Vegan Action certifies that the product does not contain any

animal products. Trademarked products may also carry warning labels such as "may contain milk," which refers to accidental low-level cross-contamination.

There are many common foods and ingredients that contain dairy, and it is important to avoid them when meal planning. The most familiar foods that contain dairy include:

- Cow's milk
- Goat's milk
- Buttermilk
- Butter
- Ghee
- Yogurt
- Ice cream
- Cheese
- Sour cream
- Pudding
- Breads, bagels, crackers
- Baked goods: cakes, cookies, pies, muffins, etc.
- Frozen waffles and pancakes
- Chocolate
- Candy
- Whipped cream
- Margarine
- Nougat

The most common ingredients that contain dairy include:

- Milk
- Whey/whey protein
- Casein
- Sodium caseinate (a milk derivative)
- Evaporated milk
- Condensed milk
- Half-and-half
- Dry milk powder

- Lactoglobulin
- Lactose
- Lactulose
- Hydrolyzed milk protein
- Hydrolyzed casein

This list is only a fraction of the most popular dairy-containing products. Just like the gluten-containing product list, the complete inventory of dairy-containing products is virtually endless. Read food labels and practice looking for keywords that can tip you off to dairy ingredients.

Why Go Gluten-Free and Dairy-Free?

If you have celiac disease, an allergy or intolerance to dairy or gluten, clearly you will begin eating gluten- and dairy-free. There are also other reasons and health benefits to try this lifestyle. It turns out that many people attribute other symptoms directly to consuming gluten and dairy, such as:

- Depression
- Fatigue
- Anxiety
- Body pain
- Inflammation
- Learning disabilities
- Attention deficit disorder (ADD)
- Leaky gut
- Autoimmune disorders

Many people have opted to remove gluten and dairy from their diets and have seen dramatic improvement in their overall heath. Why? Interestingly, research done by the National Institutes of Health estimates that only about 25 percent of the world's population is genetically able to properly digest lactose. The other 75 percent of the world's population is considered lactose intolerant. That's why even people without diagnosed gluten or dairy issues can see improvements in overall health when they take those ingredients out of their diets. For example, you might:

- **Reduce inflammation:** Many people who are sensitive to gluten find a reduction in inflammation in their joints, sinuses, and digestion system when they remove gluten from their diet.
- **Improve thyroid function:** Research has shown that patients who have removed gluten from their diets have seen a decrease in their thyroid antibody levels associated with autoimmune thyroid disease. Also, a specific protein in dairy has been linked to an increase of inflammation in the thyroid gland.
- **Experience less acne:** The hormones in milk are believed to react with the testosterone in your body and increase clogged pores. More

research is being done on the direct impact gluten has on the skin, but the connection between the gut and skin has been studied extensively. In gluten-sensitive individuals, gluten increases inflammation, which can trigger acne. Inflammation can also cause a release of insulin, which results in raised hormone levels, another cause of acne.

- **Get fewer migraines:** The protein casein, which is found in dairy, is a substantial trigger for many migraine sufferers. Gluten may also be a trigger for migraines in some people. Studies from the National Institutes of Health have shown that migraines were more prevalent in people with celiac disease and irritable bowel syndrome (IBS).
- **Relieve colitis:** Dairy products may aggravate inflammation in certain individuals with colitis. Research has also shown that following a gluten-free diet can lead to improved symptoms and fewer or less severe flare-ups between periods of remission.
- **Alleviate symptoms of irritable bowel syndrome (IBS):** Research has shown that gluten sensitivity may be a factor in the development of IBS symptoms, and gluten-free diets may improve these symptoms. Since foods that contain lactose, like milk, may cause bloating and gas in many people, those with IBS often have their symptoms worsen after eating dairy.
- **Boost energy levels:** Fatigue is one of the most frequent symptoms mentioned by those with celiac disease or gluten sensitivity. This fatigue can be caused by malnutrition and anemia, which frequently appear in people with celiac disease. Many individuals with lactose intolerance also experience symptoms of fatigue.

Gluten-Free and Dairy-Free Ingredients

Navigating a gluten-free and dairy-free world in a sea of grocery store shelves filled with gluten and dairy products takes some practice, but it does not have to be expensive, complicated, or overwhelming. Substitution is the name of the game, and finding the right alternatives to the products that you used in the past is the key to making it fast and easy.

Flour Options

The choice of flour can be what makes or breaks your gluten- and dairy-free baked goods. The most popular and widely available gluten-free flour options are:

- Rice flour
- Almond flour
- Coconut flour
- Oat Flour
- Sorghum flour

Gluten-free all-purpose flour blends contain additives that help replace the texture and binding elasticity of gluten missing from gluten-free flour, such as:

- Xanthan gum
- Potato starch
- Tapioca starch

The best choice for general baking is to use a *gluten-free all-purpose flour* that already contains xanthan gum. These types of blends are known as *cup for cup* or *1 for 1*.

Read the labels of the gluten-free flour blends because some of them contain dairy. Not all gluten-free flours are created equally, and you will get slightly different results depending on the specific blend that you choose. Visit www.mamaknowsglutenfree.com to learn more about the recommended brands of gluten-free flours.

question

How do you know which fast food on the menu has gluten and dairy?

Most large fast-food chains will provide allergen information on request or by visiting their websites. However, they do typically include a disclaimer in the fine print that explains that they will not assume liability for adverse reactions as the result of eating their food. Also, many of the ingredients are subject to substitution without notice, so be sure you communicate clearly with your server about your dietary needs.

POPULAR GLUTEN-FREE FLOURS

The flour options most commonly used in gluten-free baking include:

- **All-purpose blends:** Blends are the most popular and versatile type of gluten-free flour. Blends have a mixture of gluten-free flours with starches and xanthan gum added to them. Be sure to read the label to make sure the one you're choosing doesn't contain dairy.
- **Rice flour:** Rice flour is made from finely ground rice. Rice flour blends are useful when baking gluten-free and dairy-free because they are more cost-effective than the other options, and they produce the results closest to the taste and texture of wheat flour.
- **Almond flour:** Almond flour is a popular grain-free and gluten-free flour made from ground blanched almonds. It has a nutty flavor and produces thicker and denser results. It is commonly used in baked goods like muffins and can also be a grain-free alternative to bread crumbs.
- **Coconut flour:** Coconut flour is made from dried coconut meat and offers a mild coconut flavor. It has a light texture and absorbs a lot more liquid than rice or almond flour. It is a grain-free and gluten-free flour option that is also good for those with a nut allergy. It is often used as a supporting flour, meaning it is sometimes blended with another flour to improve texture in baked goods. It is a popular add-in for low-carb almond flour recipes.
- **Oat flour:** Oat flour is made by grinding whole-grain oats. Not everyone following the gluten-free diet can tolerate oats. It is safest to use oat flour that is certified gluten-free and from Purity Protocol oats. Purity Protocol oats ensures that oats are gluten-free and have met requirements for seed stock purity as well as criteria for harvesting, transport, storage, processing, and manufacturing. You can also make your own oat flour by processing gluten-free rolled oats in a food processor until finely ground. Oat flour is popular for making cookies and quick breads.

A NOTE ON GUMS

In gluten-free baking, gums provide elasticity and stickiness to doughs and batters. Xanthan gum is the most popular of gums and is often added to gluten-free all-purpose flour blends. Be sure to double-check your flour to see if it is already added. Adding too much gum to your recipe can result in an overly gummy texture.

If you have to add xanthan gum to your flour, these are the guidelines on amounts to add per 1 cup of gluten-free flour:

- Yeast breads: ½ teaspoon
- Cakes: ¼ teaspoon
- Cookies: ¼ teaspoon
- Muffins and quick breads: ¼ teaspoon

Dairy-Free Milk

Several different alternatives to dairy milk are readily available nowadays, and the good news is that supermarkets and even smaller stores are stocking more of these dairy-free options every day. The dairy-free milk most commonly used in cooking include:

- **Almond milk:** Unsweetened almond milk is the recommended dairy alternative when cooking and baking. It is a little thicker and darker in color than some other dairy substitutes. It has a mild nutty flavor that translates well with baked goods. However, those with tree nut allergies should not use almond milk. It is widely available.
- **Cashew milk:** Unsweetened cashew milk is thick and creamy, with a slight nutty flavor. It has a darker color than most dairy-free milks and has a consistency very similar to dairy milk. It is lower in carbohydrates and sugar than some other options. It is less widely available.
- **Coconut milk:** Unsweetened coconut milk has a slight coconut flavor and is a little thinner and lighter in color than most other dairy substitutes. The sweet coconut flavor will be present in foods that are made with coconut milk, so the unsweetened version is the best option when using coconut milk. Full-fat canned coconut milk is thick and

rich and is often substituted for heavy cream in recipes. It is widely available. Please note these two variations:

- **Coconut milk beverage:** Do not confuse the coconut milk beverage (sold in cartons) with canned coconut milk or coconut cream. Coconut milk beverage sold in cartons is similar in fat content to 2% milk.
- **Canned coconut cream:** This is the richest of all coconut milk and is often used for making dairy-free whipped cream. If you cannot find coconut cream, you can chill a can of coconut milk and skim the cream from the top to use in recipes.
- **Rice milk:** Unsweetened rice milk is one of the least allergenic of the dairy alternatives. It has a watery consistency, and the color is very light. It has a higher-than-average carbohydrate count per cup than other options. It is widely available.
- **Soy milk:** Unsweetened soy milk has a mild, creamy flavor. It has a consistency and color similar to dairy milk. It is widely available.
- **Other available options:** Flax, hemp, oat, and pea milk are used less frequently, usually more expensive, and less widely available.

Cooking Fats and Oils

Using the correct type of fat and oil in a recipe can make all the difference in making a great-tasting dish. The fats and oils most commonly used in gluten-free and dairy-free cooking include:

- **Dairy-free buttery spread:** Dairy-free buttery spread is rich, with a creamy, smooth texture. It is very much like traditional dairy-containing butter spread. It is typically made up of a combination of different vegetable oils, pea protein, and lecithin. It is good as a replacement for dairy butter in the majority of baking and cooking applications. It is widely available.

- **Canola oil:** Canola oil is a lightly flavored vegetable oil with a smooth texture. It is good for stir-frying, deep-frying, grilling, and baking. It is widely available.
- **Coconut oil:** This is recommended as a substitute for butter in recipes. It is sweet flavored and smooth textured. Add a dash of salt to reduce unwanted sweetness. It's often used for sautéing vegetables and meat over medium heat. Coconut oil has a solid consistency under 75°F. It is widely available.
- **Olive oil:** Olive oil is a good choice for sautéing vegetables and meat. It has many health benefits and a delicious flavor. It is also an excellent pick for salad dressings and can be used in place of butter for many recipes. It is widely available.
- **Shortening:** Shortening comprises a variety of fat products that are used for baking and cooking. The most common types of shortening are vegetable shortening and animal fat (lard). Vegetable shortening is often used for deep-frying, pie crusts, and flaky doughs. It has a neutral flavor and does not have to be refrigerated. It is widely available.
- **Cooking spray:** There are many varieties of gluten-free nonstick cooking sprays on the market. Some of the most popular varieties are made with canola oil, olive oil, and coconut oil. Using gluten-free nonstick cooking sprays makes greasing pans, pots, and skillets easy.

Other Ingredients

There are many additional pantry essentials that you will experiment with and quickly add to your kitchen when cooking gluten- and dairy-free. A few that might make the transition quicker include gluten-free bread crumbs, gluten-free chicken broth, gluten-free spices, and gluten-free soy sauce.

Gluten-Free and Dairy-Free for Families

Making the decision to eat gluten-free and dairy-free is often the result of a medical recommendation or in response to a health-related condition, and it often is safest and easiest to have everyone adopt the diet. To get the best results and the easiest transition, everyone at home should understand why you're doing it and do what they can to participate in the process. The first step is to educate your family and share with them the importance of why you have decided, as a family, to eat gluten-free and dairy-free. Then explain to them how they might benefit as a result, even if they do not have a medical connection to the diet. Show them all the delicious gluten-free and dairy-free recipes in this book so they see how tasty it will be.

The most important reason for the entire family to consider going gluten- and dairy-free together is to support each other. It is very difficult if one person is transitioning to a gluten-free and dairy-free diet but the person across the dinner table is eating takeout stuffed-crust, triple-cheese pizza. Families congregate around meals, and showing support to family members by sharing their diet is a great way to build strong connections and help them make the transition. Another important reason the entire family should consider following a gluten- and dairy-free lifestyle together is to avoid accidental cross contamination of foods or materials.

How to Avoid Cross Contamination and Accidental Exposure

Cross contamination can happen if different foods are prepared on the same surfaces or if cutting boards or utensils are not properly washed after coming into contact with gluten- or dairy-containing products. It is very important to consider the possibility of cross contamination anytime you prepare gluten-free and dairy-free products in the same kitchen as gluten- and dairy-containing ingredients.

When a portion of your family is gluten- and dairy-free and the other portion is not, the probability of cross contamination increases. Even the most careful family members will get their wires crossed from time to time and unknowingly dip their knife into the peanut butter jar after they spread jelly all over their gluten-filled bread! In this example, keeping different jars of peanut butter with labels identifying which is gluten-free and which is not would have been a smart way to avoid cross contamination.

Food Preparation Tips
These are some valuable tips for preparing food that will help you avoid cross contamination:

- Wash everything thoroughly, and wash your hands after handling gluten or dairy products.
- Prepare your gluten-free and dairy-free products on a different surface and different area of the kitchen than your gluten- and dairy-containing foods.
- Prepare your foods on top of barriers like foil or parchment paper.
- Use dedicated utensils and preparation equipment, such as cutting boards, knives, strainers, pots, bowls, and cooking sheets. Be especially careful with wooden items like spoons and cutting boards, which are difficult to fully sanitize.
- Do not use the same dishcloths when handling gluten-free and dairy-free products and gluten- and dairy-containing ingredients.
- Use different appliances (such as blenders or toasters) to be extra safe.
- Purchase condiments in squeezable containers.

Dealing with Crumbs
Gluten-free eaters should beware of crumbs and food that can go airborne, like flour. Cracker crumbs in the pantry, chicken nugget crumbs in the freezer, and bread crumbs in the bread basket are common culprits of accidental exposure. Ensure that everyone in the family understands the risks and knows the basics of managing and avoiding the chances of contamination and exposure. Clean often and clean well to ensure you get all those gluten crumbs!

Tips for Storing Food
Food storage is a big issue for the gluten-free and dairy-free family. Even a small trace of food on a container lid could make a person very sick if their allergy or intolerance is severe! Here are several great tips for storing your food:

- Always use tightly closed storage containers for food and ingredients.

- Label potentially confusing items "Gluten-Free," "Gluten," "Dairy-Free," or "Dairy," etc.
- Store gluten-free and dairy-free ingredients in areas separate from other ingredients.
- Organize the refrigerator to reduce risks. It's best to store gluten-free and dairy-free foods on the shelves above other foods to avoid cross contamination from accidental spills or leaks.
- Use plastic storage bags as an additional layer of protection for foods and ingredients.

Living a Gluten-Free and Dairy-Free Lifestyle

There's no one right way to make the transition to a gluten- and dairy-free way of life, so be patient and reward yourself for all your successes. Depending on you or your loved one's symptoms, it may be a slow transition or an instant one.

Most people have a negative association with the word *diet*, so try to avoid using the term *diet* with your new lifestyle. The next steps to a successful transition to living a gluten- and dairy-free lifestyle are to think about your weekly meal planning process, your eating habits when it comes to eating out at restaurants, how you eat when traveling, and what you eat at the workplace.

Meal Planning

The best way to start living a gluten-free and dairy-free lifestyle is to think about the meals that you and your family already love. What foods do you buy each week at the grocery store? Ask your family members for their input. Make a list of the meals and foods you already buy and see which ones are still safe to eat and which need substitutes.

If you are not satisfied with the meals that you are currently making for you and your family, then now is a great time to reevaluate your meal-planning preferences. There is a whole world of great meals that you may have never even considered. Have you ever made crepes for breakfast? How about chicken lettuce wraps for lunch? Have you ever made chicken piccata for dinner? If these meals sound too complicated, you might be surprised to learn that they're not. All of the recipes in this book are easy to follow, even for a beginner!

Knowing what you are making ahead of time may take some of the stress out of cooking for the week, so use your meal ideas to plan out your week. Now work on your shopping list, making sure you note everything you'll need to make the dishes on your list. Having a shopping list in hand (or on your phone) will help you manage your budget, avoid multiple stops, and stay away from impulse buying at the grocery store.

Restaurants

When you are gluten-free and dairy-free, there are some important things to understand about eating out at restaurants. The most important factor in your decision of where to eat out is your particular level of physical reaction to gluten or dairy. If you "only" get a mild headache or stuffy nose from consuming gluten or dairy, accidentally consuming some of it will be an inconvenience but not life-threatening. However, if you or your loved is prone to more serious reactions after eating gluten or dairy, then you will need to be especially careful when eating out.

Although many restaurants are well aware of food sensitivities and conduct themselves accordingly, unfortunately, many are not equipped or trained, or even fully comprehend the subject of cross contamination and food allergies. The great news is that some restaurants now have specific gluten-free and dairy-free menu items. Plus, many states are now requiring restaurants and food service establishments to provide food allergen training for their staff. Here are some questions to ask to help avoid cross contamination at a restaurant:

- Will my food be prepared in a separate area from the other food?
- Are dedicated cutting boards and utensils used to prepare my meal?
- Is there a dedicated fryer and/or grill area for allergen-free meals?
- What kind of training has the staff been given on food allergies and specialty food preparation?
- Will my meal be labeled specifically and identified in a way that segregates it from the other meals?
- Will the person preparing my food change their gloves before handling my food? (If they have been properly trained, they should not blink an eye and change their gloves.)

alert

If you can see the food storage situation in the restaurant, check to see if the food that is advertised as gluten-free and dairy-free is stored in close proximity to the same area as gluten- and dairy-containing foods. It's perfectly okay to look around at public spaces in the restaurant to see how it handles ingredients. Be sure to explain your food allergy or intolerance to the person taking your order.

Traveling

Traveling while eating gluten-free and dairy-free takes a little extra planning so you have appropriate food options while getting to and from your destination, as well as when you're there.

essential

Smart travelers with gluten-free and dairy-free food considerations pack their most dependable nonperishable gluten-free and dairy-free items. The best products to pack are gluten-free and dairy-free items like bread for sandwiches, peanut butter packets, protein/snack bars, instant oats, crackers, and just about anything that is nonperishable, gluten-free, and dairy-free that suits your fancy and can fit inside a suitcase and stay intact.

The best way to travel gluten-free and dairy-free is to plan your food needs just the same way that you plan your transportation and accommodations. Research your airline's meal availability and call ahead of time to preorder specialty meals. However, most airlines will not guarantee an allergen-free meal, so plan on bringing your own food, especially if you are highly reactive.

Similarly, thoroughly research the hotels, restaurants, and local grocery stores where you will be visiting to determine availability for your needs. Planning ahead of time will let you focus on enjoying yourself while you're away. There are also several phone apps now available that can show you gluten-free and dairy-free options to eat in the city you are visiting.

Gluten-Free and Dairy-Free at Work

In the workplace, it seems like it is always someone's birthday, and a birthday cake or donuts appear in the breakroom. You don't want to miss out on these social events either, however, so your best bet is to bring your own homemade gluten-free and dairy-free goodies to work.

Office meeting organizers are beginning to consider various dietary options when planning for meetings, and they may provide whole foods, like fruit or vegetables, in addition to donuts, cakes, and brownies. Prepackaged gluten-free and dairy-free products are always an option as well, but they will cost significantly more than making your own, and they might not be nearly as tasty or as healthy. This book has superb recipes for fresh bagels, chocolaty donuts, wonderful cakes, and many other yummy alternatives to what you see in the breakroom. Bring in one of these options—you might even discover that a coworker has the same dietary issues as you!

Let's Start Cooking!

Now that you have learned the basics for gluten-free and dairy-free living, it's time to delve into the three hundred mouthwatering recipes in this book and start living a deliciously healthy lifestyle. With these incredible dishes, you won't miss any of the gluten or dairy!

CHAPTER 2

Breakfast

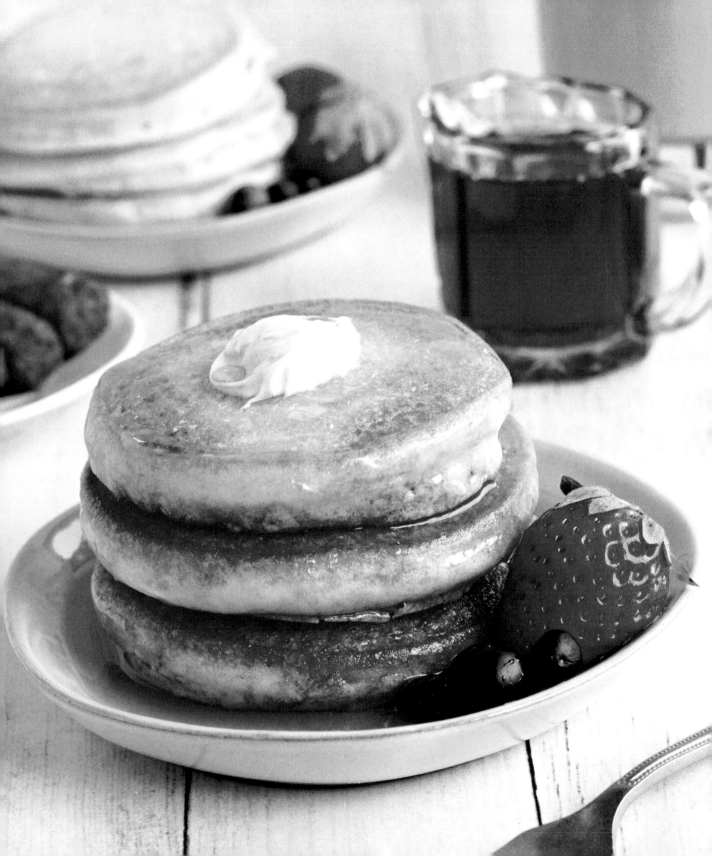

Fluffy Homemade Pancakes

What lazy weekend breakfast would be complete without a stack of fluffy, piping hot pancakes? This pancake mix is made with only a few simple ingredients but makes perfect pancakes every time! Serve with dairy-free buttery spread and maple syrup for a classic treat.

1 large egg

2 tablespoons granulated sugar

1 teaspoon pure vanilla extract

2 tablespoons vegetable oil

1 cup gluten-free all-purpose flour with xanthan gum

1 tablespoon gluten-free baking powder

¼ teaspoon salt

¾ cup unsweetened almond milk

1 In a large bowl, whisk egg, sugar, vanilla extract, and oil together.

2 Add flour, baking powder, and salt to the egg mixture and mix until fully combined.

3 Stir in milk and mix until smooth.

4 Spray a griddle or large skillet with gluten-free nonstick cooking spray. Scoop batter into a ¼-cup measuring cup and pour onto a greased griddle or large skillet for each pancake.

5 Cook pancakes for about 2–3 minutes on medium-high heat until batter starts to bubble and pancakes start to puff. Flip pancakes and cook for another 2 minutes until they are golden brown.

SERVES 4

Per Serving:

Calories	215
Fat	10g
Protein	6g
Sodium	495mg
Fiber	2g
Carbohydrates	30g
Sugar	8g

HAVE YOUR PANCAKES ALL WEEK

These pancakes can be frozen up to 2 months and reheated in the microwave. To freeze the pancakes, allow them to completely cool and place them on a parchment paper–lined baking sheet and flash freeze them for 10 minutes. (Flash freezing them keeps them from sticking together.) Once the pancakes are flash frozen, remove them from the baking sheet and place them inside a freezer-safe bag or airtight container and store for up to 1 week. When you're making the batter, stir in 2 extra tablespoons of almond milk if you prefer thinner pancakes.

Chocolate Cake Donuts

These easy Chocolate Cake Donuts are soft and cakey. Covered in a rich chocolate glaze and dunked in sprinkles, they are perfect for dessert or as a special treat.

MASTERING A PIPING BAG

Pouring batter into a piping bag can be really messy. Don't worry; there is an easy trick to ensure all of the batter gets into the bag easily. Place the bag inside a tall cup or glass, with the tip down inside the cup, and then fold the excess bag over the edges of the cup and pour in the batter.

DONUTS

1 cup gluten-free all-purpose flour with xanthan gum
1 teaspoon gluten-free baking powder
¼ teaspoon baking soda
¼ teaspoon salt
½ cup light brown sugar, packed
1 large egg
3 tablespoons dairy-free buttery spread, melted
½ cup unsweetened almond milk
1 teaspoon pure vanilla extract
¼ cup cocoa powder

GLAZE

1 cup confectioners' sugar
1 teaspoon pure vanilla extract
4 tablespoons cocoa powder
2½ tablespoons unsweetened almond milk
⅛ teaspoon ground cinnamon
½ cup gluten-free sprinkles

1 Preheat oven to 350°F. Spray a full-sized twelve-cup donut pan with gluten-free nonstick cooking spray.

2 In a small bowl, combine flour, baking powder, baking soda, and salt.

3 In a large bowl, mix together brown sugar, egg, buttery spread, milk, vanilla extract, and cocoa powder until fully combined.

4 Pour the flour mixture into the large bowl with the brown sugar mixture. Mix until fully combined and thick.

5 Add batter to a large plastic storage bag or piping bag. Seal the bag and cut a corner (or tip if using a piping bag) off. Carefully squeeze batter into donut pan. Bake for 10–12 minutes. Place pan on a cooling rack and cool for 1 minute. Remove donuts from the pan and place on rack.

6 In a small bowl, whisk together the glaze ingredients except for the sprinkles. Place the sprinkles in a small bowl. Dip each warm donut into the glaze and then into the sprinkles and place on a plate or wire rack. Store in an airtight container at room temperature for 3 days.

Banana Chocolate Peanut Butter Overnight Oats

If you're rushed for time in the morning, consider making breakfast the night before. This recipe takes only 3 minutes, but you'll get an easy, on-the-go breakfast that is creamy, chocolaty, and satisfying.

½ cup unsweetened almond milk
2 tablespoons gluten-free peanut butter
½ tablespoon unsweetened cocoa powder

1 large ripe banana, peeled and mashed
1 tablespoon pure maple syrup
½ cup gluten-free rolled oats

1 In a 12-ounce Mason jar or small container with a lid, add milk, peanut butter, cocoa powder, mashed banana, and maple syrup and stir with a spoon to combine.

2 Add oats and stir. Then press down with a spoon to make sure all the oats have been covered by the milk.

3 Cover securely with a lid or plastic wrap and set in the refrigerator overnight (or for at least 6 hours).

SERVES 1

Per Serving:

Calories	465
Fat	21g
Protein	15g
Sodium	210mg
Fiber	10g
Carbohydrates	53g
Sugar	16g

Mocha Latte Overnight Oats

If you can't get enough of a mocha latte flavor in your coffee, try it in these oats! This is an easy-to-make-ahead breakfast packed with flavor.

½ cup unsweetened almond milk
¼ cup cold coffee
1 tablespoon unsweetened cocoa powder
1 teaspoon gluten-free and dairy-free mini chocolate chips

2 tablespoons honey
1 teaspoon pure vanilla extract
½ cup gluten-free rolled oats

1 In a 12-ounce Mason jar or small container with a lid, add milk, coffee, cocoa powder, chocolate chips, honey, and vanilla extract. Stir with a spoon to combine.

2 Add oats and stir. Then press down with a spoon to ensure all the oats have been covered by the milk.

3 Cover securely with a lid or plastic wrap and set in the refrigerator overnight (or for at least 6 hours).

SERVES 1

Per Serving:

Calories	360
Fat	8g
Protein	7g
Sodium	97mg
Fiber	6g
Carbohydrates	66g
Sugar	34g

Lemon Muffins

MAKES 12 MUFFINS

**Per Serving
(Serving Size: 1 muffin):**

Calories	190
Fat	3g
Protein	2g
Sodium	235mg
Fiber	3g
Carbohydrates	40g
Sugar	27g

THE FLAVOR OF LEMON

There are a variety of excellent flavors that complement lemon without overshadowing it. Blueberries or raspberries are frequently added to lemon cakes and muffins to give them an extra special sweet flavor. Poppy seeds are also a popular savory complement. The biggest challenge may be finding something that doesn't go with the lemon!

These easy-to-make Lemon Muffins are soft and moist with a sweet and tart lemony glaze. They're easy enough for a quick breakfast or snack and special enough to serve for dessert.

MUFFINS
1½ cups gluten-free all-purpose flour with xanthan gum
1 cup sugar
½ teaspoon gluten-free baking powder
1 teaspoon baking soda
¼ teaspoon salt
½ teaspoon dried lemon peel
2 large eggs
1 teaspoon pure vanilla extract
1 tablespoon gluten-free lemon extract
⅓ cup dairy-free buttery spread, melted
1 cup unsweetened almond milk

GLAZE
1 cup confectioners' sugar
¼ cup lemon juice

1 Preheat oven to 350°F. Prepare a twelve-cup muffin tin with baking cup liners or gluten-free nonstick cooking spray.

2 In a large bowl, whisk together flour, sugar, baking powder, baking soda, salt, and lemon peel.

3 Add eggs, vanilla extract, lemon extract, buttery spread, and milk to the flour mixture.

4 Scoop batter into prepared muffin tin.

5 Bake for 20–25 minutes or until a toothpick inserted in the center of a muffin comes out clean. Place muffin tin on a cooling rack and cool for 2 minutes. Remove muffins from tin and place on rack to continue cooling.

6 In a small bowl, whisk the glaze ingredients together until smooth; drizzle over warm muffins. Store in an airtight container at room temperature for up to 3 days.

Homestyle Waffles

This classic waffle recipe makes waffles that are perfectly crisp on the outside and fluffy on the inside.

2 large eggs
¼ cup sugar
2 teaspoons pure vanilla extract
½ cup vegetable oil
2 cups gluten-free all-purpose flour with xanthan gum
4 teaspoons gluten-free baking powder
¼ teaspoon salt
1¾ cups unsweetened almond milk

SERVES 6

Per Serving:

Calories	370
Fat	22g
Protein	8g
Sodium	570mg
Fiber	2g
Carbohydrates	38g
Sugar	11g

1 Preheat waffle iron.

2 In a large bowl, whisk eggs, sugar, vanilla, and oil together. Add flour, baking powder, and salt to the egg mixture and whisk until fully combined. Stir in milk and mix until smooth.

3 Spray waffle iron with gluten-free nonstick cooking spray. Pour about ½ cup batter onto the center of the waffle iron. Close waffle iron and cook until the waffle is golden brown and crisp, about 5 minutes. Repeat with gluten-free nonstick cooking spray and remaining batter.

Corned Beef Hash

This traditional recipe turns leftover corned beef into a hearty breakfast. For a shorter cook time, substitute one 32-ounce package of frozen cubed hash browns instead of peeling, chopping, and boiling the potatoes.

3 cups peeled and diced russet potatoes
4 tablespoons dairy-free buttery spread
1 cup peeled and chopped sweet onion
½ teaspoon salt
½ teaspoon ground black pepper
2 cups chopped cooked gluten-free, dairy-free corned beef

SERVES 4

Per Serving:

Calories	340
Fat	16g
Protein	14g
Sodium	1,045mg
Fiber	16g
Carbohydrates	37g
Sugar	6g

1 Bring a large pot of salted water over high heat to a boil. Add potatoes and cook until tender but still firm, about 15 minutes.

2 In a large nonstick pan, melt buttery spread over medium-high heat. Add onions, salt, and pepper. Sauté for 5 minutes until onions are softened.

3 Stir in corned beef and cook for 3 minutes until corned beef is just starting to brown. Add potatoes and cook for 6 minutes. Then gently press the hash down, flip with a spatula, and cook for another 6 minutes until potatoes are browned and corned beef is crisp in areas. Serve warm.

Double Chocolate Muffins

MAKES 12 MUFFINS

**Per Serving
(Serving Size: 1 muffin):**

Calories	190
Fat	7g
Protein	4g
Sodium	380mg
Fiber	1g
Carbohydrates	30g
Sugar	18g

TIPS FOR THE PERFECT MUFFINS

For uniformly sized muffins, use an ice cream scoop. The scoop makes it nice and easy to get the perfect amount in the muffin tin, and you're more likely to avoid drips.

These bakery-style muffins are moist, tender, and deliciously chocolaty! They make a great lunchbox treat or just the right partner for your morning coffee.

1½ cups gluten-free all-purpose flour with xanthan gum

1 cup sugar

½ teaspoon gluten-free baking powder

1 teaspoon baking soda

¼ teaspoon salt

½ cup cocoa powder

2 large eggs

1 teaspoon pure vanilla extract

⅓ cup dairy-free buttery spread, melted

1 cup unsweetened almond milk

½ cup gluten-free and dairy-free chocolate chips

1 Preheat oven to 350°F. Prepare a twelve-cup muffin tin with baking cup liners or gluten-free nonstick cooking spray.

2 In a large bowl, add flour, sugar, baking powder, baking soda, salt, and cocoa powder and whisk together to combine.

3 Add eggs, vanilla extract, buttery spread, and milk to the flour mixture and mix until fully combined. Fold in chocolate chips.

4 Scoop batter into prepared muffin tin. Bake for 20–25 minutes or until a toothpick inserted in the center comes out clean. Place muffin tin on a cooling rack and cool for 2 minutes. Remove muffins from tin and place on rack to finish cooling. Store in an airtight container at room temperature for up to 3 days.

Baked Vanilla Cake Donuts

These soft Baked Vanilla Cake Donuts with a thick glaze are easier to make than you may think. They are wonderful for breakfast or to take along for a well-deserved snack break at work or school.

DONUTS

1 cup gluten-free all-purpose flour with xanthan gum

1 teaspoon gluten-free baking powder

¼ teaspoon baking soda

¼ teaspoon salt

⅛ teaspoon ground nutmeg

½ cup light brown sugar, packed

1 large egg

3 tablespoons dairy-free buttery spread, melted

½ cup unsweetened almond milk

1 tablespoon pure vanilla extract

GLAZE

1 cup confectioners' sugar

1 teaspoon pure vanilla extract

2 teaspoons unsweetened almond milk

MAKES 12 DONUTS

Per Serving (Serving Size: 1 donut):

Calories	125
Fat	1g
Protein	1g
Sodium	75mg
Fiber	0g
Carbohydrates	27g
Sugar	19g

1 Preheat oven to 350°F. Spray a full-sized twelve-cup donut pan with gluten-free nonstick cooking spray.

2 In a small bowl, combine flour, baking powder, baking soda, salt, and nutmeg and whisk to combine the ingredients.

3 In a large bowl, mix together brown sugar, egg, buttery spread, milk, and vanilla extract until fully combined.

4 Pour the flour mixture into the large bowl with the brown sugar mixture. Mix until fully combined.

5 Add batter to a large plastic storage bag or piping bag. Seal the bag and cut a corner (or tip if using a piping bag) off. Squeeze the bag carefully, filling the greased donut pan with batter. Bake for 10–12 minutes. Place plan on a cooling rack and cool for 1 minute. Remove donuts from the pan and place on the rack.

6 In a small bowl, whisk together the glaze ingredients. Dip each warm donut into the glaze and place on a plate or wire rack. Serve warm. Store in an airtight container at room temperature for up to 3 days.

Easy Blueberry Banana Muffins

MAKES 12 MUFFINS

**Per Serving
(Serving Size: 1 muffin):**

Calories	130
Fat	4g
Protein	3g
Sodium	330mg
Fiber	2g
Carbohydrates	25g
Sugar	13g

BENEFITS OF BLUEBERRIES

Blueberries are full of antioxidants and other chemicals that support everything from improving brain function to lowering blood pressure. Whether you eat fresh or frozen, you'll get the fiber, potassium, and vitamin C they contain!

This one-bowl wonder is so easy that you don't even need to get a mixer out! These super moist muffins will be a hit with anyone who tries one. If you have fresh blueberries, use those!

2 large very ripe bananas, peeled and mashed
1 teaspoon baking soda
⅓ cup dairy-free buttery spread, melted
½ cup sugar
⅛ teaspoon salt
2 large eggs, whisked
1 teaspoon pure vanilla extract
1½ cups gluten-free all-purpose flour with xanthan gum
½ teaspoon ground cinnamon
1 teaspoon dried lemon peel
1 cup frozen blueberries

1 Preheat oven to 350°F. Prepare a twelve-cup muffin tin with baking cup liners or gluten-free nonstick cooking spray.

2 In a medium bowl, combine bananas and baking soda. Allow the mixture to sit for at least 2 minutes. (Allowing the mashed bananas and baking soda to sit for at least 2 minutes before adding the rest of the ingredients is key to what makes these so light and fluffy.)

3 Stir buttery spread into the mashed bananas, then stir in sugar, salt, eggs, and vanilla extract.

4 Mix in flour, cinnamon, and lemon peel. Gently stir in blueberries.

5 Scoop batter into muffin tin. Bake for 20 minutes or until a toothpick inserted in the center comes out clean. Place muffin tin on a cooling rack and cool for 2 minutes. Remove muffins from tin and place on rack to finish cooling. Store in an airtight container at room temperature for up to 3 days.

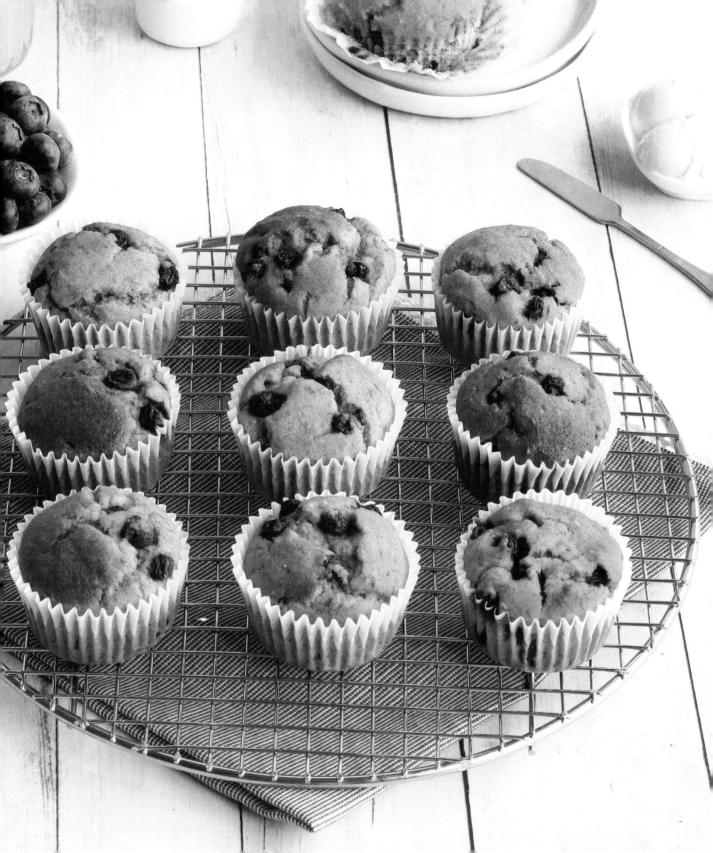

Blueberry Muffins

MAKES 12 MUFFINS

Per Serving
(Serving Size: 1 muffin):

Calories	85
Fat	3g
Protein	2g
Sodium	190mg
Fiber	0g
Carbohydrates	15g
Sugar	2g

IN A PINCH

You will often see premade gluten-free muffins in popular flavors on supermarket shelves. Before indulging, ask the store's bakery about their preparation methods to be sure they align with your needs.

These muffins are so good that you'll stop going to that bakery around the corner every morning! Transfer your cooled muffins into freezer bags to store for up to 2 months. If you have fresh blueberries, feel free to use them.

1½ cups gluten-free all-purpose flour with xanthan gum
1¼ cups granulated sugar, divided
½ teaspoon gluten-free baking powder
1 teaspoon baking soda
¼ teaspoon salt
½ teaspoon dried lemon peel
2 large eggs
1 teaspoon pure vanilla extract
⅓ cup dairy-free buttery spread, melted
1 cup unsweetened almond milk
1 cup frozen blueberries

1 Preheat oven to 350°F. Prepare a twelve-cup muffin tin with baking cup liners or gluten-free nonstick cooking spray.

2 In a large bowl, whisk together flour, 1 cup sugar, baking powder, baking soda, salt, and dried lemon peel.

3 Add eggs, vanilla extract, buttery spread, and milk to the flour mixture and mix until fully combined. Fold in blueberries.

4 Scoop batter into prepared muffin tin. Sprinkle tops of the muffins with remaining ¼ cup sugar. Bake for 20–25 minutes or until a toothpick inserted in the center comes out clean. Place muffin tin on a cooling rack and cool for 2 minutes. Remove muffins from tin and place on rack to cool completely. Store in an airtight container at room temperature for up to 3 days.

Tater Tot Breakfast Casserole

For the busy family on the go, this breakfast casserole is super easy to quickly put together and tastes amazing! It also travels well in a storage container and reheats nicely as a late-morning snack at work. Store leftovers in an airtight container in the refrigerator for up to 3 days.

1 pound gluten-free bacon

2 (9-ounce) packages gluten-free breakfast sausage links

1 (32-ounce) package Tater Tots

12 large eggs

½ cup unsweetened almond milk

1 tablespoon onion powder

½ teaspoon salt

¼ teaspoon ground black pepper

1 Preheat oven to 350°F and spray a 9" × 13" baking dish with gluten-free nonstick cooking spray.

2 Cook bacon in a large skillet over medium-high heat for 3 minutes on each side until brown and crispy. Place cooked bacon on a paper towel–lined plate and allow to cool for about 5 minutes. Crumble. Drain bacon grease from the skillet.

3 Cook sausage in the same skillet for 5 minutes on each side until cooked through. Remove to the plate with the bacon. Allow to cool for 2 minutes and cut into ½" pieces.

4 Arrange Tater Tots in a single layer in the prepared baking dish.

5 In a medium bowl, whisk together eggs, milk, onion powder, salt, and pepper. Stir in cooked bacon and sausage. Pour the mixture over Tater Tots.

6 Bake for 40–45 minutes until the egg mixture is set. Allow to stand 10 minutes before cutting.

SERVES 12

Per Serving:

Calories	500
Fat	40g
Protein	17g
Sodium	1,400mg
Fiber	2g
Carbohydrates	18g
Sugar	1g

MEET THE EGG

Eggs are considered a superfood. They are a very good source of inexpensive, high-quality protein. Eggs are also rich sources of selenium; vitamins D, B_2, B_6, and B_{12}; and minerals such as zinc, iron, and copper. As an added bonus, they are rich in nutrients that promote heart health, such as betaine and choline.

Carrot Cake Crumb Muffins

This recipe creates muffins that are super moist, deliciously spiced, and topped with a scrumptious brown sugar crumb topping and a vanilla glaze. You will have a hard time not eating more than one!

MAKES 12 MUFFINS

Per Serving
(Serving Size: 1 muffin):

Calories	220
Fat	4g
Protein	4g
Sodium	360mg
Fiber	2g
Carbohydrates	45g
Sugar	30g

INGREDIENT TEMPERATURE MATTERS

Always remember to bake with ingredients that are at room temperature when the recipe calls for it. Cold ingredients do not mix as well with room-temperature ingredients. Baking is a science, and depending on the ingredient, there are particular chemical reactions that occur as a result of temperature. Ingredients are considered room temperature if they are 70°F.

MUFFINS
- 1½ cups gluten-free all-purpose flour with xanthan gum
- ½ cup granulated sugar
- ½ teaspoon gluten-free baking powder
- 1 teaspoon baking soda
- ⅛ teaspoon salt
- 1 teaspoon ground cinnamon
- ¼ teaspoon ground nutmeg
- ½ teaspoon dried lemon peel
- ½ cup applesauce
- ½ cup undrained canned crushed pineapple
- 1 cup peeled and shredded carrots
- ¼ cup shredded sweetened coconut
- ¼ cup finely chopped pecans
- ¼ cup raisins
- 2 large eggs
- 1 teaspoon pure vanilla extract

CRUMB TOPPING
- ¼ cup light brown sugar, packed
- 2 tablespoons granulated sugar
- ⅓ cup gluten-free all-purpose flour with xanthan gum
- 2 tablespoons finely chopped pecans
- 1 tablespoon shredded sweetened coconut
- 2 tablespoons dairy-free buttery spread, melted

VANILLA GLAZE
- 1 cup confectioners' sugar
- 1 teaspoon pure vanilla extract
- 2 tablespoons unsweetened almond milk

1. Preheat oven to 350°F. Prepare a twelve-cup muffin tin with baking cup liners or gluten-free nonstick cooking spray.

2. In a small bowl, add flour, granulated sugar, baking powder, baking soda, salt, cinnamon, nutmeg, and dried lemon peel and whisk together.

3. In a large bowl, combine applesauce, pineapple, carrots, coconut, pecans, raisins, eggs, and vanilla extract. Add the flour mixture to the large bowl and mix until fully combined. Scoop batter into prepared muffin tin.

4. To make the crumb topping, add brown sugar, granulated sugar, flour, pecans, and coconut to a small bowl and stir until fully combined. Pour in buttery spread and stir until the topping looks thick and crumbly. Sprinkle 1 tablespoon of crumb topping on top of each muffin.

5. Bake for 20–25 minutes or until a toothpick inserted in the center comes out clean. Place muffin tin on a cooling rack and cool for 2 minutes. Remove muffins from tin and place on rack to continue cooling.

6. In a small bowl, whisk together the glaze ingredients. Drizzle glaze over warm muffins. Store in an airtight container for up to 3 days.

Chocolate Chip Muffins

These are easy to make but come out just as soft and moist as bakery-style chocolate chip muffins. They are the perfect breakfast to prepare ahead of time and have ready to go in the morning.

1½ cups gluten-free all-purpose flour with xanthan gum
1 cup sugar
½ teaspoon gluten-free baking powder
1 teaspoon baking soda
¼ teaspoon salt
2 large eggs
1 teaspoon pure vanilla extract
⅓ cup dairy-free buttery spread, melted
1 cup unsweetened almond milk
1 cup gluten-free and dairy-free chocolate chips

1 Preheat oven to 350°F. Prepare a twelve-cup muffin tin with baking cup liners or gluten-free nonstick cooking spray.

2 In a large bowl, add flour, sugar, baking powder, baking soda, and salt. Whisk together to combine the ingredients.

3 Add eggs, vanilla extract, buttery spread, and milk to the flour mixture and mix until fully combined. Stir in chocolate chips.

4 Scoop batter into prepared muffin tin. Bake for 20–25 minutes or until a toothpick inserted in the center of a muffin comes out clean. Place muffin tin on a cooling rack and cool for 2 minutes. Remove muffins from tin and place on rack to finish cooling. Store in an airtight container at room temperature for up to 3 days.

MAKES 12 MUFFINS

**Per Serving
(Serving Size: 1 muffin):**

Calories	240
Fat	10g
Protein	5g
Sodium	380mg
Fiber	1g
Carbohydrates	32g
Sugar	18g

THE EVOLUTION OF CHOCOLATE

If you go into your local grocer today, you will find dozens and dozens of different types, flavors, and combinations of specialty chocolate: sea salt, orange peel, cherries and almonds, Belgian, and raspberry to name just a few. Remember, even dark chocolates can contain milk, so read labels carefully!

Crepes

SERVES 4

Per Serving:

Calories	190
Fat	6g
Protein	7g
Sodium	455mg
Fiber	2g
Carbohydrates	28g
Sugar	8g

Crepes can be sweet (paired with berries and dairy-free cream) or savory (stuffed with scrambled eggs and bacon), but any way that you make them, they are delicious!

2 large eggs
¾ cup unsweetened almond milk
½ cup water
1 cup gluten-free all-purpose flour without xanthan gum

¼ teaspoon xanthan gum
2 tablespoons granulated sugar
1 teaspoon pure vanilla extract
3 tablespoons dairy-free buttery spread, melted

1 In a large bowl, whisk eggs with a mixer. Add remaining ingredients and mix on medium for 1 minute until combined and batter is smooth.

2 Spray a crepe pan with gluten-free nonstick cooking spray. Pour ¼ cup batter into the center of the pan. Pick up the pan and swirl it to spread batter evenly. Cook over medium heat for 30–45 seconds or until browned on the bottom. Flip the crepe over and cook for about 30 more seconds until brown on the other side. Repeat with remaining batter.

3 Slide the crepe onto a plate, laying it flat. Serve crepes rolled or folded into triangles.

Sausage Gravy and Biscuits

SERVES 6

Per Serving:

Calories	375
Fat	15g
Protein	20g
Sodium	1,920mg
Fiber	3g
Carbohydrates	43g
Sugar	6g

Pull up a chair at the breakfast table and enjoy this classic southern Sausage Gravy and Biscuits.

1 pound gluten-free ground sausage
1 tablespoon garlic powder
1 tablespoon onion powder
2 cups unsweetened almond milk
4 tablespoons gluten-free all-purpose flour with xanthan gum

1 teaspoon salt
1 teaspoon ground black pepper
2 tablespoons dairy-free buttery spread
1 recipe Southern Buttermilk Biscuits (see recipe in Chapter 8)

1 In a large skillet, combine sausage, garlic powder, and onion powder. Cook over medium heat for 3–5 minutes, stirring often, until sausage is browned and crumbled.

2 In a small bowl, whisk milk, flour, salt, and pepper for 1 minute until the flour dissolves. Pour the milk mixture into the skillet and cook for 10 minutes, stirring as it thickens. Stir in buttery spread.

3 Serve over biscuits.

Western Frittata

Frittatas are perfect for brunches and will reheat well for up to 3 days. They are easily customized, and you can use any combination of meats and vegetables to achieve your favorite flavor profile.

2 tablespoons olive oil
½ cup seeded and diced green bell pepper
½ cup seeded and diced red bell pepper
½ cup peeled and diced sweet onion
1½ cups diced cooked gluten-free, dairy-free ham
12 large eggs
¼ cup unsweetened almond milk
½ teaspoon salt

1 Preheat oven to 425°F.

2 Add olive oil, bell peppers, onions, and ham to a 12" oven-safe skillet. Cook over medium-high heat for 2–3 minutes until vegetables are tender.

3 Add eggs in a medium bowl and whisk until the whites and yolks are combined. (Do not overmix; whisk only enough to blend the whites and yolks.) Add milk and salt and mix until combined.

4 Pour egg mixture over vegetables. Stir with a spatula to combine and distribute the mixture evenly in the pan.

5 Cook for 1 minute on the stovetop until the edges of the frittata turn lighter in color. Place frittata in the oven and bake for 7–14 minutes until eggs puff up. Remove frittata from the oven and allow to cool for 5–10 minutes before cutting and serving.

SERVES 8

Per Serving:

Calories	94
Fat	7g
Protein	8g
Sodium	570mg
Fiber	1g
Carbohydrates	1g
Sugar	1g

FRITTATAS VERSUS OMELETS

Frittatas are normally thicker than omelets, and the ingredients are mixed into the egg instead of sprinkled on top. Frittatas also start on the stovetop and finish in the oven, unlike omelets, which are on the stovetop from start to finish.

Pumpkin Crumb Muffins

Per Serving
(Serving Size: 1 muffin):

Calories	180
Fat	3g
Protein	3g
Sodium	400mg
Fiber	2g
Carbohydrates	38g
Sugar	25g

MAKE YOUR OWN PUMPKIN PIE SPICE

It is very easy to make your own pumpkin pie spice mix—you probably already have everything you need in your pantry. In a small bowl, whisk together 3 tablespoons ground cinnamon, 3 tablespoons ground ginger, 2 teaspoons ground nutmeg, ½ teaspoon ground allspice, and ¼ teaspoon ground cloves until well combined. Store in a small jar or airtight container for up to 6 months.

These soft and moist pumpkin muffins covered with brown sugar crumb topping and vanilla maple glaze are absolutely delicious! Be sure to use regular canned pumpkin and not pumpkin pie filling.

MUFFINS

1½ cups canned pumpkin
1 teaspoon baking soda
¼ cup light brown sugar, packed
¼ cup granulated sugar
1 tablespoon pumpkin pie spice
1 teaspoon ground cinnamon
¼ teaspoon salt
2 large eggs, room temperature
1 teaspoon pure vanilla extract
1½ cups gluten-free all-purpose flour with xanthan gum
½ teaspoon gluten-free baking powder
⅓ cup dairy-free buttery spread, melted

CRUMB TOPPING

¼ cup light brown sugar, packed
2 tablespoons granulated sugar
½ teaspoon pumpkin pie spice
⅓ cup gluten-free all-purpose flour with xanthan gum
2 tablespoons dairy-free buttery spread, melted

VANILLA MAPLE GLAZE

1 cup confectioners' sugar
1 teaspoon pure vanilla extract
2 tablespoons pure maple syrup
1½ teaspoons unsweetened almond milk

1 Preheat oven to 350°F. Prepare one twelve-cup muffin tin and two wells of a 6-cup muffin tin with baking cup liners or gluten-free non-stick cooking spray.

2 In a large bowl, add pumpkin, baking soda, brown sugar, granulated sugar, pumpkin pie spice, cinnamon, and salt and mix until ingredients are fully combined. Add eggs and vanilla extract and mix until fully combined.

3 Add flour and baking powder to a small bowl, give it a quick stir, and then pour into the pumpkin mixture. Pour buttery spread into muffin batter and mix until fully combined. The muffin batter will be thick. Scoop batter into prepared muffin tins.

4 To make the crumb topping, add brown sugar, granulated sugar, pumpkin pie spice, and flour to a small bowl and stir until fully combined. Pour in buttery spread and stir until topping looks thick and crumbly. Sprinkle 1 tablespoon of crumb topping on top of each muffin.

5 Bake for 20–25 minutes or until a toothpick inserted in the center of a muffin comes out clean. Place muffin tin on a cooling rack and cool for 2 minutes. Remove muffins from tin and place on rack to continue cooling.

6 In a small bowl, add the glaze ingredients and stir until smooth. Drizzle glaze over tops of muffins. Store in an airtight container for up to 3 days.

Breakfast Burritos

Go south of the border for breakfast with these mouthwatering burritos. They are a protein-packed, grab-and-go breakfast that will satisfy even the biggest appetite!

2 tablespoons olive oil
½ pound gluten-free ground sausage
¼ teaspoon ground cumin
4 large eggs
¼ teaspoon salt
4 gluten-free and dairy-free flour tortillas
¼ cup gluten-free salsa
1 cup frozen Tater Tots, cooked
1 large avocado, peeled, pitted, and diced
¼ cup chopped fresh cilantro

1 Heat olive oil in a large skillet over medium-high heat. Add sausage and cumin and cook for 5–8 minutes until it is browned and in crumbles. Drain excess oil, reserving 1 tablespoon in the skillet.

2 Whisk eggs and salt in a small bowl and add to the sausage in the skillet. Reduce heat to low and scramble for 2–3 minutes until just cooked through.

3 Heat each tortilla in a medium pan over medium heat for 1–2 minutes or in the microwave for 10–15 seconds.

4 Spread salsa down the center of each tortilla. Top with Tater Tots, sausage, eggs, avocado, and cilantro, then roll the burrito.

SERVES 4

Per Serving:

Calories	390
Fat	25g
Protein	18g
Sodium	890mg
Fiber	8g
Carbohydrates	25g
Sugar	2g

ROLLING BURRITOS THE EASY WAY

Placing the tortilla on top of a piece of aluminum foil while building the burrito makes the burrito easier to roll, keeps it warm, and makes it easy to hold and eat. Lay out a piece of foil long enough so that you can double it over the tortilla and cover it completely. Place the tortilla in the center of the foil. After filling the tortilla, fold the foil over itself and seal it all around the edges of the bottom of the tortilla. This keeps the burrito fillings from spilling out of the tortilla.

Easy Apple Cinnamon Crumb Muffins

MAKES 12 MUFFINS

**Per Serving
(Serving Size: 1 muffin):**

Calories	157
Fat	3g
Protein	2g
Sodium	250mg
Fiber	0g
Carbohydrates	31g
Sugar	17g

These muffins are full of sweet apple cinnamon flavor! They are covered in a brown sugar crumb topping to add even more sweetness.

MUFFINS

1½ cups unsweetened applesauce

⅓ cup dairy-free buttery spread, melted

2 large eggs, room temperature

½ cup granulated sugar

⅛ teaspoon salt

1 teaspoon pure vanilla extract

1½ cups gluten-free all-purpose flour with xanthan gum

1 teaspoon baking soda

½ teaspoon gluten-free baking powder

1 tablespoon ground cinnamon

CRUMB TOPPING

¼ cup light brown sugar, packed

2 tablespoons granulated sugar

½ teaspoon ground cinnamon

⅓ cup gluten-free all-purpose flour with xanthan gum

2 tablespoons dairy-free buttery spread, melted

1 Preheat oven to 350°F. Prepare a twelve-cup muffin tin with baking cup liners or gluten-free nonstick cooking spray.

2 In a large bowl, add applesauce, buttery spread, and eggs and mix together until combined. Stir in granulated sugar, salt, and vanilla extract. Stir in flour, baking soda, baking powder, and cinnamon, and mix until all ingredients are smooth and fully combined.

3 Scoop batter into prepared muffin tin.

4 To make the crumb topping, add brown sugar, granulated sugar, cinnamon, and flour to a small bowl and stir until fully combined. Pour in buttery spread and stir until the topping looks thick and crumbly. Sprinkle 1 tablespoon of crumb topping on top of each muffin.

5 Bake for 20 minutes or until a toothpick inserted in the center comes out clean. Place muffin tin on a cooling rack and cool for 2 minutes. Remove muffins from tin and place on rack to finish cooling. Store in an airtight container at room temperature for up to 3 days.

Bacon and Egg Muffins

These muffins have all of the flavors of a hearty breakfast packed into a muffin. They're a perfect choice when you want the flavors of a big diner breakfast but need to rush out the door!

2 cups gluten-free all-purpose flour with xanthan gum

¼ cup sugar

1 tablespoon gluten-free baking powder

½ teaspoon baking soda

½ teaspoon salt

2 large eggs

1 tablespoon white vinegar

1 cup unsweetened almond milk

1 cup dairy-free buttery spread, melted

1 cup chopped cooked gluten-free bacon, divided

1 green onion, diced

2 large hard-boiled eggs, chopped

1. Preheat oven to 375°F. Prepare a twelve-cup muffin tin with baking cup liners or gluten-free nonstick cooking spray.

2. In a large bowl, add flour, sugar, baking powder, baking soda, and salt. Stir to combine. Add uncooked eggs to the flour mixture and mix until fully combined.

3. In a small bowl, add vinegar and milk and let sit for 1–2 minutes.

4. Add buttery spread and the vinegar mixture to batter and mix until fully combined.

5. Reserve 2 tablespoons bacon Add the rest of the bacon, green onions, and hard-boiled eggs to batter. Stir to fully mix everything.

6. Scoop batter into prepared muffin tin. Sprinkle the reserved bacon on top of each muffin.

7. Bake for 30 minutes or until a toothpick inserted in the center of a muffin comes out clean. Place muffin tin on a cooling rack and cool for 2 minutes. Remove muffins from tin and place on rack to finish cooling.

MAKES 12 MUFFINS

Per Serving (Serving Size: 1 muffin):

Calories	160
Fat	7g
Protein	6g
Sodium	580mg
Fiber	1g
Carbohydrates	19g
Sugar	5g

PERFECTLY CHOPPED EGGS

Use a hard-boiled egg slicer for evenly diced eggs. Place the egg vertically in the slicer, slice the egg, and then carefully turn the egg horizontally. Slice again for perfectly shaped squares.

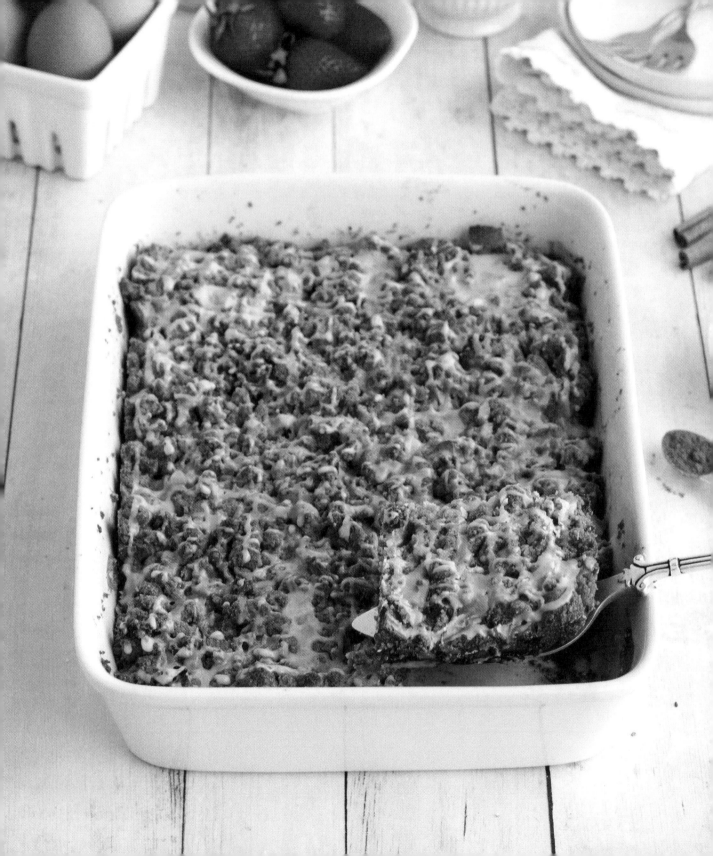

Cinnamon Roll French Toast Casserole

This Cinnamon Roll French Toast Casserole has the taste of a gooey cinnamon roll. Leftovers of this casserole heat up great, but the odds are good that there will not be any left to save for later! Store leftovers in an airtight container in the refrigerator for up to 3 days.

SERVES 12

Per Serving:

Calories	420
Fat	8g
Protein	7g
Sodium	440mg
Fiber	1g
Carbohydrates	81g
Sugar	60g

CASSEROLE

1 (14-ounce) loaf gluten-free and dairy-free bread, cut into 1" pieces

½ cup light brown sugar

1 tablespoon plus 1 teaspoon ground cinnamon, divided

6 large eggs, beaten

2 cups unsweetened almond milk

½ cup granulated sugar

1 tablespoon pure vanilla extract

CRUMB TOPPING

1 cup gluten-free all-purpose flour with xanthan gum

½ cup light brown sugar, packed

¼ teaspoon salt

1 teaspoon ground cinnamon

½ cup dairy-free buttery spread, melted

GLAZE

2 cups confectioners' sugar

1 teaspoon pure vanilla extract

2 tablespoons unsweetened almond milk

1 Preheat oven to 350°F. Spray a 9" × 13" baking dish with gluten-free nonstick cooking spray.

2 Spread bread pieces evenly on an ungreased baking sheet and bake for 5–10 minutes until nicely toasted. Remove from the oven when toasted and set aside.

3 In a small bowl, mix together brown sugar and 1 tablespoon cinnamon. Sprinkle the brown sugar mixture on the bottom of the prepared pan. Add the toasted bread pieces over the top of the brown sugar mixture.

4 In a medium bowl, whisk together eggs, milk, granulated sugar, vanilla extract, and remaining 1 teaspoon cinnamon until well blended. Pour the egg mixture evenly over the bread pieces.

5 To make the topping: In a small bowl, add flour, brown sugar, salt, cinnamon, and buttery spread and mix until crumbly. Sprinkle the crumb mixture evenly over the top of the casserole.

6 Bake on the middle rack for 1 hour or until a toothpick inserted in the center comes out clean.

7 Mix the glaze ingredients together in a small bowl until smooth. Allow casserole to cool a few minutes before drizzling glaze on it and serving.

Cinnamon Roll Muffins

MAKES 12 MUFFINS

**Per Serving
(Serving Size: 1 muffin):**

Calories	140
Fat	2g
Protein	3g
Sodium	230mg
Fiber	1g
Carbohydrates	34g
Sugar	24g

CONFECTIONERS' SUGAR VERSUS POWDERED SUGAR

Confectioners' sugar is a very fine powdered sugar that has a smooth texture that's perfect for glazes, frosting, and candies. So, what is the difference between powdered sugar and confectioners' sugar? Nothing—they are the same thing! Most brands of confectioners' sugar are gluten- and dairy-free, but always read labels to be sure.

When you don't have the time to take on made-from-scratch cinnamon rolls, whip up these muffins instead. They have the texture and the taste of a sweet, gooey cinnamon roll but come together quickly!

MUFFINS

1½ cups gluten-free all-purpose flour with xanthan gum

⅛ teaspoon salt

½ cup granulated sugar

2 teaspoons gluten-free baking powder

¾ cup unsweetened almond milk

1 large egg

1 teaspoon pure vanilla extract

¼ cup dairy-free buttery spread, melted

TOPPING

¼ cup dairy-free buttery spread, softened

¼ cup light brown sugar, packed

½ tablespoon gluten-free all-purpose flour with xanthan gum

¾ teaspoon ground cinnamon

GLAZE

1 cup confectioners' sugar

2½ tablespoons unsweetened almond milk

½ teaspoon pure vanilla extract

1 Preheat oven to 350°F. Prepare a twelve-cup muffin tin with baking cup liners or gluten-free nonstick cooking spray.

2 In a large bowl, add flour, salt, granulated sugar, baking powder, milk, egg, and vanilla and mix until fully combined. Stir in melted buttery spread. Scoop batter into prepared muffin tin.

3 In a separate large bowl, cream the topping ingredients together to make the topping.

4 Drop a teaspoonful of topping on each muffin. Use a knife to swirl the mixture through each muffin.

5 Bake for 20–25 minutes or until a toothpick inserted in the center of a muffin comes out clean. Place muffin tin on a cooling rack and cool for 2 minutes. Remove muffins from tin and place on rack to continue cooling.

6 In a medium bowl, whisk the glaze ingredients together. Drizzle over warm muffins. Store in an airtight container for up to 3 days.

Baked Pumpkin Donuts

Treat your friends with these Baked Pumpkin Donuts with maple cinnamon glaze. They are light and fluffy, and they smell heavenly!

DONUTS

¾ cup sugar

2 large eggs, room temperature

4 tablespoons vegetable oil

1 cup canned pumpkin purée

1 teaspoon pure vanilla extract

1½ cups gluten-free all-purpose flour with xanthan gum

½ teaspoon salt

1 teaspoon pumpkin pie spice

½ teaspoon ground cinnamon

1 teaspoon gluten-free baking powder

GLAZE

1 cup confectioners' sugar

¼ teaspoon ground cinnamon

1 teaspoon pure vanilla extract

4 tablespoons pure maple syrup

MAKE 12 DONUTS

**Per Serving
(Serving Size: 1 donut):**

Calories	215
Fat	6g
Protein	3g
Sodium	260mg
Fiber	6g
Carbohydrates	40mg
Sugar	28g

1 Preheat oven to 350°F. Spray a full-sized twelve-cup donut pan with gluten-free nonstick cooking spray.

2 In a large bowl, combine sugar, eggs, vegetable oil, pumpkin purée, and vanilla extract. Mix until fully combined.

3 Add flour, salt, pumpkin pie spice, cinnamon, and baking powder and mix until fully combined. The batter will be thick and sticky.

4 Add batter to a large plastic storage bag or piping bag. Seal the bag and cut a corner (or tip if using a piping bag) off. Carefully squeeze batter into donut pan. Bake for 14–16 minutes until golden brown and set. Place pan on a cooling rack and cool for 1 minute. Remove donuts from the pan and place on rack to continue cooling.

5 In a small bowl, whisk together the glaze ingredients. Dip each warm donut into the glaze and place on a plate or wire rack. Store in an airtight container for up to 3 days.

Shakshuka

Shakshuka is an Israeli and Middle Eastern meal of poached eggs in an aromatic spiced tomato sauce. It's full of flavor but very light.

SERVES 6

Per Serving:

Calories	130
Fat	9g
Protein	2g
Sodium	500mg
Fiber	4g
Carbohydrates	12g
Sugar	6g

GARDENING TOMATOES

When you think about home gardens, the first thing that often comes to mind is homegrown tomatoes. Organically grown vegetables are often more flavorful and colorful than corporately grown versions. The BushSteak tomato is ideal for growing in containers and small gardens since the compact plant grows only to 20"–24" in height but produces large, juicy tomatoes.

3 tablespoons olive oil
1 large yellow onion, peeled and chopped
2 large green bell peppers, seeded and chopped
1 tablespoon jarred minced garlic
1 teaspoon ground coriander
1 teaspoon paprika
½ teaspoon ground cumin
1 (28-ounce) can whole peeled tomatoes, including liquid
½ teaspoon salt
¼ teaspoon ground black pepper
1 teaspoon granulated sugar
6 large eggs
¼ cup chopped fresh cilantro

1   In a large skillet, heat olive oil over medium heat. Add onions and bell peppers and sauté for 5 minutes until onions become translucent. Stir in garlic and spices and cook for an additional minute until fragrant.

2   Pour in tomatoes and their juice and break down tomatoes using a spoon. Add salt, black pepper, and sugar and bring the sauce to a simmer.

3   Use a large spoon to make six small wells in the sauce and crack an egg into each well. Cover the skillet and cook for 5–8 minutes or until the eggs are poached to your liking. Spoon an egg and sauce on each plate and serve warm. Garnish with chopped cilantro.

Apple Cinnamon Baked Oatmeal Cups

Baked oatmeal cups are a variation on traditional muffins. They're packed with potassium and fiber and will keep you full all morning!

2 large bananas, peeled and mashed

2 large eggs, whisked

1 tablespoon pure vanilla extract

¼ cup honey

2 cups gluten-free oatmeal

¼ teaspoon salt

1 tablespoon plus ½ teaspoon ground cinnamon, divided

⅔ cup unsweetened almond milk

1 cup diced Gala apple, divided

½ teaspoon lemon juice

1 Preheat oven to 400°. Prepare a twelve-cup muffin tin with baking cup liners or gluten-free nonstick cooking spray.

2 In a large bowl, combine bananas, eggs, vanilla, and honey. Stir in gluten-free oatmeal, salt, and 1 tablespoon cinnamon. Add milk and stir.

3 Add chopped apples to a small bowl and toss with ½ teaspoon cinnamon and lemon juice. Add half of apple mixture to batter and stir to combine.

4 Scoop batter into muffin tin and top with remaining apple mixture. Bake for 20 minutes. Allow to cool for 1–2 minutes before serving.

MAKES 12 CUPS

Per Serving (Serving Size: 1 cup):

Calories	70
Fat	2g
Protein	2g
Sodium	110mg
Fiber	2g
Carbohydrates	31g
Sugar	7g

Sausage Balls

Sausage Balls are popular whether served for breakfast or as an appetizer. They're perfect served with toothpicks at year-end holiday parties— or at a party any month of the year.

3 cups Bisquick Gluten Free Pancake & Baking Mix

2 tablespoons dried sage

1 tablespoon paprika

4 cups shredded dairy-free Cheddar cheese

1 cup dairy-free Parmesan cheese

½ cup light brown sugar, packed

1½ cups unsweetened almond milk

2 (16-ounce) packages gluten-free sausage rolls

1 Heat oven to 350°F. Line a baking sheet with parchment paper.

2 In a large bowl, mix Bisquick, sage, paprika, cheeses, and brown sugar together. Add milk and stir until fully combined. Add sausage and stir to combine.

3 Using a teaspoon or cookie scoop, make nine dozen 1" balls. Place on prepared baking sheet.

4 Bake for 20–25 minutes until golden brown. Allow to cool for 2–3 minutes before serving.

MAKES 108 BALLS

Per Serving (Serving Size: 6 balls):

Calories	190
Fat	7g
Protein	6g
Sodium	514mg
Fiber	2g
Carbohydrates	26g
Sugar	8g

Sausage Hash Brown Egg Cups

MAKES 12 CUPS

Per Serving
(Serving Size: 1 cup):

Calories	190
Fat	14g
Protein	8g
Sodium	530mg
Fiber	1g
Carbohydrates	7g
Sugar	1g

The addition of a Tater Tot crust to these egg cups packs a big taste into a muffin-sized serving. You can also customize them by adding your favorite gluten- and dairy-free omelet fillings, such as bacon, spinach, sausage, steak, garlic, green bell peppers, onions, chicken, or tomatoes.

1 teaspoon olive oil
½ pound gluten-free ground sausage
36 frozen Tater Tots
1 teaspoon salt, divided
8 large eggs
2 tablespoons unsweetened almond milk

1 Preheat oven to 400°F and spray a twelve-cup muffin tin with gluten-free nonstick cooking spray.

2 Heat olive oil in a large skillet over medium-high heat. Add sausage and cook for 10 minutes until sausage is crumbly, evenly browned, and no longer pink; drain.

3 Microwave Tater Tots for 1–2 minutes to defrost and soften. Place three Tater Tots in each well of prepared muffin tin. Press down to make a crust and sprinkle a little salt in each well, making sure a pinch of salt is left over.

4 Bake for 10 minutes, then remove from the oven and lower the oven temperature to 350°F.

5 In a medium bowl, whisk eggs and remaining salt. Add milk and combine.

6 Sprinkle sausage on top of Tater Tots. Pour the egg mixture on top of sausage. Bake for 20 minutes. Allow to cool for 2 minutes before removing cups from muffin tin. Serve warm.

Banana Nut Muffins

This recipe offers all the nutty, sweet flavor of a traditional banana nut muffin but none of the gluten or dairy. The bananas offer lots of potassium, vitamin B_6, manganese (which can improve bone health), and copper.

2 large ripe bananas, peeled and mashed
1 teaspoon baking soda
⅓ cup dairy-free buttery spread, melted
½ cup sugar
⅛ teaspoon salt
2 large eggs, whisked
1 teaspoon pure vanilla extract
1½ cups gluten-free all-purpose flour with xanthan gum
½ teaspoon ground cinnamon
½ cup chopped walnuts

1. Preheat oven to 350°F. Prepare a twelve-cup muffin tin with baking cup liners or gluten-free nonstick cooking spray.

2. In a large bowl, combine bananas and baking soda. Allow the mixture to sit for at least 2 minutes. (Allowing the mashed bananas and baking soda to sit for at least 2 minutes before adding the rest of the ingredients is key to what makes these so light and fluffy.)

3. Stir melted buttery spread into the banana mixture. Stir in sugar, salt, eggs, and vanilla extract.

4. Mix in flour and cinnamon. Stir in walnuts.

5. Scoop batter into prepared muffin tin. Bake for 20 minutes or until a toothpick inserted in the center of a muffin comes out clean. Place muffin tin on a cooling rack and cool for 2 minutes. Remove muffins from tin and place on rack to finish cooling. Store in an airtight container at room temperature for up to 3 days.

MAKES 12 MUFFINS

**Per Serving
(Serving Size: 1 muffin):**

Calories	140
Fat	6g
Protein	4g
Sodium	340mg
Fiber	2g
Carbohydrates	21g
Sugar	10g

WALNUTS FOR WELLNESS

Walnuts are incredibly healthy because they have been found to help lower cholesterol and blood pressure. The next time you are hungry for a quick gluten- and dairy-free snack, grab a handful of walnuts!

Breakfast Cookies

MAKES 24 COOKIES

Per Serving
(Serving Size: 2 cookies):

Calories	178
Fat	7g
Protein	6g
Sodium	100mg
Fiber	3g
Carbohydrates	21g
Sugar	6g

Cookies for breakfast? You bet. These cookies have bananas, peanut butter, and oats to ensure an energy-packed start to your day.

2 large bananas, peeled and mashed
¾ cup gluten-free peanut butter
¼ cup honey
1 tablespoon pure vanilla extract
1 tablespoon ground cinnamon
¾ teaspoon salt
½ cup mini gluten-free and dairy-free chocolate chips
½ cup raisins
3 cups gluten-free oats

1. Preheat oven to 325°F. Line a baking sheet with parchment paper or spray with gluten-free nonstick cooking spray.

2. Add bananas, peanut butter, and honey to a large bowl, and stir to combine. Add vanilla extract, cinnamon, and salt and stir. Stir in the chocolate chips and raisins. Add gluten-free oats. Mix all ingredients together.

3. Use a 1½" tablespoon cookie scoop sprayed with gluten-free nonstick cooking spray to scoop out batter and place onto prepared baking sheet. Flatten the tops slightly. Bake for 15 minutes or until lightly browned. Allow to cool for 2–3 minutes before serving.

Country Breakfast Skillet

SERVES 6

Per Serving:

Calories	431
Fat	23g
Protein	25g
Sodium	1,492mg
Fiber	24g
Carbohydrates	29g
Sugar	3g

This Country Breakfast Skillet brings everything you love about a hearty breakfast into one sizzling dish. You can substitute gluten-free turkey bacon and gluten-free turkey sausage if you prefer.

2 teaspoons olive oil
6 cups frozen cubed hash browns
¾ cup seeded and chopped green bell pepper
½ cup peeled and chopped sweet onion
1 teaspoon salt
¼ teaspoon ground black pepper
6 large eggs
6 cooked gluten-free bacon strips, chopped
6 cooked gluten-free sausage links, chopped

1. Heat olive oil in a large skillet over medium heat. Add hash browns, bell peppers, onions, salt, and black pepper and cook for 2 minutes, stirring occasionally. Cover and cook for 15 minutes, stirring occasionally, until potatoes are browned and tender.

2. Make six small wells in the potato mixture with a large spoon; break one egg into each well. Cover skillet and cook on low heat for 8–10 minutes or until eggs are completely set. Sprinkle bacon and sausage all over the mixture. Spoon an egg with the potato mixture on each plate and serve warm.

Baked Apple Cinnamon Donuts

These homemade baked donuts are easily made with applesauce and are dipped in a rich maple vanilla glaze. Most store-bought applesauce is gluten- and dairy-free, but always read labels to be sure.

MUFFINS

¾ cup sugar

2 large eggs

1 cup applesauce

3 tablespoons vegetable oil

½ teaspoon pure vanilla extract

1½ cups gluten-free all-purpose flour with xanthan gum

½ teaspoon ground cinnamon

½ teaspoon salt

1 teaspoon gluten-free baking powder

GLAZE

1 cup confectioners' sugar

¼ teaspoon ground cinnamon

1 teaspoon pure vanilla extract

4 tablespoons pure maple syrup

1. Preheat oven to 350°F. Spray a full-sized sixteen-cup donut pan with gluten-free nonstick cooking spray.

2. In a large bowl, combine sugar, eggs, applesauce, vegetable oil, and vanilla extract. Mix until fully combined.

3. Add flour, cinnamon, salt, and baking powder and mix until fully combined. The batter will be thick and sticky.

4. Add batter to a large plastic storage bag or piping bag. Seal the bag and cut a corner (or tip, if using a piping bag) off. Carefully squeeze batter into donut pan. Bake for 14–16 minutes until golden brown and set. Place plan on a cooling rack and cool for 1 minute. Remove donuts from the pan and place on rack to continue cooling.

5. In a small bowl, whisk together the glaze ingredients. Dip each warm donut into the glaze and place on a plate or wire rack. Store in an airtight container at room temperature for up to 3 days.

MAKES 16 DONUTS

**Per Serving
(Serving Size: 1 donut):**

Calories	160
Fat	4g
Protein	2g
Sodium	120mg
Fiber	1g
Carbohydrates	31g
Sugar	23g

SWEET KNOWLEDGE

Maple syrup comes from tapping a hole in maple trees and boiling the sap to make thick syrup. Maple syrup is classified as either Grade A or Grade B. The lighter version is Grade A and the darker version is Grade B. Pure maple syrup is naturally gluten- and dairy-free.

Turkey Sausage Patties

MAKES 12 PATTIES

Per Serving
(Serving Size: 1 patty):

Calories	70
Fat	4g
Protein	7g
Sodium	124mg
Fiber	0g
Carbohydrates	1g
Sugar	0g

Turkey Sausage Patties are the perfect side dish for any breakfast. They can be used in making scrambles, skillets, omelets, and frittatas, and they make the best sausage and egg biscuit sandwiches.

1 teaspoon dried thyme
1 teaspoon dried sage
1 teaspoon onion powder
¼ teaspoon garlic powder

½ teaspoon salt
1 teaspoon pure maple syrup
1 pound ground turkey
1 tablespoon olive oil

1 Combine thyme, sage, onion powder, garlic powder, and salt in a large bowl. Add maple syrup and stir together to combine. Add ground turkey and mix until fully combined.

2 Heat olive oil in a large skillet over medium-high heat.

3 Form turkey sausage into twelve patties and fry 6–8 minutes total until browned on both sides and no longer pink in the center.

Classic French Toast

MAKES 8 SLICES

Per Serving
(Serving Size: 2 slices):

Calories	420
Fat	12g
Protein	9g
Sodium	532mg
Fiber	1g
Carbohydrates	68g
Sugar	33g

You might have worried that you couldn't make tasty French toast without gluten and dairy—but this recipe will change your mind. It's full of flavor and just as sweet and hearty as you'd hope.

2 large eggs
1 cup unsweetened almond milk
1 teaspoon ground cinnamon
¼ teaspoon ground nutmeg
2 teaspoons pure vanilla extract

1 tablespoon granulated sugar
8 slices gluten-free and dairy-free bread
2 tablespoons dairy-free buttery spread
½ cup pure maple syrup

1 Whisk together eggs, milk, cinnamon, nutmeg, vanilla extract, and sugar in a pie pan. Place bread slices in the egg mixture and flip to make sure both sides of bread are well coated.

2 Melt buttery spread in a large skillet. Place bread slices in skillet and cook on medium heat for 2–3 minutes on each side until golden brown. Serve warm with maple syrup.

CHAPTER 3

Lunch

Grilled Chicken Chimichurri Salad

SERVES 4

Per Serving:

Calories	430
Fat	30g
Protein	26g
Sodium	90mg
Fiber	6g
Carbohydrates	18g
Sugar	6g

MARINATING THE MEAT IS THE KEY

To make this dish full of flavor, be sure to let the meat marinate. This process allows the flavors to really seep into the meat and stay there during cooking.

This recipe is a nightshade-free twist on traditional chimichurri sauce. Because it doesn't contain peppers, it is not spicy either. The chimichurri sauce is both the marinade and dressing for this glorious grilled chicken salad.

MARINADE
1 cup fresh chopped cilantro
1 teaspoon jarred minced garlic
2 green onions, sliced
1 teaspoon ground cumin
½ cup cashew butter
4 teaspoons white vinegar
1 teaspoon balsamic vinegar
½ teaspoon ground turmeric
½ cup honey
¼ cup olive oil

CHICKEN
2 (6-ounce) boneless, skinless chicken breasts
2 tablespoons olive oil

SALAD
4 cups chopped romaine lettuce
2 large avocados, peeled, pitted, and diced
¼ cup chopped cilantro
½ cup chopped cucumbers
¼ cup chopped cashews
½ cup halved grape tomatoes
2 large hard-boiled eggs, peeled and sliced

1   In a food processor, purée cilantro, garlic, green onions, and cumin. In a medium microwave-safe bowl stir together cashew butter, vinegars, turmeric, and honey and microwave for 1 minute. Add the cilantro mixture to the cashew butter mixture and stir until fully combined. Pour olive oil into the combined mixture and stir to finish the marinade. Cover and refrigerate until ready to use.

2   Add chicken breasts and ½ cup of marinade to a sealable plastic bag. Seal the bag and allow chicken to marinate for at least 1 hour.

3   Add olive oil to a grill pan and heat over medium-high heat. Grill chicken for 6–7 minutes on each side until completely cooked (the meat is no longer pink, the juices run clear, and meat reaches an internal temperature of 165°F). Allow chicken to cool for 5 minutes before slicing.

4   Portion salad ingredients on four plates. Top with sliced chicken and drizzle with remaining sauce.

Smoked Salmon Sushi Bowls

High-quality gluten- and dairy-free sushi is becoming increasingly easier to get, but this is a simple way to enjoy all the flavors of sushi at home. Sushi bowls can be easily customized with your favorite toppings.

SUSHI RICE
2 cups sushi rice
2 tablespoons rice vinegar
1 tablespoon granulated sugar
2 teaspoons salt

SOY GINGER DRESSING
½ cup gluten-free soy sauce
¼ cup rice vinegar
2 tablespoons honey
1 teaspoon sesame oil
2 tablespoons minced ginger
½ teaspoon jarred minced garlic

BOWL TOPPINGS
8 ounces smoked salmon, sliced
1½ cups peeled and diced English cucumber
1 large avocado, peeled, pitted, and diced
2 nori sheets, chopped
½ teaspoon toasted black sesame seeds, for garnish

1 Cook sushi rice according to the package directions.

2 In a small microwave-safe bowl, mix vinegar, sugar, and salt. Heat in the microwave for 30 seconds and stir until sugar and salt are dissolved. Pour the vinegar mixture over the rice, stirring to coat.

3 In a medium bowl, stir together soy sauce, vinegar, honey, sesame oil, ginger, and garlic. Whisk until honey is dissolved.

4 Portion rice into four bowls and top with smoked salmon, cucumber, avocado, and nori. Drizzle the top with the soy ginger dressing. Sprinkle with sesame seeds.

SERVES 4

Per Serving:

Calories	394
Fat	9g
Protein	17g
Sodium	3,565mg
Fiber	4g
Carbohydrates	28g
Sugar	13g

SUSHI RICE IN MINUTES!

Make the sushi rice in a pressure cooker by using the rice setting and allowing the pressure to naturally release for 5–10 minutes. Many pressure cookers have a great warming feature that you can use to keep your rice warm for 30 minutes to an hour and still get rice with a nice texture.

Asian Chicken Lettuce Wraps

SERVES 4

Per Serving:

Calories	285
Fat	15g
Protein	24g
Sodium	1,100mg
Fiber	3g
Carbohydrates	13g
Sugar	5g

IS IT A NUT?

While most people probably think water chestnuts are nuts, they are not actually nuts. A water chestnut is an aquatic, green-stemmed vegetable that is grown in marshes. These vegetables are an excellent source of antioxidants that are believed to fight oxidative stress. They're also full of the key nutrients copper, fiber, protein, magnesium, and riboflavin.

Lettuce wraps are an easy and healthy way around gluten-based tortilla wraps. These pack a lot of flavor into a quick lunch.

1 teaspoon olive oil
1 pound ground chicken
1½ teaspoons jarred minced garlic
1 cup peeled and diced sweet onion
2 teaspoons sesame oil
¼ cup gluten-free soy sauce
1 teaspoon rice wine vinegar
1 tablespoon jarred minced ginger
¼ teaspoon sriracha
1 teaspoon light brown sugar, packed
1 tablespoon gluten-free peanut butter
1 (8-ounce) can water chestnuts, drained and chopped
3 green onions, thinly sliced
1 head butter lettuce

1 Heat olive oil in a large skillet over medium-high heat. Add ground chicken, garlic, and sweet onions and cook for 5–6 minutes until browned, making sure to crumble the chicken as it cooks. Drain excess grease.

2 In a medium bowl, whisk together sesame oil, soy sauce, vinegar, ginger, sriracha, brown sugar, and peanut butter until fully combined.

3 Add the sauce mixture to chicken and stir to combine. Bring sauce to a low boil. Stir in chestnuts and green onions and cook for 2–3 minutes until tender.

4 To serve, spoon the chicken mixture into the center of lettuce leaves, fold, and enjoy.

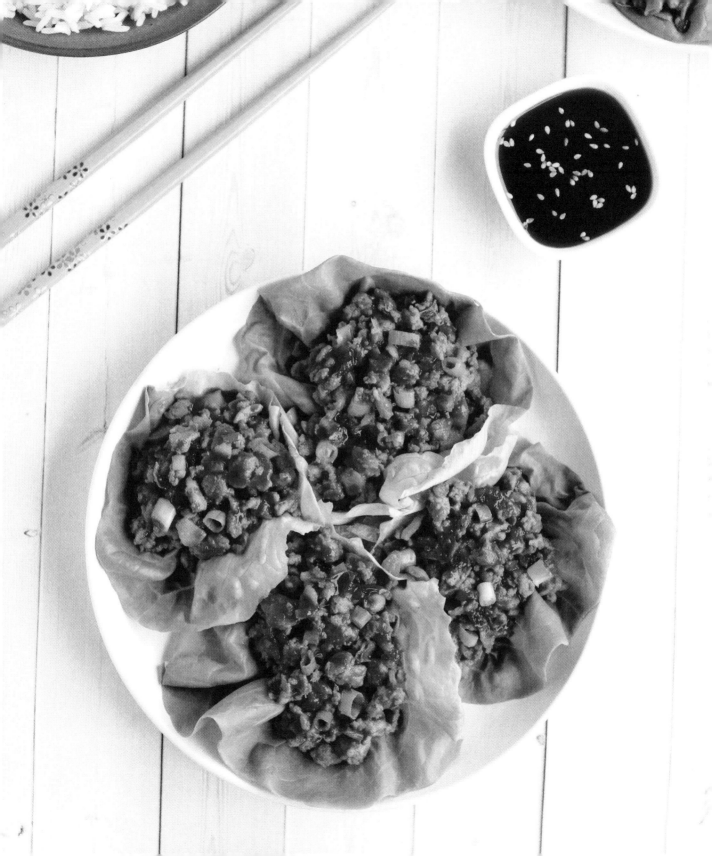

Creamy Italian Pasta Salad

SERVES 8

Per Serving:

Calories	395
Fat	24g
Protein	4g
Sodium	939mg
Fiber	1g
Carbohydrates	40g
Sugar	4g

AL DENTE

Cooking pasta or vegetables until they are al dente means that they have been cooked just long enough to where they are firm and slightly chewy but not too hard or too soft. If you prefer al dente for pasta or vegetables when dining out, you should make that request to your waiter; otherwise, you will get what the kitchen prefers! Gluten-free pasta is best al dente because if overcooked it gets really, really mushy.

This Creamy Italian Pasta Salad features artichoke hearts, black olives, grape tomatoes, roasted red peppers, and gluten-free rotini pasta to make a summer classic that everyone loves! It is a perfect gluten-free pasta salad to take to your next cookout or family get-together to ensure you have something to eat.

PASTA

1 (12-ounce) box gluten-free rotini pasta

CREAMY ITALIAN DRESSING

1 teaspoon garlic powder

1 teaspoon onion powder

1 teaspoon dried basil

1 teaspoon dried oregano

1 teaspoon dried parsley

½ teaspoon dried thyme

½ teaspoon dried marjoram

1½ teaspoons salt

½ teaspoon ground black pepper

2 tablespoons granulated sugar

1 cup mayonnaise

1 tablespoon red wine vinegar

1 tablespoon balsamic vinegar

PASTA SALAD

1 (14-ounce) can artichoke hearts, drained and chopped

1 cup sliced black olives

1 cup quartered grape tomatoes

1 cup diced roasted red peppers

¼ cup chopped fresh basil

1 Cook pasta to al dente per the box directions. After draining the pasta, rinse pasta with cold water and allow to cool, then add to a large bowl.

2 In a small bowl, add all the dressing ingredients together and stir until fully combined.

3 Add artichokes, olives, tomatoes, red peppers, and dressing to pasta and stir until fully coated. Cover and refrigerate for 30 minutes before serving. Sprinkle with basil before serving.

Tuna Salad Avocado Bowls

The traditional tuna sandwich is always wonderful, but these healthy Tuna Salad Avocado Bowls are a gluten- and dairy-free upgrade that is delicious! They are a low-carb alternative to a traditional tuna salad sandwich.

1/4 cup mayonnaise
1/2 teaspoon Old Bay Seasoning
1/2 teaspoon dried dill
2 tablespoons sweet pickle relish
1/2 teaspoon lemon juice

2 large avocados, pitted and halved
2 (5-ounce) cans tuna, drained
1 large hard-boiled egg, peeled and chopped

SERVES 4

Per Serving:

Calories	300
Fat	23g
Protein	17g
Sodium	415mg
Fiber	5g
Carbohydrates	9g
Sugar	3g

1 In a large bowl, whisk together mayonnaise, Old Bay Seasoning, dill, relish, and lemon juice.

2 Scoop out some of the avocados from the pitted areas to widen the areas. Place scooped avocado in a small bowl and mash with a fork.

3 Add mashed avocado and tuna to the mayonnaise mixture and stir until well blended. Once fully combined, add egg and stir until well blended. Add tuna salad into the center of each avocado half.

Southern Chicken Salad

This Southern Chicken Salad showcases tender chunks of chicken in a perfectly seasoned, creamy mayonnaise–honey mustard sauce with sweet and crunchy apples. Gala apples are an excellent choice for just the right sweet addition.

3/4 cup mayonnaise
1/4 teaspoon seasoned salt
2 tablespoons gluten-free and dairy-free honey mustard salad dressing

1 teaspoon lemon juice
4 cups chopped, cooked chicken breast
1 large Gala apple, peeled, cored, and chopped

SERVES 6

Per Serving:

Calories	357
Fat	29g
Protein	10g
Sodium	598mg
Fiber	1g
Carbohydrates	14g
Sugar	4g

1 In a large bowl, whisk together mayonnaise, seasoned salt, honey mustard dressing, and lemon juice.

2 Add chicken and stir until well blended, then add apples and stir until well blended.

3 Cover and refrigerate for 30 minutes before serving.

Taco Salad

Per Serving:

Calories	650
Fat	36g
Protein	35g
Sodium	1,065mg
Fiber	14g
Carbohydrates	52g
Sugar	3g

TURKEY INSTEAD OF BEEF

For most recipes, including this one, ground turkey is a great option in place of ground beef. It will often have less fat, so you may want to add some oil when browning the meat. Ground turkey is also typically less expensive than ground beef.

This salad is loaded with all the makings of tasty tacos, but without the mess! Pack the toppings in a separate container from the meat to take along to work or school.

TACO MEAT

1 teaspoon olive oil
1 pound 90/10 ground beef
1 tablespoon ground cumin
2 teaspoons onion powder
½ teaspoon garlic powder
2 teaspoons paprika
2 teaspoons dried oregano
½ teaspoon salt

SALAD

1 (15-ounce) can corn, drained
1 (15-ounce) can black beans, drained and rinsed
1 cup halved grape tomatoes
2 large avocados, peeled, pitted, and chopped
½ cup sliced black olives
½ cup chopped fresh cilantro
1 large romaine lettuce heart, chopped
½ cup crushed gluten-free tortilla chips

1 Heat olive oil in a large skillet over medium-high heat. Add ground beef and seasonings and break up ground beef into equal-sized pieces as it cooks. Cook for 5–8 minutes until browned and broken into crumbles; drain oil.

2 Add salad ingredients except tortilla chips to a large bowl and toss to combine. Top with beef and tortilla chips.

Soy Ginger Vegetable Stir-Fry

This is a quick and easy stir-fry with a rainbow of sautéed vegetables coated with a soy ginger sauce that will fill your home with the most fabulous savory scents! Serve over rice or gluten-free rice noodles.

¼ cup gluten-free soy sauce
2 tablespoons rice vinegar
2 tablespoons light brown sugar, packed
2 tablespoons cornstarch
1 tablespoon jarred minced ginger
1 teaspoon sesame oil
¼ teaspoon sriracha
2 tablespoons vegetable oil
1 tablespoon jarred minced garlic
2 cups broccoli florets
1 cup peeled and sliced carrots
1 medium sweet onion, peeled and thinly sliced
1 large red bell pepper, seeded and cut into strips
1 cup sliced white button mushrooms
2 cups sugar snap peas
1 teaspoon sesame seeds

1 In a small bowl add soy sauce, rice vinegar, brown sugar, cornstarch, ginger, sesame oil, and sriracha and whisk until combined.

2 Heat vegetable oil in a large wok or skillet over medium-high heat. Add garlic, broccoli, carrots, onions, and peppers, and cook for 2–3 minutes. Add mushrooms and snap peas and allow to cook for 2–3 minutes longer.

3 Stir in sauce and allow to cook for 1–2 minutes until vegetables are coated and sauce has thickened.

4 Sprinkle with sesame seeds.

SERVES 4

Per Serving:

Calories	290
Fat	14g
Protein	8g
Sodium	1,950mg
Fiber	6g
Carbohydrates	35g
Sugar	18g

POUR IT ON!

Sesame oil is a healthy way to add a punch of flavor to your dish. It has many health benefits, including being rich in polyunsaturated and monounsaturated fats and low in saturated fats. Sesame oil has a rich flavor, so if you have not used it before, test it a little at a time.

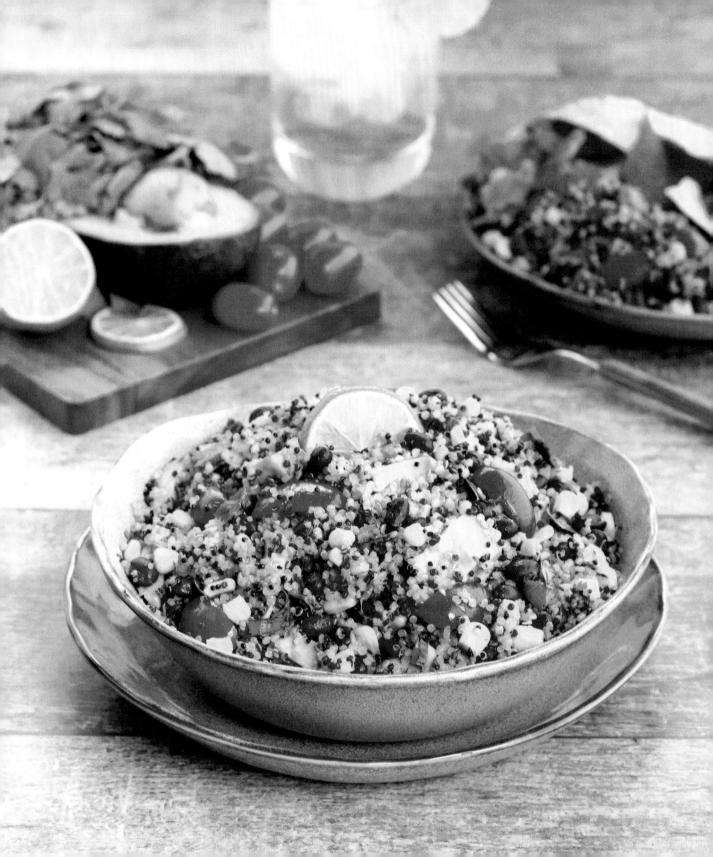

Southwest Tricolored Quinoa Salad

This healthy southwest salad is bursting with a bounty of garden-fresh flavors. The sweet and tangy flavor of the dressing pairs perfectly with the fluffy, nutty quinoa!

4 tablespoons olive oil
1 tablespoon lime juice
1 tablespoon honey
1 tablespoon ground cumin
¼ teaspoon salt
½ cup chopped fresh cilantro
1 cup tricolored quinoa
1 large avocado, peeled, pitted, and diced
1 cup canned black beans, drained and rinsed
1 cup canned corn, drained
1 cup grape tomatoes, quartered

1. In a small bowl, whisk together olive oil, lime juice, honey, cumin, and salt until fully combined. Add cilantro and stir.
2. Cook quinoa according to the package directions. Allow to cool.
3. Place cooled quinoa, avocado, beans, corn, and tomatoes in a large bowl. Pour dressing over salad and stir to fully coat and serve. Store leftovers in an airtight container for up to 3 days.

SERVES 8

Per Serving:

Calories	140
Fat	10g
Protein	2g
Sodium	82mg
Fiber	2g
Carbohydrates	11g
Sugar	3g

PROBLEM SOLVED

To keep your cilantro fresh longer, trim the stems and dry the remaining stems and leaves. Place the stems in a small water-filled jar and refrigerate. If you loosely cover the top with plastic wrap your cilantro will stay fresh for weeks.

Avocado Bacon Chicken Salad

SERVES 4

Per Serving:

Calories	340
Fat	25g
Protein	18g
Sodium	785mg
Fiber	5g
Carbohydrates	12g
Sugar	0g

The flavors of avocado and bacon combine in this zesty southwestern twist on traditional chicken salad. This recipe is an unexpected way to treat guests you entertain for lunch!

3 tablespoons lime juice
3 tablespoons olive oil
1 teaspoon salt
¼ teaspoon gluten- and dairy-free hot sauce
4 cups chopped cooked chicken breast
2 large avocados, peeled, pitted, and diced
1 cup chopped cooked gluten-free bacon
1 cup canned corn, drained
¼ cup chopped fresh cilantro

1 In a small bowl whisk together lime juice, olive oil, salt, and pepper sauce until fully combined.

2 In a large bowl add chicken, avocado, bacon, corn, and cilantro and stir to combine.

3 Drizzle dressing over chicken salad and toss to combine. Cover and refrigerate for 30 minutes before serving.

Southwestern Chicken Salad

SERVES 6

Per Serving:

Calories	385
Fat	19g
Protein	15g
Sodium	750mg
Fiber	7g
Carbohydrates	40g
Sugar	14g

Try this full-flavored and hearty chicken salad with homemade gluten-free and dairy-free bread.

¼ cup olive oil
¼ cup lime juice
¼ cup honey
2 teaspoons ground cumin
½ teaspoon garlic powder
¼ teaspoon gluten- and dairy-free hot sauce
½ teaspoon salt
4 cups chopped cooked chicken breast
1 (15-ounce) can corn, drained
1 (15-ounce) can black beans, drained and rinsed
1 cup chopped roasted red peppers
1 cup peeled and chopped red onion
1 cup chopped fresh cilantro
2 large avocados, peeled, pitted, and chopped

1 In a small bowl, whisk together olive oil, lime juice, honey, cumin, garlic powder, pepper sauce, and salt until fully combined.

2 In a large bowl, add chicken, corn, beans, red peppers, onions, cilantro, and avocado.

3 Pour lime sauce over the chicken mixture and toss to coat. Cover and refrigerate for 30 minutes before serving.

Chopped Asian Salad with Peanut Dressing

The rich peanut flavor in this salad will keep you coming back to this recipe over and over! In fact, you will want to use this peanut dressing on other proteins too, such as grilled chicken or shrimp.

PEANUT DRESSING

2 tablespoons gluten-free peanut butter
1 tablespoon gluten-free soy sauce
1 tablespoon sesame oil
2 tablespoons water
1 tablespoon rice wine vinegar
1 tablespoon lime juice
½ teaspoon jarred minced garlic
½ teaspoon jarred minced ginger
1 tablespoon honey
½ teaspoon sriracha
½ teaspoon salt
¼ teaspoon ground black pepper

SALAD

1 (14-ounce) package dairy-free coleslaw mix
2 carrots, peeled and cut into matchsticks
1 cup chopped snow peas
1 red bell pepper, seeded and finely diced
½ cup fresh chopped cilantro
¼ cup chopped green onion
1 (11-ounce) can mandarin oranges, drained
2 tablespoons sesame seeds
½ cup chopped peanuts

SERVES 4

Per Serving:

Calories	310
Fat	3g
Protein	11g
Sodium	720mg
Fiber	7g
Carbohydrates	26g
Sugar	14g

PEANUTS IN THE UNITED STATES

The peanut originated in South America, and it was later discovered that the sandy soil and warm climate in southern Georgia was particularly suitable to grow peanuts. Today, just about every county in southern Georgia grows peanuts, a location that accounts for over 50 percent of peanut production in the United States.

1 In a small bowl, add peanut butter, soy sauce, sesame oil, water, vinegar, lime juice, garlic, ginger, honey, sriracha, salt, and black pepper. Whisk together until fully combined.

2 In a large bowl, toss coleslaw mix, carrots, snow peas, bell peppers, cilantro, and green onions.

3 Add mandarin oranges, sesame seeds, and peanuts to the top of the salad and drizzle with peanut dressing.

Egg Roll Bowl

SERVES 4

Per Serving:

Calories	380
Fat	23g
Protein	26g
Sodium	1,290mg
Fiber	3g
Carbohydrates	17g
Sugar	8g

This lunch bowl has all the delicious flavors of an egg roll in a lighter, faster, and one-skillet meal. Each bite of this dish tastes like a scrumptious egg roll. Egg rolls are traditionally made with ground pork, but this recipe can be easily made with ground chicken or turkey. For an even heartier meal, serve over rice.

1 tablespoon sesame oil
1 pound ground pork
1 tablespoon jarred minced garlic
1 sweet onion, peeled and diced
½ cup sliced white button mushrooms
½ cup gluten-free chicken broth
1 tablespoon minced ginger
¼ cup gluten-free soy sauce
1 tablespoon rice wine vinegar
1 (14-ounce) bag dairy-free coleslaw mix

1. In a wok or large skillet, heat oil over medium heat. Add ground pork, garlic, onions, and mushrooms and cook for 6–8 minutes until pork is no longer pink and vegetables are tender.

2. In a small bowl, whisk together broth, ginger, soy sauce, and vinegar until fully combined.

3. Pour sauce in skillet and stir in coleslaw mix. Cover and simmer for 5–10 minutes until cabbage is wilted.

Homestyle Egg Salad

SERVES 6

Per Serving:

Calories	235
Fat	5g
Protein	13g
Sodium	525mg
Fiber	0g
Carbohydrates	1g
Sugar	1g

When you are craving a lunch sandwich from your childhood days, this light egg salad will satisfy your appetite. Egg salad goes great on toasted gluten-free and dairy-free bread (preferably homemade).

6 tablespoons mayonnaise
2 teaspoons Dijon mustard
1 tablespoon dried dill
2 tablespoons dill pickle relish
½ teaspoon salt
¼ teaspoon ground black pepper
¼ cup chopped celery
12 large hard-boiled eggs, peeled and chopped

1. In a large bowl, combine mayonnaise, mustard, dill, relish, salt, and pepper and stir to combine.

2. Add celery and eggs and stir to combines. Cover and chill for at least 1 hour before serving.

Greek Chicken Wraps

These marinated Greek Chicken Wraps topped with a creamy homemade cucumber dill sauce are a lunch indulgence that everyone will love! If you like the flavor of authentic gyros, then these will be your new favorite lunch wraps.

CHICKEN MARINADE

¼ cup olive oil
¼ cup red wine vinegar
½ cup lemon juice
2 teaspoons jarred minced garlic
1 teaspoon onion powder
1 tablespoon dried oregano
2 teaspoons dried thyme
1 teaspoon salt
1 teaspoon ground black pepper
2 (6-ounce) boneless, skinless chicken breasts, sliced into 1" pieces

CUCUMBER SAUCE

½ cup peeled and finely diced English cucumber
2 tablespoons lemon juice
1 tablespoon jarred minced garlic
2 tablespoons dried dill
1 cup mayonnaise
¼ teaspoon salt

CHICKEN WRAP

2 tablespoons olive oil
4 pieces warm gluten-free Flatbread (see recipe in Chapter 8)
½ cup diced tomatoes

SERVES 4

Per Serving:

Calories	975
Fat	77g
Protein	22g
Sodium	912mg
Fiber	1g
Carbohydrates	40g
Sugar	3g

THE GLORIOUS GYRO

The meat used for the gyro was traditionally lamb. Today, you will see roasted chicken, pork, and even beef cut into thin slices and placed atop warm flatbread. The meat is normally compressed into a form and placed on a roasting spit and slow roasted for that rich gyro flavor.

1 In a gallon-sized sealable plastic bag, add olive oil, vinegar, lemon juice, garlic, onion powder, oregano, thyme, salt, and pepper. Add chicken, seal bag, and massage ingredients to combine. Let chicken marinate in the refrigerator for 30 minutes.

2 While chicken is marinating, combine the cucumber sauce ingredients in a small bowl. Cover and refrigerate.

3 Heat olive oil in a large skillet over medium heat. Pour chicken and marinade into the skillet. Stir and cook chicken for 6–7 minutes until it is no longer pink and is fully cooked.

4 Serve over Flatbread pieces. Sprinkle with diced tomatoes and drizzle with cucumber sauce.

Mediterranean Tuna Salad

SERVES 4

Per Serving:

Calories	270
Fat	10g
Protein	22g
Sodium	920mg
Fiber	7g
Carbohydrates	25g
Sugar	6g

This is a surprising twist on traditional tuna salad that is a light, healthy, and quick lunch. The cannellini beans add flavor, texture, and extra health benefits like protein, antioxidants, iron, and magnesium.

2 tablespoons olive oil
1 tablespoon balsamic vinegar
1 teaspoon dried basil
½ teaspoon onion powder
½ teaspoon salt
2 (5-ounce) cans tuna in water, drained

1 (15-ounce) can cannellini beans, drained
1 cucumber, diced
2 large beefsteak tomatoes, diced
2 tablespoons chopped Kalamata olives

1. In a small bowl, whisk together olive oil, vinegar, basil, onion powder, and salt until fully combined.
2. In a large bowl, combine tuna, beans, cucumbers, tomatoes, and olives. Pour dressing over the tuna mixture and stir to fully combine. Refrigerate for 30 minutes before serving.

Mini Corn Dog Bites

MAKES 24 BITES

**Per Serving
(Serving Size: 4 bites):**

Calories	580
Fat	36g
Protein	15g
Sodium	1,025mg
Fiber	2g
Carbohydrates	50g
Sugar	10g

These bites are super simple to make and perfect for lunches, a snack, or a fun appetizer for your next party. Serve with ketchup and gluten-free and dairy-free honey mustard for dipping sauces.

1 box gluten-free corn bread mix with necessary gluten-free and dairy-free ingredients
6 gluten-free and dairy-free hot dogs

1. Preheat oven according to corn bread mix package directions. Spray twenty-four-cup mini muffin tin with gluten-free nonstick cooking spray.
2. Make corn bread according to the package directions. Fill muffin tin with batter.
3. Cut hot dogs into bite-sized pieces. Place hot dog pieces in the center of each cup filled with batter.
4. Bake according to the package directions.

Spinach Salad with Warm Bacon Dressing

This elegant salad is often featured on the menus at upscale restaurants. This recipe rivals any restaurant's take on it.

1 teaspoon olive oil
8 strips gluten-free bacon
1 small red onion, peeled and thinly sliced
2 cups sliced white button mushrooms
3 tablespoons red wine vinegar
2 teaspoons honey
½ teaspoon Dijon mustard
½ teaspoon salt
1 (8-ounce) package baby spinach
4 large hard-boiled eggs, peeled and sliced

1 Heat olive oil in a large skillet over medium-high heat. Add bacon and fry for 3–4 minutes on each side until brown and crispy. Remove cooked bacon to a paper towel to drain. Once cooled, crumble and set aside. Transfer 3 tablespoons bacon grease from the skillet to a small saucepan. Safely disregard the remaining oil.

2 Add onions and mushrooms to the skillet and cook on medium heat for 3–5 minutes until onions and mushrooms are caramelized and reduced.

3 Add vinegar, honey, mustard, and salt into saucepan with bacon grease. Whisk together and heat thoroughly for 2 minutes over medium-low heat.

4 Add spinach to a large bowl. Top with sautéed onions, mushrooms, and bacon. Pour hot dressing over salad and toss to combine. Place sliced eggs on top and serve.

SERVES 4

Per Serving:

Calories	185
Fat	10g
Protein	14g
Sodium	630mg
Fiber	2g
Carbohydrates	9g
Sugar	5g

HEAT IT UP!

Most people are used to cold mayonnaise-based salad dressings. However, if you get a little adventurous, you will find that hot salad dressings are a fantastic change of pace. If you are serving a large tossed salad, pour the dressing over the salad and toss just before serving, or dress the individual salad portions and serve immediately for the best results.

Crispy Southwest Wraps

SERVES 6

Per Serving:

Calories	490
Fat	28g
Protein	21g
Sodium	720mg
Fiber	9g
Carbohydrates	40g
Sugar	2g

FOOD OF THE SOUTHWEST

The food of the southwestern United States is very diverse—more so than you might imagine from chain restaurant menus. Hearty breads, rich beef dishes, smothered chicken, and sweet, milky desserts fill the menus of authentic, local diners in Arizona, New Mexico, and West Texas.

This wrap is packed with all the great flavors of the Southwest. The popular combination of seasoned beef, corn, black beans, and fresh cilantro come together in perfect harmony in this hearty lunch. Serve with chopped tomatoes and avocados and fresh lime, if desired.

1 pound 90/10 ground beef
½ large red bell pepper, seeded and chopped
½ teaspoon salt
⅛ teaspoon ground black pepper
2 teaspoons chili powder
2 teaspoons ground cumin
2 teaspoons garlic powder
2 teaspoons onion powder
1 teaspoon dried oregano
3 tablespoons water
1 (15-ounce) can black beans, drained and rinsed
1 cup canned corn, drained
½ cup chopped fresh cilantro
6 large gluten-free and dairy-free flour tortillas
1 cup cooked rice
3 tablespoons vegetable oil

1 Add beef to a large skillet and cook for 5–8 minutes over medium heat until crumbled and browned; drain grease.

2 Add bell peppers to the skillet and cook for 2 minutes until tender. Add salt, pepper, chili powder, cumin, garlic powder, onion powder, oregano, and water. Stir to combine. Add black beans, corn, and cilantro and stir to combine. Cook for 2–3 minutes.

3 Heat each tortilla in the microwave for 10 seconds to make it easier to roll. Add rice to the center of each tortilla and top with the beef mixture. Roll up, folding in the sides like a burrito.

4 Spray a large skillet with gluten-free nonstick cooking spray and place the wraps seam-side down.

5 Gently brush the tops of the wraps lightly with oil. Cook for 2 minutes on each side on medium-high heat until golden and crispy.

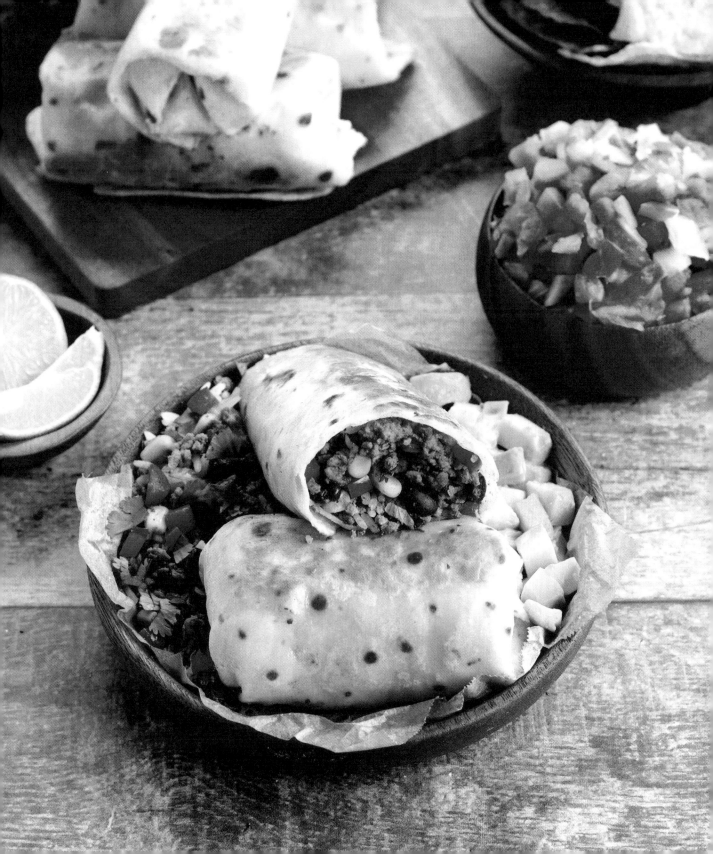

Loaded Burger Bowls

SERVES 4

Per Serving:

Calories	735
Fat	60g
Protein	33g
Sodium	1,575mg
Fiber	5g
Carbohydrates	18g
Sugar	9g

CREATIVE TOPPINGS

Mix it up and get creative with your burger toppings. Avocado, fried green tomatoes, and even a fried egg can transform a burger into a completely different meal from day to day. Do not forget about jalapeños, sun-dried tomatoes, and dairy-free mozzarella cheese.

Fill these Loaded Burger Bowls with all your favorite toppings and a "special sauce" for a great alternative to the lettuce wrap burger. It's less messy than trying to eat a lettuce-wrapped burger and is also a great low-carb substitute for traditional burgers.

BURGERS

1 pound 90/10 ground beef
1 teaspoon seasoned salt
1 teaspoon olive oil
8 strips gluten-free bacon, chopped
½ cup peeled and thinly sliced sweet onion
½ cup sliced white button mushrooms

SPECIAL SAUCE

½ cup mayonnaise
3 tablespoons ketchup
2 tablespoons sweet pickle relish
1½ teaspoons granulated sugar
1½ teaspoons white vinegar
¼ teaspoon onion powder
¼ teaspoon salt

BOWLS

1 head iceberg lettuce, chopped
1 cup halved grape tomatoes
½ cup chopped dill pickles

1. In a medium bowl, mix together beef and seasoned salt.

2. Heat olive oil in a large skillet over medium heat, then add bacon and cook for 2–3 minutes on each side until brown and crispy. Remove to a paper towel–lined plate to drain.

3. Add beef to the skillet and cook for 4–6 minutes until starting to brown and crumble. Stir in onions and mushrooms and cook for 2–3 minutes until onions and mushrooms have started to caramelize and get soft.

4. In a small bowl, whisk together the sauce ingredients until fully combined.

5. To assemble bowls, start with a layer of chopped lettuce, then spoon the beef mixture into the center. Arrange tomatoes, pickles, and bacon around the beef and drizzle with sauce and serve.

Grilled Chicken Caesar Salad

This salad has juicy, lightly seasoned chicken; crisp, fresh lettuce tossed in a creamy garlic Caesar dressing; and crunchy, homemade croutons. The rich dairy-free dressing is a showstopper!

CHICKEN

2 (6-ounce) boneless, skinless chicken breasts
2 tablespoons olive oil, divided
2 tablespoons lemon juice
½ teaspoon salt
¼ teaspoon ground black pepper
1 teaspoon jarred minced garlic

CAESAR DRESSING

½ cup mayonnaise
1 teaspoon gluten-free Worcestershire sauce
1 tablespoon lemon juice
2 teaspoons jarred minced garlic
1 teaspoon Dijon mustard
1 teaspoon olive oil
¼ teaspoon salt
⅛ teaspoon ground black pepper

CROUTONS

½ cup olive oil
1 teaspoon garlic powder
1 teaspoon onion powder
¼ teaspoon salt
4 cups cubed gluten-free and dairy-free bread

SALAD

4 large romaine lettuce hearts, chopped

SERVES 4

Per Serving:

Calories	870
Fat	65g
Protein	30g
Sodium	940mg
Fiber	14g
Carbohydrates	42g
Sugar	10g

MORE ON ANCHOVIES

Traditional Caesar dressing includes anchovies. They are high in omega-3 fatty acids. If the flavor of anchovies is something you need to complete your Caesar salad, add three chopped anchovy fillets for that "little fish" zip.

1. Place chicken in a sealable plastic bag. Add 1 tablespoon oil, lemon juice, salt, pepper, and garlic. Seal the top of the bag and massage the ingredients to combine. Let chicken marinate for 30 minutes.

2. In a small bowl, whisk together the Caesar dressing ingredients until combined. Cover and refrigerate.

3. Preheat oven to 375°F. Line a baking sheet with parchment paper.

4. In a small bowl, whisk together olive oil, garlic powder, onion powder, and salt. In a large bowl, add bread, drizzle with the olive oil mixture, and toss. Spread bread in one even layer on prepared baking sheet. Bake for 10 minutes. Remove the pan from oven, toss cubes, and return to the oven. Bake for 5 minutes until crisp and golden brown.

5. Heat remaining 1 tablespoon oil on a grill pan over medium-high heat. Grill chicken for 7 minutes per side until completely cooked; the meat should reach an internal temperature of 165°F. Allow chicken to cool before slicing it for the salad.

6. Add dressing to a large bowl, add lettuce, and toss. Add sliced grilled chicken and croutons on top of lettuce and serve.

Grilled Chicken Cobb Salad

SERVES 4

Per Serving:

Calories	530
Fat	30g
Protein	39g
Sodium	715mg
Fiber	15g
Carbohydrates	31g
Sugar	7g

ROASTED SWEET CORN

Corn can be roasted ahead of time and saved in the refrigerator for up to 3 days to add to salads for an extra flavor punch. For an even greater corn flavor blast, roast your corn on the grill. Look online to determine your favorite technique for grilling corn, and in about 10–15 minutes you'll have that great grilled corn flavor.

This traditional Cobb salad is a favorite for good reason—it tastes great and fills you up. If you marinate your chicken breasts longer, the flavors will explode even more. Drizzle with your favorite gluten-free and dairy-free salad dressing.

2 (6-ounce) boneless, skinless chicken breasts
2 tablespoons olive oil, divided
2 tablespoons lemon juice
1 teaspoon jarred minced garlic
½ teaspoon salt
¼ teaspoon ground black pepper
3 medium romaine lettuce hearts, chopped
8 strips gluten-free bacon, cooked and crumbled
1 cup canned corn, drained
4 large hard-boiled eggs, peeled and chopped
1 cup halved grape tomatoes
2 large avocados, peeled, pitted, and chopped

1 Place chicken breasts in a sealable plastic bag. Add 1 tablespoon olive oil, lemon juice, garlic, salt, and pepper. Seal the top of the bag and massage the ingredients to combine. Let chicken marinate in the refrigerator for 30 minutes.

2 Heat remaining olive oil in a large skillet over medium-high heat. Grill chicken for 6–7minutes on each side until completely cooked; the meat should no longer be pink, the juices should run clear, and it should reach an internal temperature of 165°F. Allow chicken to cool for 5 minutes before slicing it for the salad.

3 In a large bowl, add lettuce and top with chicken, bacon, corn, eggs, tomatoes, and avocado.

Broiled Romaine Salad with Balsamic Glaze

This a simple but flavorful restaurant-style salad that you can quickly make at home. Broiling romaine lettuce may sound a little unusual, but the natural flavor of the lettuce becomes more complex when you broil or grill it. Romaine lettuce is low in calories but high in minerals and packed with vitamin C, vitamin K, and folate. This salad is a perfect accompaniment to steak or grilled chicken dishes.

SERVES 2

Per Serving:

Calories	300
Fat	19g
Protein	5g
Sodium	630mg
Fiber	19g
Carbohydrates	32g
Sugar	22g

GLAZE

2 teaspoons balsamic vinegar
2 tablespoons honey
2 tablespoons olive oil
1 teaspoon garlic powder
½ teaspoon onion powder
¼ teaspoon Dijon mustard
¼ teaspoon salt
⅛ teaspoon ground black pepper

ROMAINE

1 large romaine lettuce heart, halved
½ tablespoon olive oil

1 In a small bowl, whisk together the glaze ingredients until fully combined. Microwave for 15 seconds and then whisk again. Allow to cool before drizzling on romaine.

2 Place romaine on a baking sheet sprayed with gluten-free nonstick cooking spray. Drizzle the lettuce with the olive oil and place under the broiler for 1–2 minutes. Flip when the leaves start to brown a bit, then cook for 1–2 minutes more.

3 Remove from oven, plate, and drizzle with balsamic glaze.

Sloppy Joe Baked Potatoes

SERVES 4

Per Serving:

Calories	470
Fat	17g
Protein	27g
Sodium	780mg
Fiber	5g
Carbohydrates	53g
Sugar	20g

Make lunch fun with this unique flavor combination! This plate will definitely keep you full until it's time for dinner.

4 large russet potatoes
1 teaspoon olive oil
1 pound 90/10 ground beef
¼ teaspoon salt
1 (15-ounce) can gluten-free Sloppy Joe sauce

1 With a fork, pierce each potato several times. Wrap each potato in microwaveable plastic wrap and place on a microwave-safe plate. Microwave on high for 6 minutes; turn over and microwave for an additional 5 minutes until soft. Remove and allow to cool for 5 minutes.

2 Heat olive oil in a large skillet over medium-high heat. Add beef and salt, stirring occasionally, and cook for 5 minutes until crumbled and no longer pink; then drain the oil. Add sauce. Reduce heat to low and simmer 5 minutes until hot.

3 Cut slit in top of each potato; squeeze open and fluff with fork. Top each potato with ½ cup meat mixture.

Traditional Greek Salad

SERVES 4

Per Serving:

Calories	350
Fat	32g
Protein	4g
Sodium	778mg
Fiber	6g
Carbohydrates	17g
Sugar	5g

This irresistible and refreshing salad is bursting full of all the Greek flavors that you know and love! It's perfect for a warm day when you want a light lunch.

1 romaine lettuce heart, chopped
1 large cucumber, sliced
1 green bell pepper, seeded and diced
1 pint grape tomatoes, halved
½ small red onion, peeled and thinly sliced
1 teaspoon jarred minced garlic
1 teaspoon dried oregano
½ teaspoon Dijon mustard
¼ cup red wine vinegar
1 teaspoon salt
½ teaspoon ground black pepper
½ cup olive oil
½ cup halved pitted Kalamata olives

1 Add lettuce, cucumber, bell peppers, tomatoes, and red onions in a large bowl.

2 In a small bowl, whisk together garlic, oregano, mustard, vinegar, salt, and pepper. Whisk in olive oil. Pour vinaigrette over vegetables. Add olives and toss lightly.

CHAPTER 4

Poultry

Spinach and Artichoke Chicken

SERVES 4

Per Serving:

Calories	470
Fat	20g
Protein	45g
Sodium	1,065mg
Fiber	4g
Carbohydrates	20g
Sugar	6g

THE POWER OF SPINACH

Spinach is a superfood. It is loaded with tons of nutrients and is low-calorie to boot. Spinach is full of protein, iron, vitamins, and minerals, and it contains more nutrients per serving than virtually any other vegetable.

This dish is inspired by a popular hot appetizer, and this one-pan dinner has all the best parts of spinach and artichoke dip! Plus, it's an easy skillet meal that is made in less than 30 minutes.

4 tablespoons olive oil
4 (6-ounce) boneless, skinless chicken breasts
2 tablespoons jarred minced garlic
1 small sweet onion, peeled and chopped
1 cup gluten-free chicken broth
1 tablespoon gluten-free Worcestershire sauce
1 tablespoon lemon juice
1 teaspoon salt
1 cup unsweetened almond milk
2 tablespoons gluten-free all-purpose flour with xanthan gum
4 tablespoons nutritional yeast
1 (6-ounce) bag baby spinach
1 (13-ounce) can artichoke hearts

1 Heat olive oil in a large skillet over medium-high heat. Add chicken and cook for 2 minutes on each side. Remove chicken to a plate.

2 Add garlic and onions to the skillet and stir, cooking for 30 seconds, until garlic is fragrant. Pour in broth, Worcestershire sauce, lemon juice, and salt and stir to combine. Add chicken back into the skillet and turn down the heat to medium and cook for 12–14 minutes, turning over the chicken about halfway through.

3 Transfer chicken to a plate. Combine milk, flour, and nutritional yeast in a small bowl and whisk until flour is dissolved. Pour the mixture into the skillet, stir, and bring to a low boil.

4 Add spinach to sauce and cover and cook for 2–3 minutes until wilted. Stir in artichoke hearts and cook for 2–3 minutes until heated through. Pour creamy sauce over chicken and serve.

Crispy Baked Barbecue Chicken Thighs

Crispy Baked Barbecue Chicken Thighs is a meal that is in the oven in just minutes for a delicious and budget-friendly dinner. It's covered in a homemade barbecue dry rub and gluten-free bread crumbs for a crispy and crunchy crust.

1 tablespoon light brown sugar, packed

1 tablespoon garlic powder

1 tablespoon onion powder

1 tablespoon chili powder

1 tablespoon salt

1 tablespoon paprika

1 tablespoon ground cumin

1 teaspoon mustard powder

6 (4-ounce) bone-in, skin-on chicken thighs

¾ cup gluten-free bread crumbs

½ cup dairy-free buttery spread

1 Preheat oven to 375°F. Spray a 9" × 13" glass baking dish with gluten-free nonstick cooking spray. Place chicken in baking dish.

2 In a small bowl, combine brown sugar, garlic powder, onion powder, chili powder, salt, paprika, cumin, and mustard powder together and stir until fully combined.

3 Rub 1 tablespoon seasoning mixture on each chicken thigh.

4 Sprinkle bread crumbs over chicken thighs and press onto skin.

5 Drizzle buttery spread over chicken thighs.

6 Bake for 50 minutes or until the thighs are no longer pink at the bone and the juices run clear. A meat thermometer inserted near the bone should read 165°F.

SERVES 6

Per Serving:

Calories	230
Fat	14g
Protein	12g
Sodium	700mg
Fiber	2g
Carbohydrates	14g
Sugar	3g

LOVE THAT DEEP SOUTH BARBECUE

Barbecue in the southern United States is a way of life. Just about every meat imaginable has been transformed into a barbecue version. Barbecue can be in the form of a dry rub or a sauce. You will see barbecue ribs, pork, brisket, chicken, and even seafood on the local menus.

Paleo Pesto Turkey Meatballs

SERVES 8

Per Serving
(Serving Size: 6 meatballs):

Calories	560
Fat	40g
Protein	40g
Sodium	400mg
Fiber	2g
Carbohydrates	8g
Sugar	1g

These Paleo Pesto Turkey Meatballs are incredibly tender and juicy, and come together in less than 40 minutes. They are bursting with flavor from the homemade basil pesto sauce. If you are unable to use fresh basil, substitute 4 tablespoons dried basil.

PESTO SAUCE
1 (10-ounce) package fresh basil
1 cup cashews
2 tablespoons jarred minced garlic
1 teaspoon salt
2 tablespoons lemon juice
½ cup olive oil

MEATBALLS
3 pounds ground turkey
2 large eggs, whisked
⅔ cup almond flour
2 tablespoons onion powder

1 Preheat oven to 425°F. Line two baking sheets with aluminum foil and spray with gluten-free nonstick cooking spray.

2 In a food processor, chop the basil. Add cashews to the food processor and chop until fully combined with basil. Add the garlic, salt, lemon juice and olive oil to the cashew mixture and chop until fully combined.

3 To make the meatballs, add turkey, eggs, almond flour, onion powder, and pesto sauce to a large bowl. Mix together with a large spoon or your hands until fully combined.

4 Using a 1½-tablespoons cookie scoop, scoop the meatball mixture out to form forty-eight balls and place on prepared baking sheets. Bake for 30 minutes until browned.

Crunchy Coconut Chicken Bites

These tropical bites are baked, not fried, so they're a healthier option, yet they mimic the texture and flavor of deep-fried food!

2 cups Honey Nut Chex cereal

1 cup sweetened shredded coconut

2 boneless, skinless chicken breasts, cut into 2" pieces

½ cup mayonnaise

½ cup orange marmalade, melted

SERVES 4	
Per Serving:	
Calories	580
Fat	33g
Protein	17g
Sodium	430mg
Fiber	3g
Carbohydrates	57g
Sugar	40g

1 Preheat oven to 400°F. Line a baking sheet with aluminum foil and spray with gluten-free nonstick cooking spray.

2 Crush cereal by adding it to a sealable plastic bag and crushing with a rolling pin. Add coconut to the bag.

3 Combine chicken and mayonnaise in a medium bowl and transfer to the bag with the cereal mixture. Turn the plastic storage bag over and over until the chicken pieces are coated evenly.

4 Place chicken on prepared baking sheet and bake for 18–20 minutes until the coating is a light golden brown. Serve with melted orange marmalade as a dipping sauce.

Turmeric Coconut Chicken Curry

This is a perfect recipe for those following the autoimmune protocol (AIP) or paleo diets because it is free of refined sugar and nightshade. Serve over cauliflower rice.

1 tablespoon olive oil

2 (6-ounce) boneless, skinless chicken breasts, cut into 1" pieces

1 (13-ounce) can unsweetened coconut milk

2 tablespoons honey

1 teaspoon ground cinnamon

1 teaspoon ground turmeric

½ teaspoon ground ginger

¼ teaspoon salt

½ cup raisins

2 large hard-boiled eggs, peeled and diced

½ cup chopped fresh cilantro

SERVES 4	
Per Serving:	
Calories	420
Fat	25g
Protein	45g
Sodium	230mg
Fiber	1g
Carbohydrates	27g
Sugar	23g

1 Heat the olive oil in a large skillet over medium-high heat. Sauté chicken for 5–6 minutes until golden brown.

2 Add milk and honey and stir, coating chicken. Add spices and raisins and stir to combine ingredients.

3 Bring to a low boil, then lower heat to low and simmer for 5 minutes, stirring occasionally, until sauce thickens.

4 Plate chicken and garnish with hard-boiled eggs and cilantro.

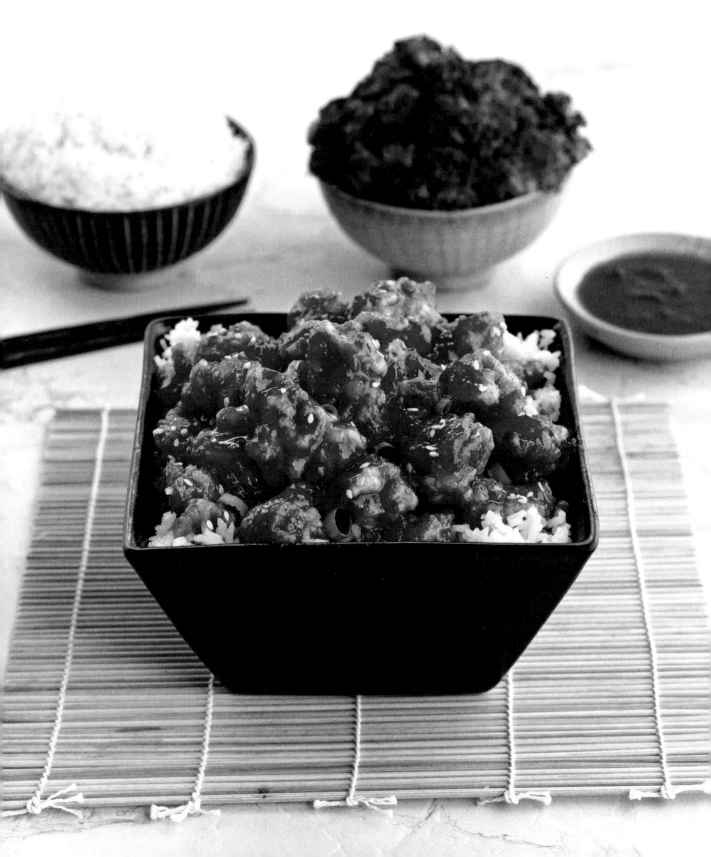

Asian Apricot Chicken

This succulent chicken recipe combines the sweetness of the apricot preserves with the saltiness of soy sauce and the complexity of the sweet but slightly spicy ginger. The chicken pieces are fried to perfect crispiness using a flour blend that makes the lightest crunchy coating. Serve over rice.

CHICKEN

½ cup gluten-free all-purpose flour with xanthan gum

½ cup gluten-free cornstarch

1 tablespoon ground ginger

2 (6-ounce) boneless, skinless chicken breasts, cut into 1" pieces

1 large egg, whisked

2 cups vegetable oil

SAUCE

2 tablespoons gluten-free soy sauce

1 teaspoon ground ginger

¾ cup apricot preserves

¼ cup water

1. Combine flour, cornstarch, and ground ginger in a large sealable plastic bag.

2. Add chicken pieces to a medium bowl with whisked egg and stir to fully coat the pieces.

3. Place all chicken pieces in the bag of flour mixture. Keep turning over the bag until chicken pieces are fully coated.

4. Heat oil in a wok or large skillet over high heat until a deep-fry thermometer inserted in the oil registers 350°F. Carefully add chicken and fry for 3–4 minutes, turning once or twice, until golden brown and crisp. Drain the chicken on a paper towel–lined plate. Carefully pour hot oil from pan into a bowl and dispose of safely once cooled.

5. Either spray your pan with a gluten-free nonstick cooking spray or put 1 teaspoon fresh oil back into wok. Add all the sauce ingredients. Stir until combined, then cook over medium heat for 1–2 minutes until sauce thickens.

6. Return fried chicken to the pan, cook for 2–3 minutes more, and stir to evenly coat chicken with the sauce.

SERVES 6

Per Serving:

Calories	330
Fat	11g
Protein	15g
Sodium	395mg
Fiber	0g
Carbohydrates	44g
Sugar	18g

CHICKEN BREASTS 101

When shopping for chicken breasts, always look at the color along with the "best by" date. The freshest chicken will have a pink color, but as it spoils, that pink color will fade to gray. If you purchase frozen chicken breasts, always look for the bag of smaller and thinner breasts. The thicker breasts will take longer to cook and tend to cook less evenly.

Oven-Fried Chicken

SERVES 8

Per Serving:

Calories	345
Fat	15g
Protein	28g
Sodium	1,100mg
Fiber	2g
Carbohydrates	22g
Sugar	0g

TIME AND THYME AGAIN

Thyme is a perennial plant in the mint family. It is used both dried and fresh and provides a distinctive and subtle minty flavor that goes well with chicken dishes, sauces, and soups. Thyme is also packed with vitamin C and is a good source of vitamin A.

This recipe is bursting with the same great tastes of traditional pan-fried chicken, but it is easier and healthier to prepare. It goes especially great with a fresh batch of Loaded Bacon Ranch Potato Salad (see recipe in Chapter 7).

1 cup unsweetened almond milk

1 tablespoon white vinegar

4 pounds chicken pieces (thighs, breasts, wings, and drum sticks)

1 cup gluten-free all-purpose flour with xanthan gum

1 cup gluten-free bread crumbs

1 tablespoon seasoned salt

1 tablespoon dried thyme

1 tablespoon onion powder

1 teaspoon garlic powder

1 teaspoon dried basil

1 teaspoon dried oregano

½ teaspoon mustard powder

1 Pour milk and vinegar in a small bowl and allow to sit for 5 minutes. Pour the mixture in a sealable plastic bag and then place chicken into the bag and seal. Massage chicken and the milk mixture with your hands to coat evenly and allow to marinate in the refrigerator for 30 minutes up to several hours.

2 Preheat oven to 375°F and spray a 9" × 13" baking dish with gluten-free nonstick cooking spray.

3 In a medium bowl, whisk together flour, bread crumbs, and seasonings. Set aside.

4 Remove chicken from the bag and dredge in the seasoned flour mixture, coating on all sides. Place chicken into prepared baking dish. Spray the tops of chicken pieces with gluten-free nonstick cooking spray. Bake for 50 minutes until internal temperature reads 165°F. Remove from oven and allow to rest 5 minutes and serve.

Chicken and Dumplings Casserole

This recipe is created in layers with shredded chicken, tasty peas and corn, creamy sauce, and a fluffy dumpling topping. The flavors meld into a classic comfort food sensation.

½ cup dairy-free buttery spread, melted
4 (6-ounce) boneless, skinless chicken breasts, cooked and shredded
½ teaspoon salt
½ teaspoon ground black pepper
1 teaspoon dried sage
½ cup frozen peas
½ cup frozen corn
2 cups unsweetened almond milk
2 cups Bisquick Gluten Free Pancake & Baking Mix
1 cup gluten-free chicken broth
3 teaspoons gluten-free chicken granules
1½ cups gluten-free and dairy-free Cream of Chicken Soup
(see recipe in Chapter 9)

SERVES 8

Per Serving:

Calories	275
Fat	8g
Protein	27g
Sodium	1,240mg
Fiber	2g
Carbohydrates	27g
Sugar	3g

1 Preheat oven to 350°F. Spray a 9" × 13" baking dish with gluten-free nonstick cooking spray.

2 Pour buttery spread into bottom of baking dish. Spread chicken over buttery spread. Sprinkle salt, pepper, and sage over chicken. Sprinkle peas and corn over chicken. Do not stir.

3 To make the second layer, mix milk and Bisquick in a small bowl. Pour the mixture on top of peas and corn. Do not stir.

4 To make the third layer, whisk together broth, chicken granules, and soup. Once blended, slowly pour over the Bisquick layer. Do not stir.

5 Bake casserole for 45–60 minutes or until the top is golden brown.

Moroccan Chicken

SERVES 4

Per Serving:

Calories	930
Fat	41g
Protein	57g
Sodium	400mg
Fiber	13g
Carbohydrates	79g
Sugar	40g

Moroccan Chicken is a savory dish made with an aromatic blend of spices alongside a bright lemon taste. The flavorful chicken thighs are smothered in a rich legume sauce. Serve over rice or quinoa.

3 tablespoons olive oil
¼ teaspoon salt
⅛ teaspoon ground black pepper
6 (4-ounce) skin-on chicken thighs
1 large sweet onion, peeled and chopped
2 tablespoons jarred minced garlic
1 tablespoon ground turmeric
1 tablespoon ground cumin
1 teaspoon ground cinnamon
1 teaspoon paprika
2 teaspoons lemon zest
1 tablespoon lemon juice
3 cups gluten-free chicken broth
4 tablespoons honey
1 tablespoon gluten-free all-purpose flour with xanthan gum
½ cup raisins
2 (10-ounce) packages frozen garbanzos and lentils
½ cup chopped fresh cilantro

1. Heat olive oil in a large skillet on medium-high.
2. Salt and pepper both sides of chicken.
3. Cook chicken for 6–7 minutes on each side until they are crispy. Remove and transfer to plate.
4. Add onions and garlic to the skillet and sauté in remaining oil for 5 minutes. Add turmeric, cumin, cinnamon, paprika, lemon zest, and lemon juice and stir until fully combined. Add broth, honey, and flour and stir until flour is dissolved.
5. Return chicken to the skillet, cover, and simmer for 15 minutes.
6. Remove lid and add raisins and packages of garbanzos and lentils. Stir to combine in sauce. Cook for an additional 15–20 minutes uncovered.
7. Sprinkle with cilantro to garnish.

Chicken Alfredo

Yes, you can even recreate the classic Chicken Alfredo dish in a gluten- and dairy-free way! This hearty meal packs the same flavor but not the ingredients you want to avoid.

1 (16-ounce) box gluten-free fettuccine

2 tablespoons olive oil, divided

2 (6-ounce) boneless, skinless chicken breasts

¾ teaspoon salt, divided

¼ teaspoon ground black pepper

4 tablespoons dairy-free buttery spread

1 tablespoon jarred minced garlic

1 tablespoon onion powder

1 cup gluten-free chicken broth

½ teaspoon dry mustard powder

2 cups unsweetened almond milk

4 tablespoons gluten-free all-purpose flour with xanthan gum

½ cup nutritional yeast

⅛ teaspoon ground nutmeg

1 Cook pasta according to package directions until al dente and toss with 1 tablespoon of olive oil.

2 In a large skillet, heat remaining olive oil over medium-high heat. Add chicken and season with ½ teaspoon salt and pepper. Cook chicken until golden and cooked through, 6–7 minutes per side. Remove from the skillet and let rest 10 minutes before slicing.

3 Add buttery spread and garlic to the skillet and sauté for 30 seconds until garlic is fragrant.

4 Add onion powder, chicken broth, mustard powder, and remaining salt and stir until combined.

5 In a small bowl, whisk together milk, flour, and nutritional yeast.

6 Pour the milk mixture into the skillet and stir until fully combined. Reduce heat to medium. Bring to a low boil and stir until sauce is thickened. Sprinkle in nutmeg and stir. Add cooked pasta and toss well to coat pasta with sauce.

SERVES 4

Per Serving:

Calories	670
Fat	37g
Protein	38g
Sodium	1,265mg
Fiber	8g
Carbohydrates	52g
Sugar	3g

CHOOSE YOUR PASTA CAREFULLY

Gluten-free fettuccine is the pasta of choice for alfredo sauce, but in a pinch, just about any gluten-free pasta will do the trick. Remember to double-check your pasta box to ensure you have a gluten-free pasta. The grocery store shelves are slammed with pastas touting various nutritional benefits, and many of the gluten-free versions are commingled with the gluten pastas, so it is easy to get them mixed up.

Chicken Piccata

If you have not tried this comforting Italian classic made with lemon, butter, and capers, then this gluten-free and dairy-free version is for you! The salty, zesty, and buttery flavors in the piccata sauce come together in a delicious yet light way.

SERVES 4

Per Serving:

Calories	250
Fat	4g
Protein	30g
Sodium	400mg
Fiber	0g
Carbohydrates	21g
Sugar	0g

CHICKEN OR VEAL?

Veal Piccata is another version of this entrée that is on the menu at many upscale restaurants. There are also piccata versions for pork and fish. Piccata dishes are usually served with pasta, but they are excellent stand-alone dishes as well.

½ cup gluten-free all-purpose flour with xanthan gum
¼ cup gluten-free cornstarch
½ teaspoon salt
¼ teaspoon ground black pepper
3 (6-ounce) boneless, skinless chicken breasts, cut into ½" medallions
2 tablespoons olive oil
1 teaspoon jarred minced garlic
1 cup gluten-free chicken broth
¼ cup lemon juice
2 tablespoons capers, drained and rinsed
2 tablespoons dairy-free buttery spread

1. Preheat oven to 200°F. Line a baking sheet with aluminum foil.
2. Add flour, cornstarch, salt, and pepper to a pie pan and whisk to combine. Dredge chicken pieces in the mixture. Heat olive oil in a large skillet. Pan-fry chicken over medium-high heat for 3 minutes on each side until golden brown. Place chicken pieces on prepared baking sheet and place in the oven to keep warm. Drain most of the oil from the skillet, reserving 1 tablespoon of oil in the skillet.
3. Add garlic to the skillet and cook for 30 seconds until fragrant. Pour in broth. Scrape and dissolve any brown bits from the bottom of the skillet. Stir in lemon juice and bring the mixture to a boil. Boil for 5–8 minutes, stirring occasionally, until the sauce reduces. Add capers and buttery spread and stir to combine until buttery spread is melted.
4. Add chicken back to the skillet and simmer for 5 more minutes until sauce is reduced and slightly thickens. Serve warm.

Tuscan Chicken

Just like Tuscany, it's easy to fall in love with the famous flavors of this mouthwatering recipe—mushrooms, spinach, and sun-dried tomatoes! Transport yourself to the famed area of Italy with this quick and easy weeknight meal.

2 tablespoons olive oil

4 (6-ounce) boneless, skinless chicken breasts

2 tablespoons jarred minced garlic

1 cup sliced white button mushrooms

1 cup gluten-free chicken broth

1 tablespoon Italian seasoning

½ teaspoon salt

4 tablespoons nutritional yeast

1 cup unsweetened almond milk

2 tablespoons gluten-free all-purpose flour with xanthan gum

1 cup chopped baby spinach

½ cup chopped sun-dried tomatoes

1　In a large skillet, add olive oil and cook chicken on medium-high heat for 3–5 minutes on each side until brown on each side. Remove chicken and set aside on a plate.

2　Add garlic and mushrooms to the skillet and sauté for 2 minutes until mushrooms start to soften.

3　Add chicken broth, Italian seasoning, salt, and nutritional yeast and whisk together.

4　Add milk and flour to a small bowl and whisk until flour has dissolved. Add the milk mixture to the skillet and whisk until it starts to thicken, about 2 minutes.

5　Add spinach and tomatoes to the skillet and let simmer for 2–4 minutes until spinach starts to wilt. Add chicken back to the skillet and simmer for 4–5 minutes.

SERVES 4

Per Serving:

Calories	365
Fat	14g
Protein	44g
Sodium	460mg
Fiber	2g
Carbohydrates	10g
Sugar	3g

TOP TUSCAN DISHES

The cuisine of the central region of Italy is described as *Tuscan*. Tuscan food is known for being simple, seasonal, and incredibly fresh and for using the finest quality locally grown produce. Tiramisu and bruschetta are two of the most well-known Tuscan foods.

Crispy Baked Chicken Thighs

SERVES 6

Per Serving:

Calories	275
Fat	17g
Protein	27g
Sodium	505mg
Fiber	1g
Carbohydrates	151g
Sugar	0g

This easy one-pan meal with its simple spice blend has tons of flavor, and the crispy skin and moist, juicy thigh meat is as healthy as it is delicious! Leaving the skin on keeps the chicken moist and flavorful. The chicken skin also has omega-6 fatty acids and heart-healthy unsaturated fats. Try roasting vegetables alongside the chicken for a side dish.

6 (4-ounce) bone-in, skin-on chicken thighs
1 teaspoon garlic powder
1 tablespoon onion powder
1 tablespoon dried oregano
1 tablespoon dried thyme
1 tablespoon dried sage
1 teaspoon salt

1 Preheat oven to 350°F. Spray a 9" × 13" glass baking pan with gluten-free nonstick cooking spray.

2 Place chicken thighs in greased baking pan.

3 In a small bowl, combine garlic powder, onion powder, oregano, thyme, sage, and salt together and stir until fully combined. Sprinkle the spice mixture over chicken thighs.

4 Bake chicken for 1 hour until skin is crispy, thighs are no longer pink at the bone, and the juices run clear. A meat thermometer inserted near the bone should read 165°F.

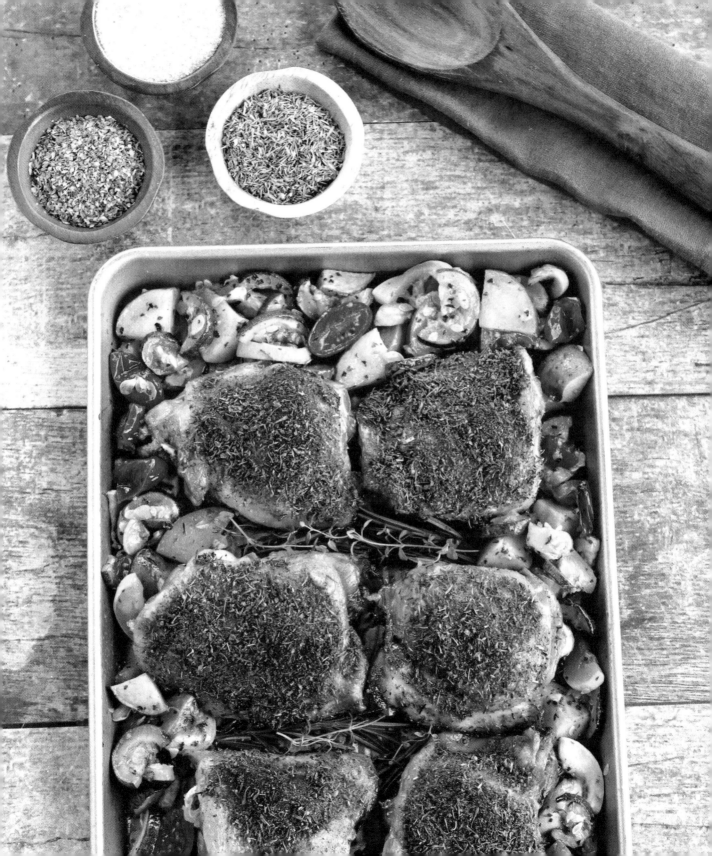

Rosemary Roasted Chicken

Don't be intimidated by cooking a whole chicken. It usually requires minimal prep, and the cooking time is hands-off. Plus, whole chickens are less expensive than buying separate chicken parts, so it's easier on your wallet as well.

SERVES 6

Per Serving:

Calories	565
Fat	31g
Protein	63g
Sodium	1,300mg
Fiber	1g
Carbohydrates	6g
Sugar	3g

1 large lemon, halved
1 (3-pound) whole chicken, rinsed and patted dry
1 tablespoon salt
1 teaspoon ground black pepper
1 small sweet onion, peeled and quartered
¼ cup chopped fresh rosemary

1. Preheat oven to 350°F. Spray a medium roasting pan with a rack with gluten-free nonstick cooking spray.
2. Squeeze lemon juice directly over chicken skin. Season chicken with salt and pepper and stuff the inside of chicken with onion, rosemary, and lemon halves. Place chicken with breast-side up on a rack in prepared roasting pan.
3. Roast for 2 to 2½ hours until cooked through, the juices run clear, and internal temperature reaches 165°F.

Honey Garlic Chicken

This is an easy chicken dish with a unique sticky honey garlic sauce. It pairs well with homestyle mashed potatoes and freshly steamed green beans.

SERVES 4

Per Serving:

Calories	405
Fat	18g
Protein	30g
Sodium	600mg
Fiber	0g
Carbohydrates	31g
Sugar	22g

3 (6-ounce) boneless, skinless chicken breasts, cut into 1" pieces
¼ cup gluten-free all-purpose flour with xanthan gum
¼ cup gluten-free cornstarch
½ teaspoon salt
¼ teaspoon ground black pepper
4 tablespoons olive oil
1 teaspoon jarred minced garlic
⅓ cup honey
1 tablespoon gluten-free soy sauce
1½ tablespoons rice vinegar

1. Put chicken pieces in a large sealable plastic bag. Add flour, cornstarch, salt, and pepper to the bag and shake to coat the chicken.
2. Heat oil in a large skillet over medium-high heat and add garlic and sauté for 30 seconds. Add chicken and cook for 3 minutes per side.
3. In a small microwave-safe bowl, whisk together honey, soy sauce, and vinegar and microwave for 15 seconds.
4. Turn heat down to medium. Add honey sauce to the skillet and stir to coat chicken with sauce. Cook for 3–4 minutes more, then serve.

Chicken Scaloppine

This recipe is a delicious dish of thin breaded chicken breasts and white wine lemon sauce. Remember to find gluten-free bread crumbs and avoid cross contamination with other bread crumbs. Serve over rice or gluten-free and dairy-free pasta.

4 (6-ounce) boneless, skinless chicken breasts
1 tablespoon lemon juice
¼ teaspoon salt
¼ teaspoon ground black pepper
½ cup gluten-free bread crumbs
1 teaspoon garlic powder
1 teaspoon onion powder
1 tablespoon Italian seasoning
2 tablespoons olive oil
½ cup gluten-free chicken broth
¼ cup white wine
2 tablespoons capers
1 tablespoon dairy-free buttery spread

1 Place each chicken breast between two sheets of heavy-duty plastic wrap; pound to ¼" thickness using a meat mallet or rolling pin. Brush chicken with lemon juice and sprinkle with salt and pepper.

2 In a pie pan, add bread crumbs, garlic powder, onion powder, and Italian seasoning and whisk to combine. Dredge chicken in the bread crumb mixture.

3 In a large skillet, heat olive oil over medium-high heat. Add chicken to pan; cook 3 minutes on each side until chicken is cooked through. Remove chicken from the skillet and cover with aluminum foil to keep warm.

4 Add chicken broth and wine to the skillet and cook for 30 seconds, stirring constantly. Stir in capers and buttery spread.

5 Add chicken back into the skillet, cover with sauce and simmer for 2–4minutes.

SERVES 4

Per Serving:

Calories	360
Fat	15g
Protein	40g
Sodium	465mg
Fiber	2g
Carbohydrates	12g
Sugar	1g

CREATE PIZZAZZ WITH CAPERS

Capers are small flower buds from the caper bush that grows in the Mediterranean. Once picked, capers are pickled in vinegar or cured in salt. They add a burst of flavor to savory dishes and make this recipe a flavor-packed event!

Baked Balsamic Chicken

SERVES 4

Per Serving:

Calories	455
Fat	11g
Protein	39g
Sodium	91mg
Fiber	0g
Carbohydrates	45g
Sugar	43g

DELIVER AUTHENTIC TASTE

Balsamic vinegar is a kitchen staple that every good cook needs to keep in stock. It goes great with both meat and seafood. The flavor is rich, complex, and a little acidic and can complement many dishes. Balsamic vinegar is made from grapes and is naturally gluten- and dairy-free.

This juicy and tender baked chicken is a versatile entrée. Serve it alongside garlic roasted potatoes.

4 (6-ounce) boneless, skinless chicken breasts
1 teaspoon salt, divided
¼ teaspoon ground black pepper
1 teaspoon Italian seasoning
2 tablespoons olive oil
1 cup balsamic vinegar
½ cup granulated sugar
2 tablespoons honey

1 Preheat oven to 400°F and spray a 9" × 13" baking dish with gluten-free nonstick cooking spray.

2 Season chicken with ½ teaspoon salt, pepper, and Italian seasoning.

3 Add olive oil to a large skillet and cook chicken on medium-high heat for 2 minutes on each side.

4 Transfer chicken to prepared dish, cover with aluminum foil, and bake for 15 minutes.

5 While chicken is baking, add balsamic vinegar, sugar, honey, and remaining salt to a medium saucepan. Bring to a boil over medium-high heat, then reduce to medium-low heat and allow to simmer 10–15 minutes. The sauce should reduce by half. Remove from heat.

6 Uncover chicken and brush balsamic glaze on top of chicken. Return chicken to the oven and bake uncovered for another 5–10 minutes until chicken is completely cooked through and reaches an internal temperature of 165°F. Drizzle remaining balsamic glaze over chicken and serve.

Sesame Chicken

If you love Chinese takeout, this is the recipe for you! Once you master this technique, you won't miss the restaurant version at all. Your home-made variety will taste fresher too.

½ cup gluten-free all-purpose flour with xanthan gum
½ cup gluten-free cornstarch
2 (6-ounce) boneless, skinless chicken breasts, diced into ½" pieces
1 large egg, whisked
2 cups vegetable oil
¼ cup honey
⅓ cup gluten-free soy sauce
½ cup ketchup
¼ cup light brown sugar, packed
¼ cup rice vinegar
1 teaspoon jarred minced ginger
2 teaspoons cornstarch
1 tablespoon sesame oil
2 teaspoons jarred minced garlic
2 tablespoons sesame seeds
2 green onions, sliced

1 Combine flour and cornstarch in a large sealable plastic bag. Add chicken to a medium bowl with egg and stir to fully coat pieces. Place chicken in the bag with the flour mixture. Keep turning over the bag until chicken pieces are fully coated.

2 Heat vegetable oil in a large skillet or wok over medium-high heat. Add chicken to hot oil and fry for 6–8 minutes until light golden brown. Drain chicken on a paper towel–lined plate. Discard oil from wok. Allow oil to completely cool before disposing of it.

3 In a small bowl, whisk together honey, soy sauce, ketchup, sugar, vinegar, ginger, and cornstarch until fully combined.

4 Heat sesame oil in the same skillet or wok over medium heat. Add garlic and cook for 30 seconds. Add sauce and bring to a simmer. Cook for 3–4 minutes or until just thickened. Add chicken to the skillet and toss to coat with sauce and cook for 1–2 minutes. Sprinkle with sesame seeds and green onions and serve.

SERVES 4

Per Serving:

Calories	545
Fat	19g
Protein	24g
Sodium	1,700mg
Fiber	1g
Carbohydrates	72g
Sugar	38g

THE MANY USES FOR CORNSTARCH

While best known as a thickening agent for sauces and gravy, cornstarch has a whole list of other very impressive uses. It has been used for many years to treat insect bites when applied as a paste. Cornstarch also comes in handy for removing oil stains in fabric and for reducing irritation from sunburns.

Savory Roasted Milk Chicken Thighs

SERVES 6

Per Serving:

Calories	160
Fat	10g
Protein	13g
Sodium	360mg
Fiber	0g
Carbohydrates	3g
Sugar	0g

Chicken thighs are less expensive than other parts of the chicken, and this slow-simmering dish will make them delicious too. Roasting meat in milk helps tenderize the meat and turns into a delicious sauce.

6 (4-ounce) bone-in, skin-on chicken thighs
1 teaspoon ground cumin
1 teaspoon paprika
½ teaspoon salt
¼ teaspoon ground black pepper
4 tablespoons dairy-free buttery spread, divided
1½ teaspoons jarred minced garlic
1 cup unsweetened almond milk
¾ cup gluten-free chicken broth
1 teaspoon dried thyme
1 tablespoon lemon juice
2 tablespoons gluten-free all-purpose flour with xanthan gum

1 Preheat oven to 400°F.

2 Season both sides of chicken with cumin, paprika, salt, and pepper.

3 In a large ovenproof skillet over medium-high heat, melt 3 tablespoons buttery spread. Place chicken skin-side down first and sear each side of chicken until crispy brown, about 2–3 minutes each. Remove chicken from pan.

4 Add garlic to the skillet and cook for 30 seconds until fragrant. Add milk, broth, thyme, and lemon juice. Bring liquid to a low simmer.

5 Place chicken back into the skillet and transfer to oven. Roast chicken for 25–30 minutes or until fully cooked and internal temperature of chicken is 165°F.

6 Remove chicken from the skillet. Heat up milk sauce over a medium to high heat and bring to a low simmer. Whisk in remaining buttery spread and flour until flour dissolves. Cook until gravy is thick and creamy, about 2–3 minutes. Remove from heat, pour on top of chicken thighs, and serve.

Hawaiian Chicken Kebabs

Simple, sweet, and tangy marinated chicken is accented with fresh pineapple, bell peppers, and onions in this dish. This a great recipe choice for cookouts or a nice, quiet evening on the back porch!

⅓ cup ketchup

¼ cup light brown sugar, packed

⅓ cup gluten-free soy sauce

¼ cup pineapple juice

1½ tablespoons rice vinegar

1 tablespoon jarred minced garlic

1 tablespoon jarred minced ginger

½ teaspoon sesame oil

4 (6-ounce) boneless, skinless chicken breasts, chopped into 1¼" cubes

1 large red onion, peeled and diced into 1¼" pieces

1 large green bell pepper, seeded and diced into 1¼" pieces

3 cups cubed fresh pineapple

2 tablespoons olive oil

½ teaspoon salt

¼ ground black pepper

1. In a small bowl, whisk together ketchup, brown sugar, soy sauce, pineapple juice, vinegar, garlic, ginger, and sesame oil.

2. Place chicken in a gallon-sized sealable plastic bag. Save ½ cup marinade in the refrigerator, then pour remaining marinade into bag with chicken. Seal bag and refrigerate 1 hour. Soak ten wooden skewer sticks in water for 1 hour.

3. Preheat a gas grill to 400°F. In a medium bowl, add red onions, bell peppers, and pineapple and drizzle with olive oil and toss. Season with salt and pepper. Thread marinated chicken, onions, bell peppers, and pineapple onto skewers.

4. Place skewers on a greased grill. Grill 5 minutes, then brush marinade along tops with reserved ¼ cup marinade. Turn skewers over and brush remaining ¼ cup marinade on opposite side.

5. Grill 4–5 more minutes, or until chicken registers 165°F on a meat thermometer. Serve warm.

SERVES 5

Per Serving:

Calories	375
Fat	10g
Protein	34g
Sodium	1,535mg
Fiber	3g
Carbohydrates	35g
Sugar	28g

JUST SAY ALOHA!

Hawaii has historically had a very distinctive type of cuisine. Many dishes include locally native plants, fruits, and vegetables like yams and bananas. More modern-day Hawaiian food is greatly influenced by the foods that immigrants from Japan, Korea, and Vietnam brought.

Teriyaki Chicken

You will love this light and sweet Teriyaki Chicken that tastes just like your favorite restaurant's! Serve this dish with steamed rice and Sautéed Garlic Green Beans (see recipe in Chapter 7) for a satisfying meal.

SERVES 4

Per Serving:

Calories	280
Fat	10g
Protein	27g
Sodium	1,060mg
Fiber	0g
Carbohydrates	17g
Sugar	15g

1 tablespoon vegetable oil

1 pound boneless, skinless chicken thighs, cut into 1½" pieces

1 teaspoon cornstarch

2 teaspoons water

¼ cup gluten-free soy sauce

3 tablespoons light brown sugar, packed

1 tablespoon honey

3 tablespoons rice wine vinegar

1 tablespoon jarred minced garlic

1 teaspoon jarred minced ginger

1 tablespoon sesame oil

1. Heat vegetable oil in a large skillet over medium heat. Cook chicken for 6–8 minutes, stirring occasionally, until lightly browned and crisp.

2. In a small bowl, whisk together cornstarch and water. In another small bowl, whisk together soy sauce, brown sugar, honey, vinegar, ginger, sesame oil, and the cornstarch mixture to combine.

3. Add the garlic to the skillet, stir, and sauté for 30 seconds, until fragrant. Pour in sauce and stir to coat chicken. Simmer for 2–3 minutes until sauce thickens.

Baked Honey Mustard Chicken

The tangy and sweet flavor of honey mustard makes this quick meal a great choice when you're short on time.

SERVES 4

Per Serving:

Calories	385
Fat	9g
Protein	40g
Sodium	500mg
Fiber	0g
Carbohydrates	35g
Sugar	32g

4 (6-ounce) boneless, skinless chicken breasts

½ teaspoon salt

¼ teaspoon ground black pepper

1 tablespoon olive oil

¼ cup stone-ground mustard

2 tablespoons Dijon mustard

½ cup honey

2 tablespoons dairy-free buttery spread

1. Preheat oven to 375°F. Spray a 9" × 13" baking dish with gluten-free nonstick cooking spray.

2. Season chicken with salt and pepper. Heat oil in a large skillet over medium-high heat. Sear chicken on both sides until golden brown, 2–3 minutes per side.

3. In a small bowl, whisk together mustards, honey, and buttery spread. Pour half of the sauce into prepared baking pan. Top with chicken, then pour rest of sauce over top of chicken.

4. Cover with aluminum foil, then bake for 20 minutes. Uncover and bake for 10 more minutes or until chicken measures 165°F on a meat thermometer.

Pasta Primavera with Chicken

This light and fresh dish is best made with fresh vegetables. See what's local in your area and vary your choices throughout the year based on what's in season.

1 (12-ounce) box gluten-free penne pasta
2 tablespoons plus ¼ cup olive oil, divided
2 (6-ounce) boneless, skinless chicken breasts
½ teaspoon salt
¼ teaspoon ground black pepper
1 teaspoon jarred minced garlic
½ medium red onion, peeled and sliced
1 large carrot, peeled and sliced into matchsticks
1 medium red bell pepper, seeded and sliced into matchsticks
1 medium yellow squash, sliced and halved
1 large zucchini, sliced and halved
1 cup halved grape tomatoes
1 tablespoon Italian seasoning
1 tablespoon lemon juice

1 Cook pasta according to the package directions.

2 Heat 2 tablespoons of olive oil in a large skillet over medium-high heat. Add chicken and season with salt and black pepper. Cook for 6–7 minutes on each side until golden and cooked through and a meat thermometer reaches 165°F. Remove from the skillet and let rest 10 minutes before slicing.

3 Add the ¼ cup of olive oil and garlic to the skillet and sauté for 30 seconds until fragrant. Add red onions, carrots, and bell peppers and sauté 2 minutes. Add squash and zucchini and sauté 2 minutes until softened. Add tomatoes, Italian seasoning, and lemon juice and sauté 2 minutes longer.

4 Toss pasta with the vegetable mixture in a large bowl to combine. Top with sliced chicken and serve.

SERVES 6

Per Serving:

Calories	365
Fat	16g
Protein	6g
Sodium	215mg
Fiber	4g
Carbohydrates	52g
Sugar	4g

KEEP LEMON JUICE IN YOUR REFRIGERATOR

Lemon juice is high in vitamin C, aids in digestion, and has dozens of other impressive household uses. It is a smart idea to keep a fresh bottle in the refrigerator for recipes or just to add to your afternoon tea.

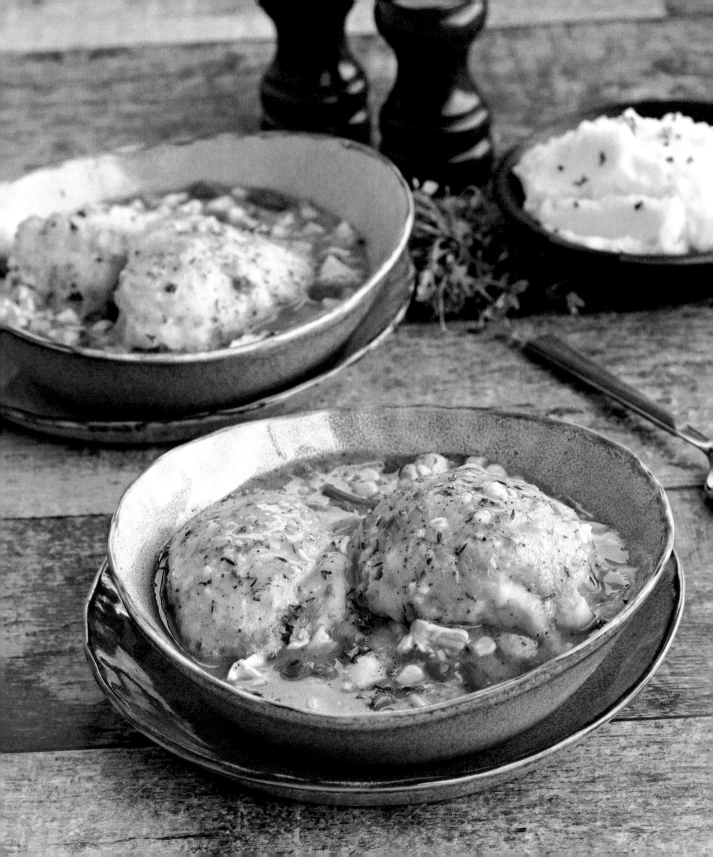

Chicken and Dumplings

This easy gluten-free Chicken and Dumplings is the perfect wrap-up-in-a-blanket southern comfort dish. The creamy sauce and fluffy dumplings go perfectly with homemade mashed potatoes.

SERVES 6

Per Serving:

Calories	385
Fat	12g
Protein	26g
Sodium	1,350mg
Fiber	3g
Carbohydrates	33g
Sugar	5g

CHICKEN

4 cups gluten-free chicken broth

4 cups diced cooked skinless chicken breasts

2 cups frozen mixed vegetables

1 tablespoon dried sage

1 tablespoon dried thyme

1 tablespoon onion powder

½ teaspoon salt

2 cups unsweetened almond milk

6 tablespoons gluten-free cornstarch

DUMPLINGS

2 large eggs

1½ cups Bisquick Gluten Free Pancake & Baking Mix

4 tablespoons dairy-free buttery spread, melted

⅔ cup unsweetened almond milk

1 In a large pot, add chicken broth, chicken, vegetables, sage, thyme, onion powder, and salt. Bring to a low boil over medium heat.

2 In a small bowl, add milk and cornstarch together and stir until cornstarch is dissolved. Pour the milk mixture into the large pot with chicken broth and stir until fully combined. Continue to boil.

3 In a medium bowl, whisk eggs. Add Bisquick and stir. Add the buttery spread and milk to the Bisquick mixture and stir until fully combined. The batter will be sticky.

4 Using a greased ice cream scoop, drop dumpling batter into the chicken broth mixture. Reduce the heat to low and cook for 10 minutes. Cover and cook for an additional 15 minutes. Remove from heat and serve.

SAVE TIME AND STILL HAVE CHICKEN AND DUMPLINGS

One of the shortcuts to making chicken and dumplings so easy is using a gluten-free rotisserie chicken. Most grocery stores and even big box stores now have ready-made, piping hot fresh rotisserie chickens available. Always remember to make sure that the spices and marinades they use are gluten-free and dairy-free.

Buffalo Turkey Burgers

SERVES 4

Per Serving:

Calories	216
Fat	15g
Protein	24g
Sodium	445mg
Fiber	0g
Carbohydrates	1g
Sugar	0g

This recipe brings all the flavors of buffalo wings to a turkey burger! Brush your favorite gluten-free and dairy-free burger bun with melted dairy-free buttery spread and place in the skillet for 1–3 minutes to serve up the perfect restaurant-quality burger.

1 pound ground turkey

1 stalk celery, finely diced

2 teaspoons gluten-free and dairy-free hot wing sauce

½ teaspoon salt

¼ teaspoon ground black pepper

2 tablespoons olive oil

1 In a large bowl, mix ground turkey, celery, wing sauce, salt, and pepper. Form four patties.

2 Heat olive oil in a large skillet over medium heat. Place turkey burgers in the skillet and cook on one side for 4–5 minutes until browned, then flip. Cook another 4–5 minutes or until burgers are cooked all the way through and the internal temperature is 165°F.

Easy Chicken Fried Rice

SERVES 6

Per Serving:

Calories	280
Fat	7g
Protein	23g
Sodium	630mg
Fiber	2g
Carbohydrates	27g
Sugar	2g

Since eating out might become more challenging, instead make your favorite takeout flavors at home! Chicken fried rice is much easier to prepare than you might think, and it will quickly become a dish that you will make over and over.

3 tablespoons sesame oil

2 (6-ounce) boneless, skinless chicken breasts, diced into 1" pieces

1 tablespoon jarred minced garlic

2 tablespoons jarred minced ginger

1 cup frozen peas

½ cup peeled and diced carrots

6 large eggs, whisked

3 cups cooked white rice

3 tablespoons gluten-free soy sauce

1 Add oil to a large skillet or wok and heat over medium-high heat. Add chicken and cook for 3–5 minutes, flipping so all sides cook evenly.

2 Add garlic, ginger, peas, and carrots and cook for 2 minutes.

3 Push the chicken mixture to one side of the skillet, then add eggs and scramble for 1–2 minutes. Stir eggs and the chicken mixture together.

4 Add rice to the skillet and stir to combine with the chicken mixture.

5 Pour soy sauce over rice and stir to combine. Fry the rice for another 3–5 minutes. Serve warm.

Chicken Marsala

This is a delicious dish that is special enough for a romantic date or dinner party. This dish goes well with Italian Roasted Vegetables, Roasted Garlic Potatoes, or Ratatouille (see recipes in Chapter 7).

½ cup gluten-free all-purpose flour with xanthan gum
¼ cup gluten-free cornstarch
½ teaspoon salt
¼ teaspoon ground black pepper
3 (6-ounce) boneless, skinless chicken breasts cut into ½" pieces
2 tablespoons olive oil
1 teaspoon jarred minced garlic
1 tablespoon onion powder
2 cups sliced white button mushrooms
½ cup Marsala wine
½ cup gluten-free chicken broth
2 tablespoons dairy-free buttery spread

1 Preheat oven to 200°F. Line a baking sheet with aluminum foil and spray with gluten-free nonstick cooking spray.

2 Add flour, cornstarch, salt, and pepper to a pie pan and whisk to combine. Dredge chicken pieces in flour.

3 Heat olive oil in a large skillet over medium-high heat. Pan-fry chicken for 3 minutes on each side until golden brown. Place chicken onto prepared baking sheet and place in the oven to keep warm. Drain most of the oil from the skillet, reserving 1 tablespoon in the skillet.

4 Add garlic and onion powder to the skillet and sauté for 30 seconds until fragrant. Add mushrooms to the skillet and sauté for 5 minutes until nicely browned. Pour Marsala and broth into the skillet and simmer for 1 minute to reduce sauce slightly. Stir in the buttery spread and return chicken to the skillet and simmer for 5 more minutes until sauce is reduced and slightly thickened.

SERVES 4

Per Serving:

Calories	355
Fat	12g
Protein	32g
Sodium	430mg
Fiber	0g
Carbohydrates	23g
Sugar	2g

MORE ON MARSALA

Marsala is a Sicilian wine that includes various types and ranges of flavors. The most common flavors are vanilla, brown sugar, fruit, and nuts. Marsala wine ranges from a dry to a sweet style of wine. You can substitute a dry Marsala for a sweet Marsala, but generally it is not the other way around. Dry Marsala has more versatility in cooking. A typical bottle of Marsala wine usually costs less than $15, and it will bring all of the beautiful flavors of this recipe to life. You can also easily find Marsala cooking wine at grocery stores as well.

Melt-in-Your-Mouth Chicken Breasts

SERVES 4

Per Serving:

Calories	580
Fat	46g
Protein	39g
Sodium	425mg
Fiber	0g
Carbohydrates	0g
Sugar	0g

This is a simple yet fantastic combination that many people have never tasted. It's perfect when you're in a pinch for a weeknight dinner. Serve alongside Easy Rice Pilaf, Honey-Glazed Carrots, or Balsamic-Roasted Brussels Sprouts (see recipes in Chapter 7).

1 cup mayonnaise
1 tablespoon seasoned salt
4 (6-ounce) boneless, skinless chicken breasts, sliced in half

1 Preheat oven to 375°F. Spray a 9" × 13" baking dish with gluten-free nonstick cooking spray.

2 In a small bowl, mix mayonnaise and salt together.

3 Place chicken in the dish and spread with the mayonnaise mixture.

4 Bake for 45 minutes until the internal temperature is 165°F.

Easy Homemade Chicken Nuggets

SERVES 4

Per Serving:

Calories	400
Fat	12g
Protein	41g
Sodium	610mg
Fiber	2g
Carbohydrates	28g
Sugar	1g

Many store-bought nuggets contain gluten and dairy ingredients, so making these at home is often your best bet. Your kids will eat these as fast as you can pull them out of the oven!

¾ cup gluten-free all-purpose flour with xanthan gum
½ cup gluten-free bread crumbs
1 tablespoon paprika
½ teaspoon garlic

½ teaspoon salt
4 (6-ounce) boneless, skinless chicken breasts, cut into 1½" pieces
1 large egg, beaten
¼ cup dairy-free buttery spread, melted

1 Preheat oven to 450°F. Spray a baking sheet with gluten-free nonstick cooking spray.

2 Place flour, bread crumbs, paprika, garlic, and salt in a large sealable plastic bag. Place chicken and egg in a large bowl and stir until pieces are fully covered in egg.

3 Place chicken in the plastic bag with the flour mixture and toss to coat.

4 Place coated chicken on the greased baking sheet. Drizzle buttery spread over chicken. Bake for 20 minutes until golden brown.

Baked Bacon Ranch Chicken Breasts

Bacon and ranch are a popular combination, and with good reason. This creamy homemade ranch dressing complements the salty bacon just right. If you want an alternative to pork bacon, turkey bacon is an excellent choice, and you won't miss any flavor.

1 cup mayonnaise
1 tablespoon dried dill
1½ teaspoons garlic powder
1½ teaspoons onion powder
2 teaspoons dried parsley
1½ teaspoons salt

½ teaspoon ground black pepper
1 tablespoon granulated sugar
4 (6-ounce) boneless, skinless chicken breasts, sliced in half
½ cup crumbled cooked gluten-free bacon

SERVES 4

Per Serving:

Calories	625
Fat	48g
Protein	42g
Sodium	1,400mg
Fiber	0g
Carbohydrates	5g
Sugar	4g

1 Preheat oven to 375°F. Spray a 9" × 13" baking dish with gluten-free nonstick cooking spray.

2 In a small bowl, mix mayonnaise, seasonings, and sugar together.

3 Place chicken in the dish and spread with the mayonnaise mixture.

4 Bake for 45 minutes until the internal temperature is 165°F. Remove from oven and top with crumbled bacon before serving.

Chicken Fajitas

Enjoy the sensational experience of a sizzling, hot pan of Chicken Fajitas without leaving your house.

3 tablespoons olive oil, divided
2 tablespoons lime juice
2 tablespoons ground cumin
1 teaspoon garlic powder
1 teaspoon paprika
1 tablespoon dried oregano

1 teaspoon salt
2 (6-ounce) boneless, skinless chicken breasts, cut into thin strips
3 large red, green, and yellow bell peppers, seeded and cut into strips
1 large sweet onion, peeled and thinly sliced

SERVES 4

Per Serving:

Calories	255
Fat	13g
Protein	21g
Sodium	625mg
Fiber	3g
Carbohydrates	11g
Sugar	7g

1 In a large bowl, combine 2 tablespoons olive oil, lime juice, and seasonings, then add the chicken. Toss chicken to coat; cover and marinate in the refrigerator for 30 minutes.

2 In a large skillet over medium-high heat, heat remaining 1 tablespoon oil, then sauté peppers and onions for 5 minutes until soft. Remove from skillet and keep warm.

3 In the same skillet, cook marinated chicken over medium-high heat for 5–6 minutes or until no longer pink. Return peppers and onions to skillet and cook for another 5–6 minutes before serving.

Bruschetta Chicken Bake

The flavors of fresh Roma tomatoes and basil take this chicken to another place and time. This has the great taste of the bruschetta appetizer but without the gluten and dairy ingredients.

SERVES 4

Per Serving:

Calories	450
Fat	5g
Protein	40g
Sodium	970mg
Fiber	1g
Carbohydrates	56g
Sugar	53g

HOMEGROWN BASIL

It is so fulfilling to grow your own basil because the flavor of basil that you grow yourself just always seems to taste better. Basil will grow well in your windowsill with some sunshine and water, so it's easy to plant even if you don't have a lot of space.

CHICKEN

6 large Roma tomatoes, diced
½ cup chopped fresh basil
1 tablespoon jarred minced garlic
2 teaspoons light brown sugar, packed
2 tablespoons balsamic vinegar
1 teaspoon salt, divided
4 (6-ounce) boneless, skinless chicken breasts
¼ teaspoon ground black pepper

GLAZE

1 cup balsamic vinegar
½ cup granulated sugar
2 tablespoons honey
½ teaspoon salt

1. Preheat oven to 375°F and spray a 9" × 13" baking dish with gluten-free nonstick cooking spray.

2. In a large bowl, toss tomatoes, basil, garlic, brown sugar, vinegar, and ½ teaspoon salt.

3. Lay chicken breasts flat in the bottom of the baking dish and season with remaining salt and pepper. Pour the tomato mixture over chicken.

4. Bake for 35–45 minutes or until chicken reaches an internal temperature of 165°F.

5. While chicken is baking, add the glaze ingredients to a medium saucepan. Bring to a boil over medium-high heat, then reduce to medium-low heat and allow to simmer 10–15 minutes. The sauce should reduce by half. Remove from heat.

6. Remove chicken from the oven when done and drizzle with glaze.

Homestyle Chicken and Rice Casserole

This is the classic American version of the tried-and-true chicken casserole. There are many variations of this dish, but no matter which one you choose, nothing says comfort more than a piping hot, heaping mound of chicken and rice casserole.

12 tablespoons dairy-free buttery spread, divided
1 cup chopped white button mushrooms
1 cup chopped celery
½ teaspoon jarred minced garlic
½ cup gluten-free all-purpose flour with xanthan gum
1 teaspoon dried thyme
1 teaspoon onion powder
3 cups gluten-free chicken broth
½ teaspoon salt
⅛ teaspoon ground black pepper
⅛ teaspoon ground nutmeg
1½ cups unsweetened almond milk
4 (6-ounce) boneless, skinless chicken breasts, cubed
2 cups water
2 cups instant white rice

1 Preheat oven to 400°F. Spray a 9" × 13" baking pan with gluten-free nonstick cooking spray.

2 In a large skillet, heat 4 tablespoons buttery spread over medium-high heat; sauté mushrooms, celery, and garlic until tender, about 2–3 minutes. Sprinkle with flour, thyme, and onion powder. Stir to coat vegetables. Stir in broth, salt, pepper, and nutmeg. Stir the mixture until flour dissolves. Bring soup to a boil and stir for 2 minutes until thickened. Reduce the heat to a low simmer and stir in milk. Simmer uncovered for 10–15 minutes. Add chicken, water, and rice to the mixture and stir to combine.

3 Pour the mixture into prepared baking pan. Place remaining buttery spread evenly over the top of the chicken mixture.

4 Bake for 60 minutes to 75 minutes until rice is tender and chicken is cooked through. Cool 15 minutes before serving.

SERVES 6

Per Serving:

Calories	325
Fat	11g
Protein	30g
Sodium	565mg
Fiber	1g
Carbohydrates	25g
Sugar	1g

MAKE THIS AHEAD OF TIME

Casseroles have been go-to family meals for so many years because they are time savers and taste great. Casseroles can often be made a day ahead of time and refrigerated until it is time to bake them.

Honey Lemon Ginger Chicken

SERVES 4

Per Serving:

Calories	425
Fat	11g
Protein	40g
Sodium	480mg
Fiber	1g
Carbohydrates	41g
Sugar	33g

This uncomplicated dish is full of sweet and tangy flavor, and once you try it, you will make it again and again. Serve over rice or zucchini noodles.

2 teaspoons sesame oil, divided
1½ teaspoons jarred minced garlic
1 tablespoon jarred minced ginger
¼ teaspoon salt
½ cup honey
4 tablespoons lemon juice
½ teaspoon lemon zest

1 tablespoon apple cider vinegar
1 tablespoon gluten-free soy sauce
3 teaspoons cornstarch
4 (6-ounce) boneless, skinless chicken breasts, diced
¼ cup peeled and shredded carrots
¼ cup chopped cashews

1. In a medium saucepan, add 1 teaspoon sesame oil, garlic, and ginger. Sauté over medium heat for 2–3 minutes. Add salt, honey, lemon juice, lemon zest, vinegar, soy sauce, and cornstarch. Bring to a boil and then reduce to a simmer. Simmer to thicken while cooking chicken.

2. Heat remaining sesame oil in a large skillet over medium-high heat. Sauté chicken for about 5–8 minutes until lightly browned and no longer has pink in centers. Add carrots and cashews. Add sauce to chicken and toss to coat. Simmer for 2–3 minutes.

Easy Baked Lemon Pepper Chicken

SERVES 4

Per Serving:

Calories	265
Fat	10g
Protein	39g
Sodium	405mg
Fiber	0g
Carbohydrates	1g
Sugar	0g

Expect to get compliments for these zesty and succulent chicken breasts! This recipe is perfect for a quick, refreshing, and light dinner.

4 (6-ounce) boneless, skinless chicken breasts
1 tablespoon lemon pepper seasoning
1 tablespoon olive oil
3 tablespoons dairy-free buttery spread, melted

1 teaspoon jarred minced garlic
¼ cup gluten-free chicken broth
¼ cup lemon juice
1 tablespoon chopped fresh parsley

1. Preheat oven to 400°F and spray a 9" × 13" baking dish with gluten-free nonstick cooking spray.

2. Season chicken on both sides with lemon pepper seasoning.

3. Heat olive oil in a large skillet over medium-high heat. Add chicken and cook for 3–5 minutes on each side until browned. Transfer chicken to prepared baking dish.

4. In a small bowl, mix together buttery spread, garlic, chicken broth, and lemon juice. Pour the buttery spread mixture over chicken.

5. Bake for 25–30 minutes until internal temperature reaches 165°F. Spoon sauce from the pan over chicken and sprinkle with parsley.

CHAPTER 5

Beef and Pork

Southern Chicken-Fried Steak

SERVES 4

Per Serving:

Calories	750
Fat	52g
Protein	35g
Sodium	440mg
Fiber	0g
Carbohydrates	49g
Sugar	0g

If this is a dish you often get at a restaurant, you might want to make it at home now, where you can better control the ingredients and preparation. The crunchy breading and tender steak are a match made in culinary heaven.

STEAK

1 cup gluten-free all-purpose flour with xanthan gum

½ cup cornstarch

2 tablespoons seasoned salt

4 (4-ounce) cube steaks

¼ teaspoon salt

⅛ teaspoon ground black pepper

2 large eggs

½ cup unsweetened almond milk

¾ cup vegetable oil

GRAVY

6 tablespoons gluten-free all-purpose flour with xanthan gum

3 cups unsweetened almond milk

½ teaspoon seasoned salt

¼ teaspoon ground black pepper

1 Combine flour, cornstarch, and seasoned salt in a pie pan. Sprinkle both sides of steaks with salt and pepper, then place in the flour mixture. Turn to coat. Whisk eggs and milk together in a separate pie pan. Place steaks into the egg mixture, turning to coat. Place steaks back in flour and turn to coat. Place breaded meat on a clean plate.

2 Heat oil in a large skillet over medium-high heat. Add two steaks to hot oil and fry until browned, about 3–5 minutes per side. Remove each steak to a paper towel–lined plate to drain and cover with aluminum foil to keep warm. Repeat with remaining steaks.

3 After all the meat is cooked, pour the grease into a heatproof bowl. Add 2 tablespoons of grease back to the skillet and heat over a medium-low heat.

4 Whisk flour with grease until a paste forms. Pour in the milk, whisking constantly. Add seasoned salt and pepper and cook for 5–10 minutes, whisking, until gravy is smooth and thick. Serve steaks topped with gravy.

Mongolian Beef

This flavorful take on flank steak cooks quickly, so it's a good choice for a weeknight dinner. For a little extra heat, add a ½ teaspoon of your favorite hot chili sauce.

1 pound flank steak, sliced thin
¼ cup cornstarch
3 tablespoons vegetable oil
⅓ cup gluten-free soy sauce
½ cup light brown sugar, packed

¼ cup water
1 tablespoon jarred minced ginger
1 tablespoon jarred minced garlic
2 green onions, sliced for garnish

SERVES 4	
Per Serving:	
Calories	522
Fat	22g
Protein	42g
Sodium	1,415mg
Fiber	1g
Carbohydrates	36g
Sugar	27g

1 In a large sealable plastic bag, add steak and cornstarch and keep turning over the bag until meat is fully coated.

2 Heat oil in a large skillet over high heat. Add steak in a single layer and cook on each side for 1 minute until the edges are starting to brown. Remove and set aside on a plate.

3 In a small bowl, combine soy sauce, brown sugar, water, ginger, and garlic. Add sauce to the skillet and bring to a boil. Add steak back to the skillet and allow sauce to thicken for 2–3 minutes. Toss with green onions.

Brown Butter Filet Mignon

Take your filet mignon to the next level with this simple technique of cooking it in a savory brown butter sauce. This recipe will make the average cut of meat taste like the finest restaurant steak.

1 (6-ounce) filet mignon
½ teaspoon salt
1 tablespoon olive oil

1 tablespoon dairy-free buttery spread
1 teaspoon dried sage

SERVES 1	
Per Serving:	
Calories	450
Fat	27g
Protein	52g
Sodium	1,375mg
Fiber	0g
Carbohydrates	0g
Sugar	0g

1 Cover fillet on both sides with salt and allow steak to come to room temperature.

2 In a small sauté pan, heat olive oil over high heat until 350°F. (The oil needs to be really hot to make a perfect crust.)

3 Place fillet in the pan and cook over high heat for 3 minutes. Turn steak over and add buttery spread and sage. Spoon buttery spread and sage from the pan over steak as it cooks for 3 more minutes. Remove steak from the pan and allow it to rest before serving.

Cottage Pie

This is the ultimate comfort casserole with layers of meat, vegetables, and creamy potatoes. Make it on a cold or rainy night for just the right meal.

SERVES 6

Per Serving:

Calories	355
Fat	20g
Protein	35g
Sodium	1,050mg
Fiber	3g
Carbohydrates	20g
Sugar	4g

MAKING MASHED POTATOES

If you're in a rush, you can buy gluten-free and dairy-free instant mashed potatoes and use dairy-free milk and dairy-free buttery spread to make them. If you have time, make homemade mashed potatoes using the cooked potatoes and the same dairy-free ingredients (see Pressure Cooker Mashed Potatoes recipe in Chapter 11).

½ cup dairy-free buttery spread, divided
1 medium sweet onion, peeled and chopped
1½ pounds 90/10 ground round beef
1 teaspoon gluten-free Worcestershire sauce
2 teaspoons salt, divided
¼ teaspoon ground black pepper
1 teaspoon dried thyme
½ teaspoon dried rosemary
½ cup gluten-free beef broth
2 cups mixed frozen vegetables, such as corn, peas, and carrots
3 large potatoes, peeled, quartered, and boiled

1 Preheat oven to 400°F. Spray a 9" × 13" baking dish with gluten-free nonstick cooking spray.

2 In a large skillet, melt 4 tablespoons buttery spread over medium heat. Add onions and cook for 5–10 minutes until tender.

3 Add ground beef and Worcestershire sauce. Season with 1 teaspoon salt, pepper, thyme, and rosemary. Cook for 3–5 minutes until beef is no longer pink. Add beef broth and mixed vegetables and simmer for 10 minutes.

4 Add boiled potatoes and remaining buttery spread and salt in a large bowl and mash with a potato masher or hand mixer.

5 Spread the beef mixture in an even layer in prepared baking dish. Spread mashed potatoes over the top of the beef mixture. Use a fork to poke the surface all over the top of the potatoes.

6 Bake for 30 minutes until browned and bubbling. Broil for 1–2 minutes to brown the mashed potatoes before serving.

Mini Meatloaves

These quick and easy individual meatloaves cook in half the time of traditional meatloaf.

1 pound 90/10 ground beef

1 tablespoon onion powder

1 teaspoon garlic powder

1 teaspoon salt

2 tablespoons gluten-free
Worcestershire sauce

½ cup gluten-free bread crumbs

1 large egg, whisked

¼ cup unsweetened almond milk

¼ cup light brown sugar, packed

1 teaspoon mustard

⅓ cup ketchup

1 Preheat oven to 350°F and spray a twelve-cup muffin tin with gluten-free nonstick cooking spray.

2 In a large bowl, combine beef, seasonings, Worcestershire sauce, bread crumbs, egg, and milk. Press mixture into muffin tin.

3 In a small bowl, whisk brown sugar, mustard, and ketchup. Spoon sauce over the meat.

4 Bake for 30 minutes until internal temperature reaches 160°F. Remove from muffin tin and serve.

SERVES 6	
Per Serving **(Serving Size: 2 mini meatloaves):**	
Calories	370
Fat	13g
Protein	17g
Sodium	685mg
Fiber	1g
Carbohydrates	20g
Sugar	12g

Sautéed Beef with Broccoli

The warm, caramelized steak in this dish is a classic favorite and makes this a go-to meal for busy families. Serve over rice for a filling meal.

½ cup gluten-free soy sauce

¼ cup cornstarch

3 tablespoons rice wine vinegar

3 tablespoons light brown sugar, packed

1 tablespoon gluten-free peanut butter

1 tablespoon jarred minced ginger

1 tablespoon jarred minced garlic

1 pound flank steak, sliced thin

2 teaspoons sesame oil

2 cups broccoli florets

¼ cup gluten-free beef broth

1 In a small bowl, mix together soy sauce, cornstarch, vinegar, brown sugar, peanut butter, ginger, and garlic. Pour half the liquid over sliced meat in a bowl and toss. Reserve the other half of the sauce and set aside.

2 Heat oil in a large skillet or wok over high heat. Add broccoli and stir-fry for 1 minute. Remove to a plate.

3 Add meat in a single layer and cook for 1 minute. Turn meat over and cook for another 30 seconds. Remove to a plate.

4 Pour reserved sauce and beef broth into the skillet. Stir and cook for 2–3 minutes until sauce starts to thicken. Add beef and broccoli back to the skillet and toss to coat and simmer for another 2 minutes.

SERVES 4	
Per Serving:	
Calories	440
Fat	16g
Protein	45g
Sodium	2,135mg
Fiber	2g
Carbohydrates	25g
Sugar	12g

Swedish Meatballs

These savory meatballs in a creamy sauce are perfect for potlucks and family dinners and as a party appetizer. If you'd rather make them into a weeknight dinner, enjoy them over your favorite rice or gluten-free and dairy-free pasta.

MAKES 24 MEATBALLS

Per Serving
(Serving Size: 4 meatballs):

Calories	275
Fat	18g
Protein	16g
Sodium	595mg
Fiber	1g
Carbohydrates	9g
Sugar	1g

KNOW YOUR BEEF BROTH

Several broth manufacturers are now producing gluten-free beef and chicken broth. Always carefully check your labels to catch any ingredients that may be added to your broth. The certified gluten-free stamp is a good, quick indicator of safety.

MEATBALLS

1 pound 90/10 ground beef
⅓ cup gluten-free bread crumbs
¼ teaspoon ground allspice
¼ teaspoon ground nutmeg
1 teaspoon onion powder
1 teaspoon garlic powder
½ teaspoon salt
⅛ teaspoon ground black pepper
1 large egg, whisked
½ cup unsweetened almond milk
2 tablespoons olive oil

SAUCE

2 tablespoons dairy-free buttery spread
4 tablespoons gluten-free all-purpose flour with xanthan gum
2 cups gluten-free beef broth
1 cup unsweetened almond milk
½ teaspoon salt
¼ teaspoon ground black pepper
1 tablespoon gluten-free Worcestershire sauce
1 teaspoon Dijon mustard

1. In a medium bowl, combine beef, bread crumbs, allspice, nutmeg, onion powder, garlic powder, salt, pepper, egg, and milk. Mix until combined.

2. Roll meat into twenty-four small meatballs. In a large skillet, heat olive oil over medium-high heat. Add meatballs and cook for 7–12 minutes, turning to brown on each side and to cook throughout. Transfer to a plate and cover with aluminum foil.

3. Add buttery spread to the skillet and melt. Whisk in flour until it dissolves and turns brown. Pour in broth, milk, salt, pepper, Worcestershire sauce, and mustard. Stir to combine ingredients. Bring to a simmer. Add meatballs back to the skillet and simmer for another 1–2 minutes.

Easy Homemade Beef Stroganoff

This dish will take you back to your grandmother's house on Sunday afternoon! The gluten- and dairy-free version doesn't miss any of the taste...or the memories. Serve over cooked gluten-free and dairy-free pasta.

1½ pounds beef round steak, cut into thin strips
½ teaspoon salt, divided
4 tablespoons dairy-free buttery spread
1 medium sweet onion, peeled and sliced
1 teaspoon jarred minced garlic
2 cups sliced white button mushrooms
4 tablespoons gluten-free all-purpose flour with xanthan gum
1 cup unsweetened almond milk
¼ teaspoon ground black pepper
1 tablespoon gluten-free Worcestershire sauce
1 teaspoon Dijon mustard
2 cups gluten-free beef broth
½ cup dairy-free sour cream

1. Sprinkle steak strips with ¼ teaspoon salt. Heat buttery spread in a large skillet over medium-high heat and add steak and quickly brown for 1 minute. Remove steak and place on a plate. Add onions, garlic, and mushrooms to the skillet. Sauté for 2 minutes until tender.

2. Sprinkle the skillet with flour. Put steak back into the skillet with onion and mushrooms. Add milk, remaining salt, pepper, Worcestershire sauce, Dijon mustard, and beef broth and stir to combine. Cook covered for 15 minutes.

3. Stir in sour cream the last few minutes, right before you serve.

SERVES 4

Per Serving:

Calories	488
Fat	32g
Protein	37g
Sodium	915mg
Fiber	1g
Carbohydrates	10g
Sugar	5g

ADD SOME KICK WITH DIJON MUSTARD

It is always smart to have a bottle of quality Dijon mustard in your house for recipes. Its rich and distinctive flavor goes great with everything from turkey sandwiches to potato salad. The added kick it brings boosts the flavor of whatever you're making.

Stuffed Peppers

SERVES 6

Per Serving:

Calories	310
Fat	14g
Protein	18g
Sodium	700mg
Fiber	4g
Carbohydrates	29g
Sugar	9g

This dish is beautiful, filling, healthy, and delicious. Stuffed Peppers are also a great leftover option for lunch—they're already in neat serving sizes!

2 tablespoons olive oil
1 small sweet onion, peeled and diced
1 tablespoon jarred minced garlic
½ pound 90/10 ground beef
½ pound gluten-free Italian sausage
2 (8-ounce) cans tomato sauce, divided
½ cup white rice, uncooked
1¼ cups water
1 tablespoon gluten-free Worcestershire sauce
1 cup gluten-free beef broth
6 green bell peppers, cut in half, with stem and seeds removed
1 tablespoon Italian seasoning

1 Preheat oven to 350°F. Spray a 9" × 13" baking dish with gluten-free nonstick cooking spray.

2 Heat olive oil in large skillet on medium-high heat and add the onions and garlic and cook for 1–2 minutes. Add in beef and sausage and cook for 3–5 minutes until brown and crumbled.

3 Stir in one can of tomato sauce, rice, water, and Worcestershire sauce. Bring to a simmer, reduce heat, and cover. Cook 15–20 minutes or until rice is tender.

4 Pour broth into the baking dish. Fill each pepper with the rice mixture and place in prepared dish. Mix remaining can of tomato sauce and Italian seasoning in a bowl and pour over stuffed peppers. Cover with aluminum foil and bake 1 hour.

Salisbury Steak

This rich dish comes together quickly, even with homemade gravy. Serve it over your rice or mashed potatoes.

SERVES 4

Per Serving:

Calories	435
Fat	27g
Protein	26g
Sodium	1,000mg
Fiber	2g
Carbohydrates	17g
Sugar	5g

PATTIES

- 1 pound 90/10 ground beef
- ¼ cup gluten-free bread crumbs
- 1 large egg, beaten
- 1 tablespoon gluten-free Worcestershire sauce
- 1 teaspoon onion powder
- ½ teaspoon garlic powder
- ¼ teaspoon salt
- ¼ teaspoon ground black pepper
- 2 tablespoons olive oil
- 2 tablespoons dairy-free buttery spread
- 1 tablespoon jarred minced garlic
- 1½ cups sliced white button mushrooms
- 1 small sweet onion, peeled and thinly sliced

GRAVY

- 1 tablespoon cornstarch
- 2 tablespoons cold water
- 2 cups gluten-free beef broth
- 2 tablespoons ketchup
- 2 tablespoons gluten-free Worcestershire sauce

1. In a large bowl, mix together beef, bread crumbs, egg, Worcestershire sauce, onion powder, garlic powder, salt, and pepper. Shape into four oval patties.

2. Heat olive oil in a large skillet over medium-high heat. Cook patties for 5–6 minutes on each side and then remove from the skillet.

3. Add buttery spread, garlic, mushrooms, and onions to the skillet and cook for 5–10 minutes until onions are golden and mushrooms are softened.

4. In a small bowl, mix cornstarch with cold water. Add beef broth, ketchup, Worcestershire sauce, and the cornstarch mixture to the skillet and whisk until smooth.

5. Reduce heat to medium, stirring often, and simmer for 1–2 minutes until gravy starts to thicken. Add patties back into the skillet and cook for 5 minutes.

Oven-Baked St. Louis–Style Ribs

SERVES 4

Per Serving:

Calories	1,120
Fat	79g
Protein	51g
Sodium	1,500mg
Fiber	1g
Carbohydrates	67g
Sugar	58g

These are perfectly seasoned, slow-baked, tender, fall-off-the-bone beef ribs! Don't go out for ribs when you can make these at home and control your ingredients!

1 tablespoon gluten-free liquid smoke
1 tablespoon Dijon mustard
½ teaspoon apple cider vinegar
4 pounds St. Louis–style ribs, membranes removed
1 tablespoon garlic powder
1 tablespoon onion powder
2 tablespoons light brown sugar, packed
1 teaspoon paprika
1 teaspoon seasoning salt
½ tablespoon dry mustard
2 cups gluten-free barbecue sauce

1 Preheat oven to 325°F. Line a baking sheet with aluminum foil and spray with gluten-free nonstick cooking spray.

2 In a small bowl, mix liquid smoke, mustard, and vinegar. Rub sauce over both sides of ribs.

3 In another small bowl, mix all dry spices and seasonings and stir to combine. Sprinkle dry mix over both sides of ribs and rub into meat.

4 Place ribs on prepared baking sheet and cover with another piece of aluminum foil and seal tightly to making a pouch for ribs to cook in.

5 Bake on the middle rack for 1 hour.

6 Turn the heat down to 250°F and unwrap the ribs. Baste each side with barbecue sauce every 10 minutes for a total of 30 minutes until the internal temperature is 145°F. Allow to rest 5–10 minutes before cutting.

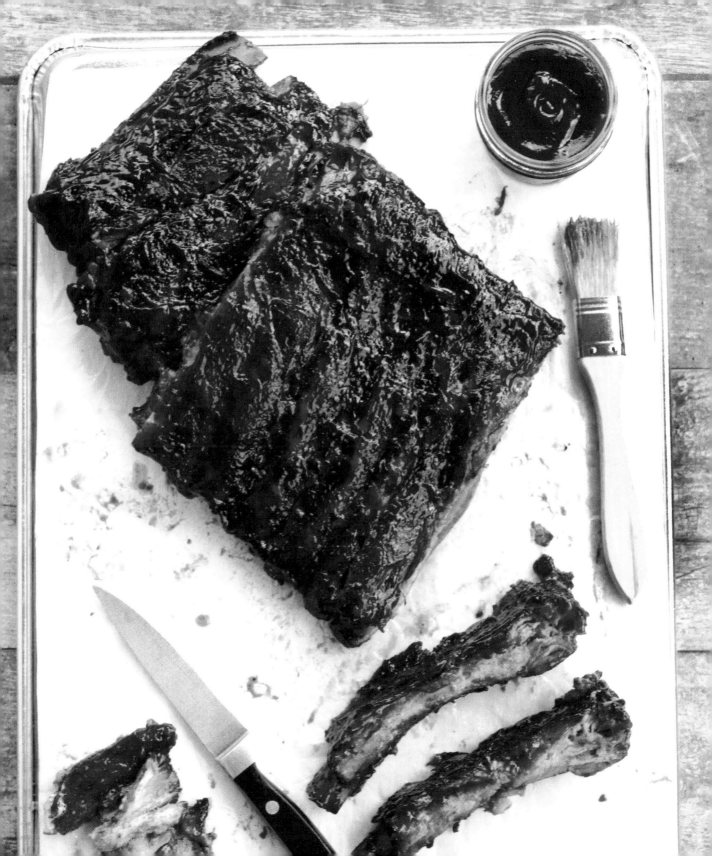

Beef Tenderloin

SERVES 8

Per Serving:

Calories	1,000
Fat	80g
Protein	68g
Sodium	735mg
Fiber	0g
Carbohydrates	0g
Sugar	0g

A CUT ABOVE THE REST

There are eight basic cuts of beef, and butchers are developing and testing new cuts every day. The eight are loin, shank, flank, brisket, rib, chuck, round, and short plate. Be cautious of pre-seasoned packaged meat. Meat is naturally gluten- and dairy-free, but not all seasonings are. Make sure to check the label for any gluten- or dairy-containing ingredients.

This juicy Beef Tenderloin is slathered with rosemary and garlic dairy-free buttery spread. The savory combination of tender beef and garlic butter is exceptional!

5 pounds beef tenderloin, trimmed and cut in half
2 teaspoons salt
2 teaspoons ground black pepper
2 tablespoons vegetable oil
3 tablespoons dairy-free buttery spread
2 teaspoons jarred minced garlic
1 tablespoon dried rosemary

1 Preheat oven to 450°F. Spray a large roasting pan with gluten-free nonstick cooking spray.

2 Season each beef tenderloin roast with salt and pepper. Heat oil in a large skillet over medium-high heat until hot. Sear roasts for 3 minutes on all four sides until well browned.

3 In a small bowl, combine buttery spread, garlic, and rosemary together. Rub the buttery spread mixture on beef.

4 Transfer beef to prepared roasting pan. Roast for 20–25 minutes for medium-rare or until a meat thermometer inserted in the thickest part registers 135°F. For medium doneness, cook until thermometer reaches 145°F. (Temperature will continue to rise about 5 degrees while meat rests.) Transfer the roasts to a carving board and let rest for 15 minutes. Carve beef tenderloin into ½"-thick slices and serve.

Prime Rib

This slow-roasted herb and garlic–crusted Prime Rib makes the perfect holiday or special-occasion dinner! The restaurant-quality taste will impress your guests.

5 pounds beef prime rib
2 teaspoons salt
½ teaspoon ground black pepper
4 tablespoons jarred minced garlic
2 teaspoons dried rosemary
2 teaspoons dried thyme
¼ cup olive oil

1   Allow prime rib to come to room temperature for 1 hour before cooking. Season it on all sides with salt and cover it loosely with plastic wrap.

2   Preheat oven to 500°F with the rack in the lower third of the oven. In a small bowl, stir together pepper, garlic, rosemary, thyme, and olive oil. Rub all over top and sides with the herb mixture.

3   Place meat into a large roasting pan bone-side down. Bake at 500°F for 15 minutes, then reduce the oven temperature to 325°F and continue baking until desired doneness. (Note: The meat will continue to cook once it's taken out of the oven, so remove the meat from the oven 5 degrees before it reaches your optimal temperature.)

   ▪ For rare, cook until thermometer reaches 125°F (10–12 minutes/pound)
   ▪ For medium-rare, cook until thermometer reaches 135°F (13–14 minutes/pound)
   ▪ For medium, cook until thermometer reaches 145°F (14–15 minutes/pound)
   ▪ For medium-well, cook until thermometer reaches 150°F (17–20 minutes/pound)

4   Remove meat from the oven and allow it to rest for 30 minutes before carving. Carve your roast by slicing against the grain at about ½" thickness.

SERVES 8

Per Serving:

Calories	1,090
Fat	86g
Protein	69g
Sodium	760mg
Fiber	0g
Carbohydrates	0g
Sugar	0g

PRIME RIB OR ROAST BEEF?

What is the difference between prime rib and roast beef? Not much, really. In some countries, *prime* refers to the grade quality of the cut, so the term *prime rib* is used to differentiate a higher quality cut. In the United States, some menus associate roast beef with adding gravy as a topping, while prime rib will be served with a side of au jus.

Easy Bacon Burger Pie

SERVES 4

Per Serving:

Calories	440
Fat	27g
Protein	34g
Sodium	1,020mg
Fiber	1g
Carbohydrates	13g
Sugar	1g

This family-friendly meal has all the flavors of a juicy bacon burger, but in pie form. It's so filling that it doesn't even need any side dishes!

1 tablespoon olive oil
1 pound 90/10 ground beef
2 teaspoons seasoned salt
1 cup chopped cooked gluten-free bacon
½ cup chopped dill pickles

½ cup halved grape tomatoes
½ cup Bisquick Gluten Free Pancake & Baking Mix
1 cup unsweetened almond milk
3 large eggs, whisked

1 Heat oven to 400°F. Spray a 9" pie pan with gluten-free nonstick cooking spray.

2 Heat oil in a large skillet and cook beef over medium-high heat for 5–7 minutes, stirring frequently, until beef is brown and crumbled; drain. Stir in seasoned salt, bacon, pickles, and tomatoes and cook for 2 minutes. Spread beef mixture in prepared pie pan.

3 In a medium bowl, stir Bisquick, milk, and eggs until combined. Pour on top of the beef mixture.

4 Bake 25–30 minutes until a knife inserted in the center comes out clean.

Taco Beef

SERVES 4

Per Serving:

Calories	245
Fat	17g
Protein	22g
Sodium	365mg
Fiber	0g
Carbohydrates	0g
Sugar	0g

Keep driving past the taco stand and instead make tacos at home on Taco Tuesday! Be ready for everyone to have seconds or thirds. Tacos are always better topped with homemade Easy Guacamole and Pico de Gallo (see recipes in Chapter 10).

1 teaspoon olive oil
1 pound 90/10 ground beef
1 tablespoon ground cumin
2 teaspoons onion powder

½ teaspoon garlic powder
2 teaspoons paprika
2 teaspoons dried oregano
½ teaspoon salt

1 Heat olive oil in a large skillet over medium heat and cook beef 6–8 minutes until browned and crumbled; drain excess oil.

2 In a small bowl, mix seasonings together.

3 Stir seasoning mix into beef and simmer for 2 minutes until heated through.

Korean Beef

This recipe tastes just like Korean barbecue from a restaurant! The unique sweet and spicy Korean sauce will make your taste buds sing.

1 tablespoon vegetable oil
1 pound 90/10 ground beef
2 teaspoons jarred minced garlic
¼ cup light brown sugar, packed
¼ cup gluten-free soy sauce
2 teaspoons sesame oil

½ teaspoon jarred minced ginger
¼ teaspoon crushed red pepper flakes
2 green onions, thinly sliced
¼ teaspoon sesame seeds
4 cups cooked rice

SERVES 4	
Per Serving:	
Calories	560
Fat	22g
Protein	29g
Sodium	1,080mg
Fiber	1g
Carbohydrates	60g
Sugar	13g

1 Heat vegetable oil in a large skillet over medium heat and cook beef and garlic for 6–8 minutes until beef is browned and crumbled.

2 In a small bowl, mix brown sugar, soy sauce, sesame oil, ginger, and red pepper flakes.

3 Stir sauce into beef and simmer for 2 minutes until heated through. Sprinkle with green onions and sesame seeds. Serve over rice.

Pork Chop Suey

This dish combines the sweet, nutty flavors of chestnuts and bamboo shoots to bring a unique and mouthwatering taste to your dinner table.

3 tablespoons vegetable oil
1 pound pork tenderloin, cut into 1½" strips
1 cup peeled and diced sweet onion
1 cup sliced white button mushrooms
1 cup diced celery
1 teaspoon jarred minced ginger
1 cup gluten-free chicken broth
½ teaspoon salt
½ teaspoon ground black pepper

1 (14.5-ounce) can bean sprouts, drained and rinsed
1 (5-ounce) can water chestnuts, drained and sliced
5 (5-ounce) cans bamboo shoots
2 teaspoons cornstarch
⅓ cup water
¼ cup gluten-free soy sauce
1 teaspoon granulated sugar

SERVES 4	
Per Serving:	
Calories	350
Fat	15g
Protein	33g
Sodium	1,570mg
Fiber	5g
Carbohydrates	22g
Sugar	12g

1 Heat oil in a large skillet over medium-high heat and sear pork 2–3 minutes, then add onions and mushroom and sauté for 5 minutes. Add celery, ginger, chicken broth, salt, and pepper, cover and simmer for 5 minutes. Add sprouts, water chestnuts, and bamboo shoots. Bring to a boil.

2 In a small bowl, combine cornstarch, water, soy sauce, and sugar. Mix together and add to skillet. Cook for 5 minutes until thickened.

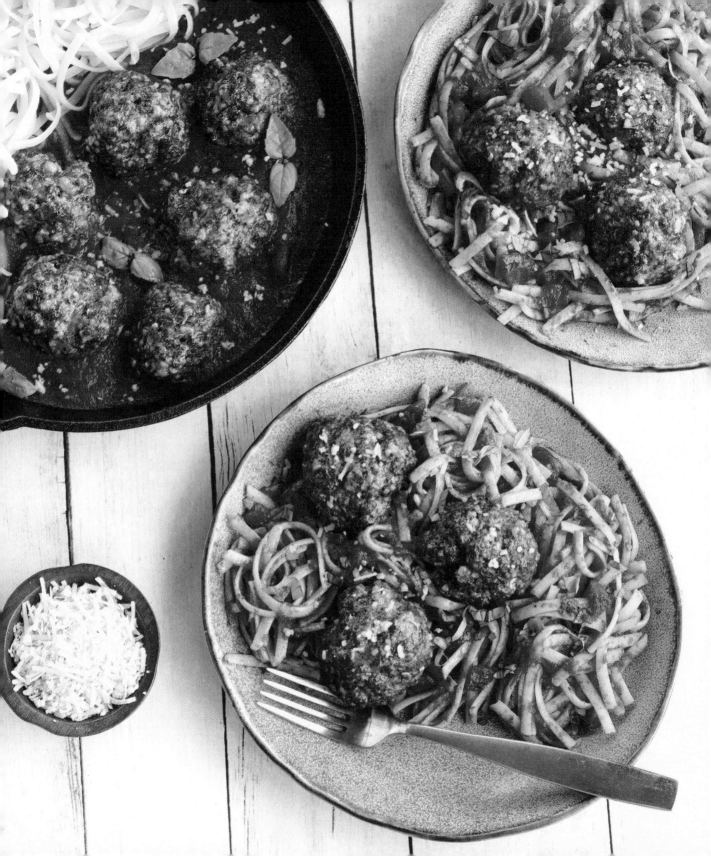

Italian Meatballs

These gluten-free and dairy-free Italian Meatballs are perfectly seasoned and ready for anything—a family meal, a potluck, or even a dinner party. Pair them with your favorite gluten-free and dairy-free pasta and sauce or eat them as is; either way, they are delightful!

1 cup gluten-free bread crumbs
2 tablespoons jarred minced garlic
2 tablespoons Italian seasoning
1 tablespoon onion powder
1 teaspoon salt
¾ cup unsweetened almond milk
2 pounds 90/10 ground beef
2 large eggs, whisked

1 Preheat oven to 375°F. Line two baking sheets with aluminum foil and spray with gluten-free nonstick cooking spray.

2 In a small bowl, add bread crumbs, garlic, Italian seasoning, onion powder, salt, and milk and stir to fully combine.

3 In a large bowl, mix beef and eggs together. Stir in the bread crumb mixture. Form the meatball mixture into thirty-six 2" balls and place onto prepared baking sheets.

4 Bake for 20–25 minutes until browned and cooked through.

SERVES 6

Per Serving
(Serving Size: 6 meatballs):

Calories	450
Fat	27g
Protein	33g
Sodium	670mg
Fiber	3g
Carbohydrates	14g
Sugar	1g

MEATBALLS ON YOUR TIME FRAME

If you're busy at dinnertime, you can plan ahead and form meatballs earlier in the day and refrigerate. Pull them out and put them in the oven when you are preparing the rest of your dinner. You can also freeze meatballs after cooking for up to 3 months and reheat them for adding to your pasta dishes. Reheat the frozen meatballs on the stove in sauces, in a slow cooker with sauce on high for 1–3 hours, or in the oven at 350°F for 20 minutes.

Southwestern Tamale Pie

This recipe tastes just like the great flavors of the Southwest without the stress of making handmade tamales. This version is mild, but if you prefer a little more heat, add gluten- and dairy-free hot sauce.

SERVES 6

Per Serving:

Calories	480
Fat	23g
Protein	29g
Sodium	1,270mg
Fiber	3g
Carbohydrates	38g
Sugar	6g

UNDERSTANDING TAMALES

Handmade tamales are delicious, but they take some time and practice to get just right. They are usually filled with meat, cheese, and chiles. Across the Southwest and particularly in New Mexico, they almost always include flame-roasted Hatch green chiles. These chiles are grown in the Hatch Valley in New Mexico. They can be either green or red chiles. When eating at restaurants in New Mexico, you are always asked if you want red or green.

1 teaspoon olive oil
1½ pounds 90/10 ground beef
1 small sweet onion, peeled and chopped
½ cup seeded and chopped green bell pepper
1 teaspoon jarred minced garlic
1 (14.5-ounce) can diced tomatoes, including liquid
1 (8-ounce) can tomato sauce
1 (11-ounce) can corn, drained
½ cup sliced black olives
1 teaspoon salt
1 tablespoon chili powder
1 teaspoon ground cumin
¼ teaspoon ground black pepper
1½ cups unsweetened almond milk
1 tablespoon granulated sugar
½ teaspoon salt
2 tablespoons dairy-free buttery spread
1 cup gluten-free cornmeal
2 large eggs, whisked

1 Preheat oven to 375°F. Spray a 9" × 13" baking pan with gluten-free nonstick cooking spray.

2 Heat olive oil in a large skillet over medium-high heat and cook beef with onions and peppers for 6–8 minutes until beef is browned and crumbled; drain oil.

3 Stir in garlic, tomatoes with juice, tomato sauce, corn, olives, salt, chili powder, cumin, and black pepper and bring to a low boil. Reduce heat to medium-low and simmer for 5 minutes. Transfer to the prepared pan.

4 In a large saucepan over medium heat, add milk, sugar, salt, and buttery spread. Reduce heat to low and stir in cornmeal, stirring constantly, until thickened.

5 Slowly add in whisked eggs, stirring until combined. Pour the milk mixture over the meat mixture, smoothing over the surface.

6 Bake 30–40 minutes until golden brown. Allow to cool for 5–10 minutes before serving.

Baked Ham with Brown Sugar Glaze

Making this delightful ham is a snap, even though it looks fancy! Enjoy this brown sugar-glazed ham with fresh, hot gluten-free and dairy-free dinner rolls.

1 (10-pound) fully cooked bone-in, spiral-cut ham
1 (20-ounce) can pineapple tidbits with juice
¾ cup light brown sugar, packed
½ teaspoon ground cinnamon
¼ teaspoon ground ginger
¼ teaspoon ground cloves

1 Allow ham to come to room temperature for 1–2 hours before baking.

2 In a medium saucepan over medium heat, combine pineapple, brown sugar, cinnamon, ginger, and cloves and cook for 3–5 minutes, stirring frequently.

3 Preheat oven to 300°F. Line a large roasting pan with aluminum foil and spray with gluten-free nonstick cooking spray.

4 Place ham cut-side down in prepared pan.

5 Brush 2 tablespoons glaze onto ham. Reserve remaining glaze for later. Cover ham tightly with a tent of aluminum foil. Bake at 300°F for 1½–2 hours. Remove ham from the oven and remove aluminum foil.

6 Increase the oven temperature to 400°F. Brush remaining glaze over ham. Return to the oven and continue to bake for 15 minutes until internal temperature reaches 140°F. Allow to rest for 15 minutes before slicing and serving.

SERVES 14

Per Serving:

Calories	88
Fat	1g
Protein	5g
Sodium	205mg
Fiber	0g
Carbohydrates	17g
Sugar	16g

Pork Tenderloin

Making this succulent Pork Tenderloin is easier than you might think. With only a few simple steps, it will be in the oven and filling your kitchen with the most lovely, hearty aroma! Serve it with roasted carrots and potatoes for a full meal.

1 tablespoon olive oil
1 pound pork tenderloin
2 teaspoons seasoned salt
½ cup mayonnaise

1   Preheat oven to 450°F. Spray a large roasting pan with gluten-free nonstick cooking spray.

2   Heat olive oil in a large skillet over medium-high heat and cook tenderloin for 10 minutes, searing each side.

3   Transfer meat to prepared roasting pan. Sprinkle seasoned salt all over tenderloin and coat with mayonnaise. Bake 20 minutes until a thermometer reads an internal temperature of 145°F.

SERVES 4

Per Serving:

Calories	365
Fat	28g
Protein	25g
Sodium	575mg
Fiber	0g
Carbohydrates	0g
Sugar	0g

KEEP THE TENDER IN YOUR TENDERLOIN

The pork tenderloin is a tender cut of meat, but it is very susceptible to becoming dry from being overcooked. Beginners often do not coat the tenderloin with any oil, and they quickly get a very dry and chewy piece of meat. That's why this recipe makes sure to coat and sear the meat to avoid drying out.

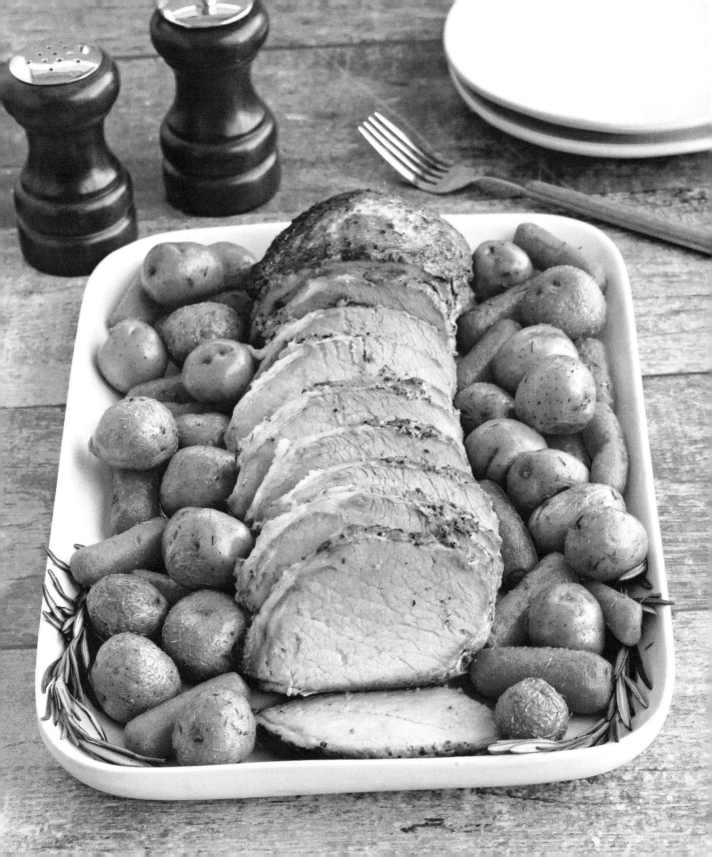

Smothered Pork Chops

SERVES 4

Per Serving:

Calories	755
Fat	47g
Protein	54g
Sodium	820mg
Fiber	0g
Carbohydrates	24g
Sugar	0g

AVOID OVERCOOKING PORK

Pork chops are fairly lean, so they can be prone to overcooking, and the finished result will be a tough, leathery piece of meat. The perfectly cooked pork chop will be tender and very juicy. For the best results, cook them to 145°F. They will have just a very light touch of pink.

Put the applesauce back in the cabinet because these smothered pork chops are so tender and juicy that you will not need anything else! Savory Stuffing and Southern-Style Sweet Potato Casserole (see recipes in Chapter 7) are perfect side dishes to go along with these savory chops.

1 cup gluten-free all-purpose flour with xanthan gum
2 tablespoons garlic powder
2 tablespoons onion powder
½ teaspoon cayenne pepper
1 teaspoon salt
½ teaspoon ground black pepper
4 (4-ounce) bone-in pork chops, ¾" thick
¼ cup olive oil
¼ teaspoon white vinegar
½ cup unsweetened almond milk
1 cup gluten-free chicken broth

1 Add flour, garlic powder, onion powder, cayenne pepper, salt, and black pepper in a pie pan and whisk to combine. Pat pork chops dry with paper towels and then dredge them in seasoned flour, shaking off the excess.

2 In a large skillet, heat olive oil over medium heat. Place pork chops in the pan in a single layer and fry for 3 minutes on each side until golden brown. Remove pork chops from the skillet and add a teaspoon of the seasoned flour mixture to the skillet.

3 To make buttermilk, add white vinegar to milk in a small bowl and let sit for 5 minutes in the refrigerator. Whisk flour into skillet grease and then pour in chicken broth. Cook for 5 minutes to reduce and thicken slightly. Stir in buttermilk and return pork chops to the skillet, covering them with sauce. Simmer for 5 minutes before serving.

German Pork Chops

Your family will be delighted with the rich and distinctive flavor of German Pork Chops. This dish goes great with Potato Pancakes (see recipe in Chapter 7).

1 teaspoon olive oil
4 (4-ounce) boneless pork chops
2 cups sauerkraut, drained
2 medium apples, sliced
1 cup peeled and chopped sweet onion

1 cup light brown sugar, packed
½ teaspoon salt
¼ teaspoon ground black pepper

SERVES 4	
Per Serving:	
Calories	425
Fat	4g
Protein	25g
Sodium	845mg
Fiber	4g
Carbohydrates	70g
Sugar	64g

1   Preheat oven to 350°F. Spray a 9" × 13" baking dish with gluten-free nonstick cooking spray.

2   Heat olive oil in a large skillet over medium-high heat. Brown pork chops for 5 minutes per side. Place chops into prepared baking dish.

3   In a large bowl, mix sauerkraut, apples, onions, brown sugar, salt, and pepper. Spread sauerkraut mixture over pork chops. Cover with aluminum foil. Bake for 45 minutes until internal temperature reaches 145°F.

Honey Garlic Pork Chops

The unique flavor combination in this recipe is just the right mix of sweet and savory.

4 (4-ounce) boneless pork chops
¼ teaspoon salt
⅛ teaspoon ground black pepper
1 teaspoon garlic powder
2 tablespoons olive oil
1 tablespoon dairy-free buttery spread

3 tablespoons jarred minced garlic
2 teaspoons jarred minced ginger
¼ cup honey
¼ cup water
2 tablespoons rice vinegar

SERVES 4	
Per Serving:	
Calories	310
Fat	12g
Protein	26g
Sodium	250mg
Fiber	0g
Carbohydrates	18g
Sugar	16g

1   Season chops with salt, pepper, and garlic powder on both sides.

2   Heat olive oil in a large ovenproof skillet over medium-high heat. Sear chops for 4–5 minutes per side until cooked through. Transfer to a plate.

3   Reduce heat to medium. Add buttery spread, garlic, and ginger to the skillet and sauté for 30 seconds until fragrant. Stir in honey, water, and vinegar. Increase heat to medium-high and continue to cook for 3–5 minutes, stirring occasionally, until sauce reduces and thickens.

4   Add pork back into the pan and baste with the sauce. Place the skillet in the oven to broil for 2 minutes or until edges are slightly charred.

Sweet and Sour Pork

SERVES 4

Per Serving:

Calories	510
Fat	5g
Protein	32g
Sodium	1,150mg
Fiber	4g
Carbohydrates	83g
Sugar	45g

THE WONDERS OF PINEAPPLE

Fresh pineapple not only tastes wonderful, but it also has many health benefits. Pineapple is the only source of the enzyme called *bromelain* that is an anti-inflammatory that is particularly beneficial for the sinuses. It is also an incredible source of riboflavin, vitamin B_6, and folate.

Try this delicious Sweet and Sour Pork instead of calling for takeout tonight. It keeps well overnight and will make another great meal for lunch! Serve over rice.

- ½ cup gluten-free all-purpose flour with xanthan gum
- ½ cup gluten-free cornstarch
- 1 pound boneless pork loin, cut into 1" cubes
- 1 large egg, beaten
- 2 cups plus 1 tablespoon vegetable oil, divided
- ½ cup honey
- 6 tablespoons rice vinegar
- 4 teaspoons gluten-free soy sauce
- 3 tablespoons tomato paste
- 1 tablespoon jarred minced garlic
- 1 tablespoon jarred minced ginger
- 1 cup peeled and chopped (1" pieces) white onion
- 1 cup seeded and chopped (1" pieces) red bell pepper
- 1 cup seeded and chopped (1" pieces) green bell pepper
- 1 cup canned pineapple chunks, drained (in juice)
- 1 tablespoon cornstarch
- 2 tablespoons water
- 2 tablespoons sliced green onion
- ½ teaspoon sesame seeds

1. Combine flour and cornstarch in a large sealable plastic bag. Add pork to a medium bowl with egg and stir to fully coat pieces. Place pork in the bag of flour mixture. Keep turning over the bag until pork is fully coated.

2. Heat 2 cups oil in a large skillet or wok over medium-high heat. Add pork to the skillet and fry for 6–8 minutes until light golden brown. Drain pork on a paper towel–lined plate. Carefully discard oil from skillet. Allow oil to completely cool before disposing.

3. In a medium bowl, combine honey, vinegar, soy sauce, and tomato paste.

4. Heat the skillet over medium-high heat and add in remaining 1 tablespoon oil. Add garlic, ginger, and onions and stir-fry for 30 seconds. Add in bell peppers and stir-fry for 1 minute. Add in pineapple and stir-fry for 1 minute. Add in pork and sauce, stir to combine, and allow sauce to come to a boil.

5. In a small bowl, whisk together cornstarch and water to make a slurry. Add slurry to the skillet, stirring constantly for 1 minute until sauce thickens. Mix the ingredients with the sauce to coat the pork. Top with green onions and sesame seeds.

CHAPTER 6

Seafood

Crispy Salmon Cakes

SERVES 4

Per Serving:

Calories	770
Fat	73g
Protein	8g
Sodium	880mg
Fiber	4g
Carbohydrates	24g
Sugar	4g

These easy gluten-free and dairy-free Crispy Salmon Cakes are full of flavor from the Old Bay Seasoning and dill. They're crispy on the outside and soft on the inside.

DILL SAUCE
½ cup mayonnaise
1 tablespoon dried dill
1 teaspoon horseradish sauce
1 teaspoon lemon juice
¼ teaspoon garlic salt

SALMON CAKES
2 large eggs, whisked
1 tablespoon Old Bay Seasoning
1 tablespoon dried dill
1 cup gluten-free bread crumbs
2 tablespoons sweet relish
2 (5-ounce) cans salmon, drained
1 cup vegetable oil

1 In a small bowl stir together all the ingredients for the creamy dill sauce.

2 In a medium bowl, add eggs, Old Bay Seasoning, dill, bread crumbs, and relish. Mix until all ingredients are combined.

3 Add salmon to the bread-crumb mixture and stir to combine ingredients well.

4 Form eight 1"-thick salmon cakes.

5 Heat vegetable oil in a large skillet over medium-high heat.

6 Fry cakes for 3–4 minutes on each side until golden brown. Drain on a paper towel–lined plate before serving with dipping sauce.

Cajun Catfish

Cajun cooking is all about finding the right balance between the flavors of the dish and level of spiciness. Adding cornmeal to the Cajun season mix not only balances the spice but also gives the fish a nice light crust to keep it moist and flavorful.

½ teaspoon ground black pepper
½ teaspoon ground white pepper
1 tablespoon garlic powder
1 tablespoon onion powder
1 tablespoon paprika
1 teaspoon dried parsley
½ teaspoon cayenne pepper
1 teaspoon salt
1 tablespoon dried oregano
1 tablespoon dried thyme
½ cup gluten-free cornmeal
4 (6-ounce) boneless catfish fillets
½ cup dairy-free buttery spread

1 In a pie pan, mix together black pepper, white pepper, garlic powder, onion powder, paprika, parsley, cayenne pepper, salt, oregano, thyme, and cornmeal until thoroughly combined. Press catfish fillets into the spice mixture on both sides to thoroughly coat.

2 Melt buttery spread in a large cast-iron pan or skillet over high heat. Allow the pan to heat up for 2–3 minutes.

3 Add fillets to the pan. The pan will sizzle up and smoke. Cook the fillets for 2–3 minutes. Using a spatula, carefully flip fillets over and cook on the other side for another 2–3 minutes.

SERVES 4

Per Serving:

Calories	330
Fat	16g
Protein	27g
Sodium	970mg
Fiber	1g
Carbohydrates	16g
Sugar	0g

MAKE THE PERFECT FISH FILLETS

Overcooking fish fillets will make them dry and tough and lead them straight to the wastebasket. Carefully watch your fish as it cooks and test doneness by inserting a fork into the thickest part of the fillet and gently twisting. If it easily flakes, then your fish fillet should be done.

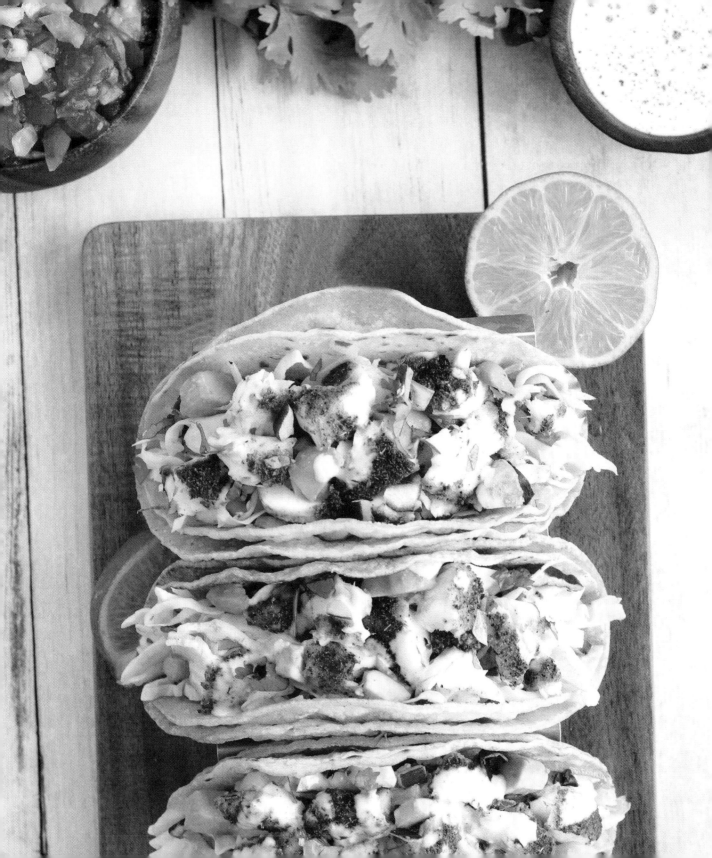

Fish Tacos

Fish Tacos are great for lunch or dinner, and they are perfectly seasoned and topped with homemade lime sauce. These tacos are even better topped with diced avocado, red onion, and chopped cilantro, and served with Southwestern Black Bean and Corn Salad (see recipe in Chapter 7).

FISH

1 tablespoon ground cumin
½ teaspoon chili powder
½ teaspoon garlic powder
1 teaspoon dried oregano
½ teaspoon onion powder
1 teaspoon paprika
½ teaspoon salt
½ teaspoon ground black pepper
1 pound tilapia
1 tablespoon olive oil

SAUCE

⅓ cup mayonnaise
¼ cup lime juice
½ teaspoon garlic powder
½ teaspoon ground cumin
¼ teaspoon salt
¼ teaspoon gluten-free and dairy-free hot sauce

TACOS

8 white corn tortillas

SERVES 4

Per Serving:

Calories	330
Fat	20g
Protein	24g
Sodium	630mg
Fiber	2g
Carbohydrates	13g
Sugar	1g

FISH OPTIONS FOR TACOS

Tilapia is the perfect fish option for tacos, but many other fish varieties will work great. Whiting, cod, and grouper are lean and delicate choices. If you prefer fish with higher fat content, catfish, trout, or mullet would be more your style.

1 Preheat oven to 400°F. Line a baking sheet with parchment paper.

2 In a small bowl, add cumin, chili powder, garlic powder, oregano, onion powder, paprika, salt, and pepper and stir to combine. Rub seasoning mix onto fish fillets. Place fish on prepared baking sheet and drizzle with olive oil. Bake for 12–15 minutes until flaky and cooked through.

3 In small bowl, whisk together mayonnaise, lime juice, garlic powder, cumin, salt, and hot sauce.

4 Heat tortillas according to package directions. Break fish into large chunks and divide among tortillas. Drizzle with sauce.

Classic Shrimp Scampi

SERVES 4

Per Serving:

Calories	230
Fat	15g
Protein	15g
Sodium	1,330mg
Fiber	0g
Carbohydrates	2g
Sugar	0g

This garlic buttery scampi sauce has a hint of white wine and can be made in minutes! You can serve it with toothpicks as an appetizer or for dinner served over rice or gluten-free pasta.

2 tablespoons jarred minced garlic, divided
1 teaspoon salt
3 tablespoons olive oil, divided
1 pound large raw shrimp, peeled and deveined
¼ cup white wine
1 tablespoon lemon juice
¼ cup dairy-free buttery spread
1 tablespoon chopped fresh parsley

1 In a medium bowl, whisk together 1 tablespoon garlic, salt, and 1 tablespoon olive oil. Add shrimp, toss to coat, and chill for 30 minutes up to 1 hour.

2 Heat remaining olive oil in a large skillet over medium heat and cook shrimp mixture for 1 minute on each side until shrimp is pink but not fully cooked. Transfer shrimp to a plate with a slotted spoon to leave as much oil in pan as possible.

3 Add remaining garlic to the skillet and cook for 1 minute until fragrant. Add wine and lemon juice and cook for 2 minutes, stirring occasionally, until sauce is reduced by half. Add buttery spread and cook for 5 minutes. Continue stirring until buttery spread is melted and sauce is thickened.

4 Add shrimp back into the skillet. Toss shrimp to coat with sauce and cook for 2 minutes until shrimp are fully cooked and the flesh is totally pink and opaque. Garnish with parsley.

Maryland-Style Crab Cakes

These crab cakes are full of sweet crabmeat and perfectly seasoned. They have just the right balance of breading to not hide the flavors of the crabmeat.

1 pound jumbo lump crabmeat

1 large egg, beaten

½ cup mayonnaise

½ teaspoon Dijon mustard

1 teaspoon gluten-free Worcestershire sauce

1 teaspoon Old Bay Seasoning

⅛ teaspoon garlic powder

¼ teaspoon dried parsley

⅛ teaspoon tarragon

½ cup gluten-free bread crumbs

6 teaspoons dairy-free buttery spread

1 Drain crabmeat and pick through it for shells, if necessary. Try not to break up the lumps. Put crabmeat in a medium bowl and set aside.

2 In a small bowl, add egg, mayonnaise, mustard, Worcestershire sauce, Old Bay Seasoning, garlic powder, parsley, and tarragon and stir to combine ingredients. Add bread crumbs to the mixture and stir to combine.

3 Gently stir the wet mixture into crabmeat, one spoonful at a time; avoid breaking up lump meat. Do not overmix.

4 Gently form the mixture into six crab cakes. Lightly grease the bottom of a baking sheet with gluten-free nonstick cooking spray and place crab cakes on prepared sheet. Place 1 teaspoon buttery spread on top of each of the cakes.

5 Broil crab cakes on low for 12–15 minutes until golden brown and cooked through. If they are browning too fast, lower the oven rack so that crab cakes can still cook for the allotted time. Remove crab cakes from the oven and allow to cool slightly before serving them.

SERVES 6

Per Serving:

Calories	250
Fat	18g
Protein	14g
Sodium	650mg
Fiber	1g
Carbohydrates	7g
Sugar	1g

CRAB CAKE VARIATIONS

Maryland crab cakes are not the only crab cake around. There are several different crab cake variations, including some from Maine and Florida. The main differences are often the bread crumb to crabmeat ratio and which seasonings are used. Maryland crab cakes are known for their use of Old Bay Seasoning, Maine crab cakes are known for their use of yellow mustard, and Florida crab cakes often have cornmeal added to the mix.

Country Shrimp and Grits

Shrimp and grits is a traditional dish in the Low Country of coastal South Carolina and Georgia. It can also be a breakfast, though many consider it more of a lunch or dinner dish.

SERVES 4

Per Serving:

Calories	340
Fat	8g
Protein	23g
Sodium	1,100mg
Fiber	2g
Carbohydrates	42g
Sugar	5g

ARE GRITS GLUTEN-FREE?

Traditional grits, in their pure form, come from corn and do not contain any gluten ingredients. Still, be careful choosing the brand of grits because of the possibility of cross con-tamination in production. It is always safe to choose a brand that is labeled gluten-free.

4 cups cooked gluten-free, dairy-free grits
1 pound raw shrimp, peeled and deveined
1 tablespoon olive oil
½ cup chopped gluten-free bacon
¼ cup peeled and chopped sweet onion
2 tablespoons seeded and chopped green bell pepper
1 teaspoon jarred minced garlic
2 tablespoons white wine
1 cup unsweetened almond milk
½ teaspoon salt
¼ teaspoon ground black pepper
2 tablespoons gluten-free all-purpose flour with xanthan gum

1 Cook grits according to the package directions; set aside and keep warm.

2 Rinse shrimp and pat dry. In a large skillet, heat olive oil over medium heat and fry bacon for 2–3 minutes on each side until browned; remove to a paper towel–lined plate. Drain the skillet, reserving 1 tablespoon of bacon grease in the skillet. Add onions, bell peppers, and garlic and sauté 2–3 minutes until onions are translucent.

3 Add shrimp and sauté for 4–5 minutes or until pink. Remove the shrimp mixture from the skillet, set aside, and cover to keep warm. Add white wine to the skillet and cook for 30 seconds to deglaze.

4 Add milk, salt, black pepper, and flour to a small bowl or glass measur-ing cup and whisk together until flour dissolves. Slowly pour the milk mixture into the skillet, stirring, and let reduce for 2–3 minutes until thickened. Serve the shrimp mixture and gravy over cooked grits.

Honey Soy–Glazed Salmon

This salmon has a mouthwatering glaze of caramelization that keeps the fish moist and tender. The salmon has rich flavor from the marinade and can be on the table in minutes.

1 cup gluten-free soy sauce
¼ cup honey
2 tablespoons lemon juice

1 tablespoon jarred minced ginger
1 tablespoon jarred minced garlic
4 (4-ounce) salmon fillets

1 In a large bowl, whisk soy sauce, honey, lemon juice, ginger, and garlic together until honey dissolves. Place salmon fillets in marinade skin-side up. Cover the bowl with plastic wrap and marinate for 30 minutes in the refrigerator.

2 Preheat broiler to high. Put salmon on an aluminum foil–lined baking sheet sprayed with gluten-free nonstick cooking spray. Place under the broiler skin-side down and broil without turning for 7–10 minutes until fish is well caramelized and is cooked through.

SERVES 4

Per Serving:

Calories	250
Fat	15g
Protein	24g
Sodium	470mg
Fiber	0g
Carbohydrates	2g
Sugar	2g

Steamed Mussels with Marsala Wine and Garlic

This is an elegant, yet easy, recipe that makes a dinner at home a special occasion! This dish goes great with freshly baked gluten-free and dairy-free dinner rolls.

2 tablespoons olive oil
1 tablespoon jarred minced garlic
1 small onion, peeled and thinly sliced
4 pounds mussels, rinsed

½ cup Marsala cooking wine
¼ cup lemon juice
1 cup gluten-free chicken broth

1 Heat oil in a 6- to 8-quart stockpot over medium-high heat. Sauté garlic and onions for 1–2 minutes. Add mussels and toss.

2 Add wine, lemon juice, and chicken broth; cover the pot and steam over medium-high heat for 5–7 minutes until mussels open. Serve with broth.

SERVES 4

Per Serving:

Calories	235
Fat	11g
Protein	18g
Sodium	410mg
Fiber	0g
Carbohydrates	10g
Sugar	2g

Cajun Jambalaya

Jambalaya is an easy one-pot recipe with chicken, sausage, shrimp, rice, and Creole seasoning. It is customizable with your favorite meats and full of bold and zesty flavors. This is an easy recipe to make gluten-free and dairy-free because you control the ingredients.

SERVES 4

Per Serving:

Calories	860
Fat	30g
Protein	63g
Sodium	3,900mg
Fiber	4g
Carbohydrates	77g
Sugar	8g

PREPARING FRESH SHRIMP

Make sure to keep your shrimp on ice from the supermarket to home. When peeling shrimp, use a sharp, small pointed knife and cut a shallow line along the outside of the shrimp. Always remove the black veins and wash thoroughly. Then you're ready to follow the recipe's instructions.

3 tablespoons olive oil, divided

2 (6-ounce) boneless, skinless chicken breasts, cut into 1" pieces

1 pound gluten-free andouille sausage, thinly sliced

1 small green bell pepper, seeded and diced

1 small red bell pepper, seeded and diced

1 cup diced celery

1 small white onion, peeled and diced

2 tablespoons jarred minced garlic

1 (14-ounce) can crushed tomatoes, including liquid

3 cups gluten-free chicken broth

1½ cups uncooked white rice

2 tablespoons Cajun seasoning

1 teaspoon dried thyme

¼ teaspoon cayenne pepper

1 bay leaf

1 pound raw large shrimp, peeled and deveined

1 cup thinly sliced okra

2 teaspoons salt

¼ teaspoon ground black pepper

1 Heat 1 tablespoon oil in a large stockpot over medium-high heat. Add chicken and sausage and sauté for 5–7 minutes, stirring occasionally, until chicken is cooked through and sausage is lightly browned. Transfer to a plate.

2 Add remaining 2 tablespoons oil to the stockpot and add bell peppers, celery, onions, and garlic. Sauté the mixture for 6 minutes, stirring occasionally, until onions are softened.

3 Add tomatoes, chicken broth, rice, Cajun seasoning, thyme, cayenne pepper, and bay leaf and stir to combine. Bring the mixture to a simmer. Reduce heat to medium-low, cover, and simmer for about 25–30 minutes until rice is nearly cooked through, stirring every 5 minutes to keep rice from burning. Add shrimp and okra and stir to combine. Continue to simmer for 5–6 minutes until shrimp are cooked through and pink. Stir in chicken, sausage, salt, and pepper. Remove and discard bay leaf. Remove from heat and serve warm.

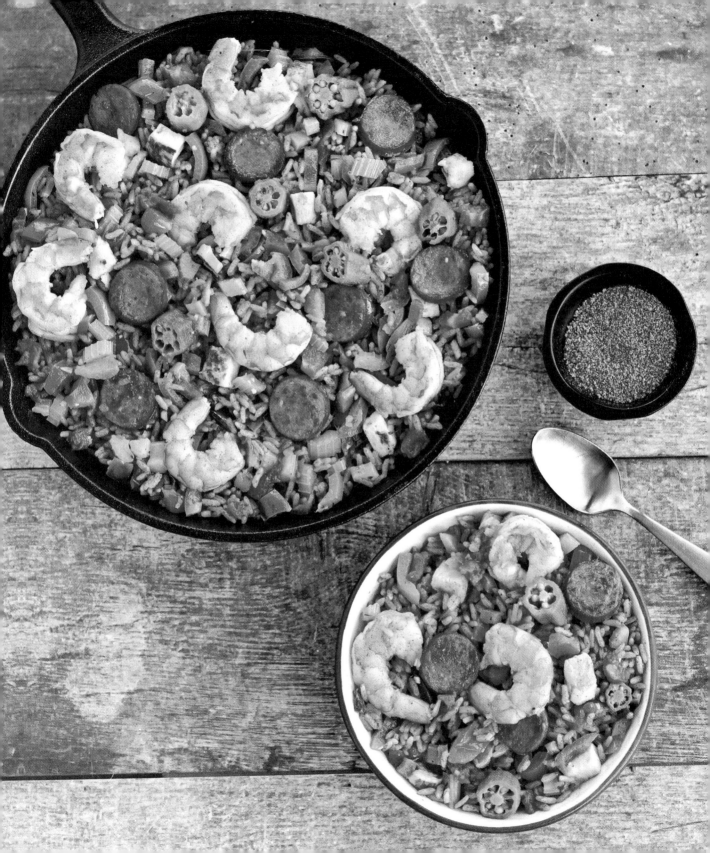

Stuffed Jumbo Shrimp

It is not as hard as you might think to make restaurant-quality baked stuffed shrimp at home! This gluten- and dairy-free version still packs in all the classic flavors.

SERVES 4

Per Serving:

Calories	220
Fat	11g
Protein	16g
Sodium	740mg
Fiber	2g
Carbohydrates	13g
Sugar	2g

TIPS FOR BUYING SHRIMP

When buying shrimp, look for shrimp that have shiny, firm shells with a faint sea smell. They should not have an ammonia smell. If you are fortunate enough to live in a coastal area where shrimp are harvested, always buy local shrimp. If not, look for wild-caught shrimp. If you are buying frozen, look at the ingredients to ensure they list only shrimp and water (avoid shrimp with additives).

1 tablespoon olive oil
¼ cup minced celery
1 tablespoon jarred minced garlic
½ cup peeled and minced onion
20 fresh jumbo shrimp, peeled and deveined but with tails on
1 large egg, beaten
½ cup gluten-free bread crumbs
1 tablespoon mayonnaise
½ teaspoon lemon juice
1 teaspoon seasoned salt
¼ teaspoon ground black pepper
½ pound fresh lump crabmeat, picked over for shells and cartilage
2 tablespoons dairy-free buttery spread, melted

1 Preheat oven to 375°F. Spray a 9" × 13" baking pan with gluten-free nonstick cooking spray.

2 In a medium skillet, heat olive oil over medium-high heat. Add celery, garlic, and onions and cook for 4 minutes, stirring until softened. Remove from heat and allow to cool.

3 Butterfly each shrimp along the outside curve. Open shrimp flat and place butterflied-side up in prepared baking dish.

4 In a small bowl, combine egg, bread crumbs, mayonnaise, lemon juice, salt, and pepper. Stir in crabmeat.

5 Place 2 tablespoons stuffing onto each shrimp, pressing gently. Drizzle buttery spread over shrimp and bake 20 minutes or until stuffing is golden brown and shrimp are pink.

Lemon Garlic Sautéed Scallops

These seared scallops have a perfect golden-brown crust, just like at the restaurants! This light dish is great paired with roasted asparagus and Easy Rice Pilaf (see recipe in Chapter 7).

2 tablespoons olive oil

1¼ pounds scallops

½ teaspoon salt

¼ teaspoon ground black pepper

3 tablespoons dairy-free buttery spread, divided

2 teaspoons jarred minced garlic

¼ cup white wine

2 tablespoons lemon juice

¼ cup chopped fresh parsley

1 Heat olive oil in a large skillet over medium-high heat. Season scallops with salt and pepper. Add scallops in a single layer to the skillet and fry for 1½ minutes on one side until a golden crust forms underneath. Turn over and fry for 1½ minutes until crisp, lightly browned, cooked through, and opaque. Remove from the skillet and transfer to a plate.

2 Melt 2 tablespoons buttery spread in the skillet. Add in garlic and cook 1 minute until fragrant. Pour in wine and bring to a simmer for 2 minutes until wine reduces by half. Stir in the remaining tablespoon buttery spread and lemon juice.

3 Remove the skillet from the heat and add scallops back into the skillet to warm up. Garnish with parsley and serve.

SERVES 4

Per Serving:

Calories	170
Fat	18g
Protein	1g
Sodium	310mg
Fiber	0g
Carbohydrates	1g
Sugar	0g

BUYING FRESH SCALLOPS

The best all-natural scallops should be translucent, and the meat should be firm. The meat of the scallop should not be split, and avoid dark meat around the edges.

Baked Salmon with Lemon

SERVES 4

Per Serving:

Calories	375
Fat	25g
Protein	35g
Sodium	390mg
Fiber	0g
Carbohydrates	0g
Sugar	0g

This baked salmon is elegant, full of flavor, and easy to prepare. Serve with Creamy Dill Sauce, Roasted Garlic Potatoes, and Honey-Glazed Carrots (see recipes in Chapter 7).

2 tablespoons olive oil
2 teaspoons lemon zest
2 tablespoons fresh lemon juice
4 (6-ounce) salmon fillets
½ teaspoon salt
¼ teaspoon ground black pepper
1 small lemon, sliced

1. Preheat oven to 400°F degrees and grease a 9" × 13" baking dish with gluten-free nonstick cooking spray.
2. In a large bowl, whisk together olive oil, lemon zest, and lemon juice.
3. Place salmon fillets in baking dish. Season tops of salmon with salt and pepper. Drizzle tops evenly with the lemon mixture and gently rub over salmon.
4. Let salmon rest at room temperature for 10 minutes. Place a lemon slice on top of each fillet, then bake 12–16 minutes or until salmon has cooked through.

Cilantro Lime Shrimp Bake

SERVES 4

Per Serving:

Calories	220
Fat	6g
Protein	31g
Sodium	1,540mg
Fiber	1g
Carbohydrates	8g
Sugar	0g

If you want a simple and flavor-packed seafood dish, try this Cilantro Lime Shrimp Bake! This recipe will work fine with any size of shrimp you buy.

2 pounds raw shrimp, peeled and deveined
2 teaspoons jarred minced garlic
¼ cup lime juice
1 teaspoon ground cumin
¼ teaspoon salt
¼ teaspoon ground black pepper
2 tablespoons dairy-free buttery spread, melted
¼ cup gluten-free panko bread crumbs
¼ cup chopped fresh cilantro

1. Preheat oven to 425°F. Spray a 9" × 13" baking dish with gluten-free nonstick cooking spray.
2. In a medium bowl, add shrimp, garlic, lime juice, cumin, salt, and pepper and toss to combine. Transfer the mixture to prepared baking dish.
3. In a separate medium bowl, stir together melted buttery spread, panko, and cilantro until combined. Sprinkle the panko mixture evenly on top of shrimp.
4. Bake for 15–18 minutes or until shrimp are pink and no longer opaque.

Clams Casino

This recipe will wow your dinner guests and introduce them to a new and exciting clam dish! Be sure to discard any broken or open clams.

1 teaspoon olive oil
¾ cup finely diced gluten-free bacon
1 cup seeded and finely diced red bell pepper
2 teaspoons jarred minced garlic
⅓ cup white wine
1 tablespoon onion powder
½ teaspoon salt
¼ ground black pepper
18 medium (2½") littleneck clams, shucked and bottom shells reserved

1 Heat olive oil in a large skillet over medium heat. Add bacon and sauté 3 minutes until crisp. Using a slotted spoon, transfer bacon to a paper towel–lined plate. Add bell peppers and garlic to the skillet and sauté for 5 minutes until peppers are softened. Add wine and simmer for 2 minutes until it is almost evaporated. Remove the skillet from the heat and cool completely. Stir bacon into the vegetable mixture. Season with onion powder, salt, and black pepper.

2 Preheat oven to 500°F. Line a large baking sheet with aluminum foil and spray with gluten-free nonstick cooking spray. Arrange clams in their shells on the baking sheet. Spoon the vegetable mixture atop the clams, dividing equally and mounding slightly. Bake for 10 minutes until topping is golden brown and cooked thoroughly.

SERVES 4

Per Serving:

Calories	120
Fat	5g
Protein	15g
Sodium	1,000mg
Fiber	0g
Carbohydrates	2g
Sugar	0g

SIMPLE STEAMED CLAMS

Fresh clams are also wonderful steamed and served with just melted (and still hot) dairy-free buttery spread. If you do not have a clam steamer, place your clams in a 6-quart Dutch oven, add an inch of boiling water, and tightly cover. Steam for 6–8 minutes or until the clams open up a little.

New England Clam Bake

Give your family the traditional tastes of New England with this wonderful clam bake! If possible, purchase fresh seafood, but if not, frozen will work well too. Serve with melted dairy-free buttery spread for dipping and lemon wedges.

DON'T OVERCOOK YOUR SEAFOOD

Overcooked seafood can ruin its unique flavor. Always watch your seafood carefully when it's cooking. For example, when you see lobster turn bright red, it is properly cooked. Another tip is to not eat any clams that do not open. It is always best to discard any clams that didn't open while cooking.

1 teaspoon olive oil

4 gluten-free chorizo sausages

1 cup cold water

2 cups white wine

3 tablespoons Old Bay Seasoning

1 teaspoon salt

2 tablespoons jarred minced garlic

2 bay leaves

2 tablespoons dried thyme

1 red onion, peeled and chopped

2 pounds new potatoes, halved

2 (2-pound) lobsters

2 dozen clams

4 ears fresh corn, cut into quarters

1 In a large stockpot or lobster pot, heat olive oil over medium heat. Pierce sausages in several places with the tip of knife, then add them to the pot with hot oil. Cook for 5 minutes or until golden brown. Transfer to a plate.

2 In the same stockpot, bring the water, wine, Old Bay Seasoning, salt, garlic, bay leaves, and thyme to a boil.

3 Add onions and potatoes, cover, and cook over medium-high heat for 15 minutes. Add lobsters on top, cover, and cook for 3 minutes. Add clams and corn and continue to cook covered for 8–10 minutes until clams open. Carefully remove seafood and vegetables from the pot and transfer to a large platter. Discard bay leaves.

Oven-Fried Orange Roughy

The mild flavor of this dish will please even the pickiest seafood critic at your table! This lean fish is tender and flaky and widely available.

¼ cup gluten-free cornmeal
¼ cup gluten-free bread crumbs
2 teaspoons seasoned salt
½ teaspoon dried dill
⅛ teaspoon ground black pepper
¼ cup unsweetened almond milk
1 pound orange roughy, cut into 1½" × 2" pieces
3 tablespoons dairy-free buttery spread, melted

1 Preheat oven to 500°F and move oven rack to the position slightly above the middle of oven. Spray a 9" × 13" baking dish with gluten-free nonstick cooking spray.

2 Mix cornmeal, bread crumbs, seasoned salt, dill, and pepper together in a pie pan. Pour milk into a separate pie pan.

3 Dip fish pieces into milk and then press into the bread-crumb mixture to coat on all sides. Place breaded fish into the baking dish. Drizzle buttery spread over breaded fish pieces.

4 Bake for 10 minutes until fish flakes easily with a fork.

SERVES 4

Per Serving:

Calories	180
Fat	5g
Protein	20g
Sodium	570mg
Fiber	1g
Carbohydrates	13g
Sugar	0g

Grilled Grouper with Lemon Butter Sauce

Grouper is a lean and mild, sweet-tasting fish that has a firm texture. The light lemon butter sauce is a perfect complement.

4 (8-ounce) grouper fillets, skin removed
½ teaspoon salt
¼ teaspoon ground black pepper
2 tablespoons olive oil
1 teaspoon jarred minced garlic
1 cup gluten-free chicken broth
¼ cup lemon juice
2 tablespoons capers, drained and rinsed
2 tablespoons dairy-free buttery spread

1 Place fillets on an aluminum foil–lined baking sheet sprayed with gluten-free nonstick cooking spray. Salt and pepper fillets. Broil 4" from the heat for 6–7 minutes on each side or until fish flakes easily with a fork. Remove from oven.

2 Heat olive oil in a medium skillet over medium heat. Add garlic and cook for 30 seconds until fragrant. Pour in broth and lemon juice and bring the mixture to a boil. Boil for 5–8 minutes, stirring occasionally, until sauce reduces. Add capers and buttery spread to the pan and stir to combine; cook 2–3 minutes until buttery spread is melted.

3 Serve with sauce poured over fillets.

SERVES 4

Per Serving:

Calories	320
Fat	12g
Protein	51g
Sodium	600mg
Fiber	0g
Carbohydrates	2g
Sugar	1g

Pecan-Crusted Honey Mustard Salmon

SERVES 4

Per Serving:

Calories	375
Fat	27g
Protein	25g
Sodium	530mg
Fiber	2g
Carbohydrates	11g
Sugar	9g

WHERE'S THE SALMON?

When you think about where most salmon are harvested, you might first think about Alaska thanks to television shows that follow fishing there. The United States does export a sizable salmon harvest each year but imports a larger amount from Norway, Canada, and Chile. Under the Country of Origin Labeling law, the US Department of Agriculture (USDA) requires all grocery stores and retailers to clearly list product origins and method of production (farm-raised or wild-caught) for fish and shellfish.

This baked salmon has a tangy and sweet honey mustard glaze and a crunchy pecan crust topping. Serve with Easy Rice Pilaf and Roasted Butternut Squash (see recipes in Chapter 7).

4 (4-ounce) salmon fillets
½ teaspoon salt
¼ teaspoon ground black pepper
2 tablespoons stone-ground mustard
2 tablespoons honey
½ teaspoon paprika
½ cup pecans

1 Preheat oven to 375°F. Line a baking sheet with aluminum foil and spray with gluten-free nonstick cooking spray.

2 Place salmon fillets on prepared baking sheet skin-side down and sprinkle with salt and pepper.

3 In a small bowl, mix mustard and honey. Pour the mixture over each salmon piece and rub the mixture into salmon on all sides.

4 Add pecans to a food processor and finely chop. Stir paprika into pecans. Evenly distribute the pecan mixture on top of each salmon fillet. Press the mixture into salmon to create a crust. Bake for 9–13 minutes.

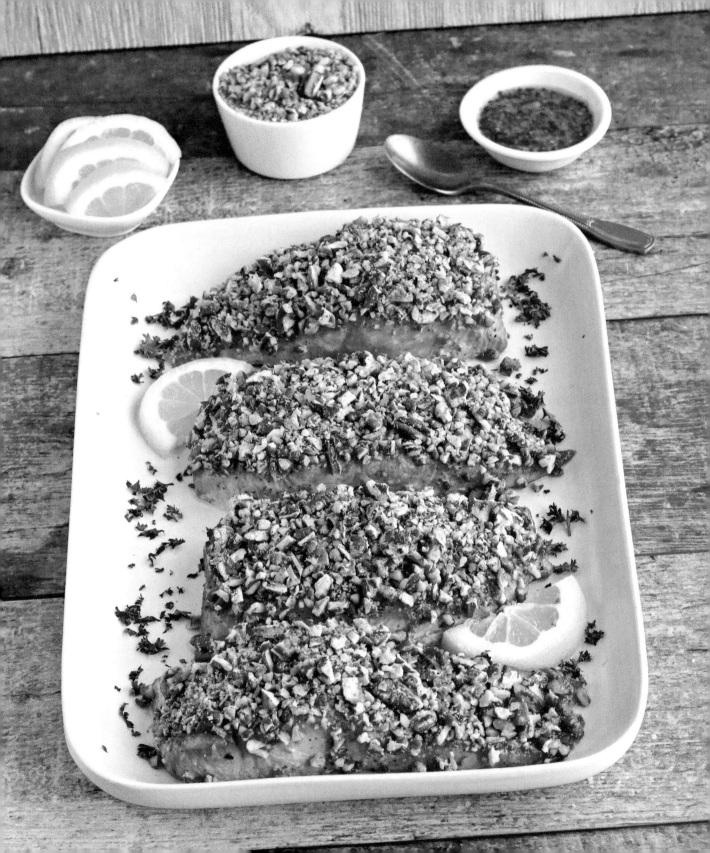

Chili Lime Tilapia with Fresh Mango Salsa

SERVES 4

Per Serving:

Calories	370
Fat	17g
Protein	35g
Sodium	390mg
Fiber	2g
Carbohydrates	18g
Sugar	14g

MORE ON MANGO SALSA

Mango salsa has become very popular in recent years. Flavor variations range from the mild and expected to the spicy and unpredictable. Store-bought options might be gluten- and dairy-free, so check the label!

This light and tender tilapia dish is a bright combination of fresh and fruity flavors with just a hint of chili. Tilapia fish has a sweet and mild taste, is lean and has a flaky texture. It is the perfect fish to complement all the flavors of this dish.

MANGO SALSA

1 small mango, peeled, pitted, and diced
2 tablespoons seeded and finely diced red bell pepper
2 tablespoons peeled and finely diced red onion
½ cup chopped fresh cilantro
1 tablespoon seeded and finely chopped jalapeño
¼ cup lime juice
¼ teaspoon salt

TILAPIA

2 teaspoons chili powder
1 teaspoon garlic powder
1 teaspoon onion powder
¾ teaspoon salt
1 teaspoon light brown sugar, packed
¼ cup lime juice
¼ cup olive oil
4 (6-ounce) tilapia fillets

1. In a medium bowl, combine the mango, bell peppers, onions, cilantro, and jalapeño. Add lime juice and salt and mix well. Cover and refrigerate for at least 1 hour.

2. Preheat oven to 350°F. Line a baking sheet with aluminum foil and spray with gluten-free nonstick cooking spray.

3. In a small bowl, whisk together chili powder, garlic powder, onion powder, salt, brown sugar, lime juice, and olive oil.

4. Pat tilapia fillets dry with a paper towel and place on prepared baking sheet. Pour sauce over fish and bake for 15–20 minutes. When finished, plate and top with mango salsa.

Marinated Grilled Tuna Steaks

These delicious East Coast-style grilled tuna steaks will make your next Friday night seafood night one to remember! Tuna is rich in omega-3 fatty acids and is a heart-healthy food. Tuna steaks are different than canned tuna, and is often served cooked rare.

8 tablespoons olive oil, divided
4 teaspoons Old Bay Seasoning
1 tablespoon lime juice
1 tablespoon lemon juice
4 (6-ounce, 1"-thick) fresh tuna steaks

1 In a large bowl, combine 4 tablespoons of olive oil, Old Bay Seasoning, lime juice, and lemon juice.

2 Add tuna steaks to the bowl. Cover and place in the refrigerator for 20 minutes, turning tuna occasionally.

3 Add 2 tablespoons oil to a stove-top cast-iron grill and heat over high heat. Brush tuna with 2 tablespoons of oil. Grill tuna on each side for 2–2½ minutes. The center should be bright pink. Allow tuna to rest for 5–10 minutes before serving.

SERVES 4

Per Serving:

Calories	235
Fat	7g
Protein	25g
Sodium	440mg
Fiber	2g
Carbohydrates	13g
Sugar	7g

Greek-Style Snapper

Bring the flavors of the Mediterranean home tonight with this Greek-Style Snapper! This recipe goes great with baked potatoes and Ratatouille (see recipe in Chapter 7).

1 tablespoon olive oil
1 small sweet onion, peeled and chopped
1 tablespoon jarred minced garlic
1 (14.5-ounce) can diced tomatoes, drained
½ cup gluten-free chicken broth
1 tablespoon red wine vinegar
2 tablespoons lemon juice
⅓ cup sliced Kalamata olives
1 teaspoon dried oregano
1 teaspoon dried dill
1 pound red snapper fillet
2 tablespoons chopped fresh parsley

1 Preheat oven to 425°F. Spray a 9" × 13" baking dish with gluten-free nonstick cooking spray.

2 Heat olive oil in a large skillet over medium-high heat. Sauté onions and garlic for 2 minutes. Stir in tomatoes, broth, vinegar, lemon juice, olives, oregano, and dill; simmer for 5 minutes.

3 Place fillets in prepared baking dish. Spoon tomato mixture over fillets. Bake for 10–15 minutes until fish flakes with a fork. Remove from oven, plate, and sprinkle with parsley.

SERVES 4

Per Serving:

Calories	450
Fat	29g
Protein	42g
Sodium	360mg
Fiber	0g
Carbohydrates	1g
Sugar	0g

New Orleans–Style Barbecue Shrimp

SERVES 4

Per Serving:

Calories	290
Fat	14g
Protein	31g
Sodium	3,000mg
Fiber	0g
Carbohydrates	5g
Sugar	1g

The bold flavors of New Orleans come alive with this easy barbecue shrimp recipe. These zesty shrimps are great served with dairy-free cole-slaw and Easy Oven-Roasted Corn on the Cob (see recipe in Chapter 7). The shrimp aren't peeled because the shells help keep the shrimp tender and moist and add flavor to the sauce.

1 cup dairy-free buttery spread
¼ cup lemon juice
2 tablespoons gluten-free Worcestershire sauce
1 tablespoon jarred minced garlic
1 tablespoon onion powder
1 teaspoon dried oregano
1 teaspoon dried thyme
1 teaspoon dried basil
1 teaspoon paprika
¼ teaspoon cayenne pepper
2 teaspoons salt
½ teaspoon ground black pepper
2 pounds large shrimp, not peeled

1 In a large skillet, melt the buttery spread over medium-high heat. Reduce the heat to medium-low and add lemon juice, Worcestershire sauce, garlic, onion powder, oregano, thyme, basil, paprika, cayenne pepper, salt, and black pepper. Stir and simmer for about 5 minutes.

2 Add shrimp and increase the heat to medium. Cook for 4–5 minutes, occasionally turning shrimp, until shrimp to turn pink. Cover the skillet and remove it from the heat. Let sit for 15 minutes, stirring every 5 minutes. Serve.

Spaghetti with White Clam Sauce

This white clam sauce is a southern Italian dish that can be easily made at home in 15 minutes. Its light base of olive oil, garlic, and white wine lets the flavor of the clams shine through.

1 (12-ounce) package gluten-free spaghetti

3 tablespoons olive oil

2 tablespoons jarred minced garlic

1 teaspoon dried thyme

¼ teaspoon crushed red pepper flakes

½ cup white wine

1 (15-ounce) can whole baby clams in juice

¼ teaspoon salt

¼ cup chopped fresh parsley

SERVES 4

Per Serving:

Calories	480
Fat	14g
Protein	12g
Sodium	810mg
Fiber	3g
Carbohydrates	72g
Sugar	0g

1 Cook pasta to al dente according to the package directions.

2 Add olive oil to a large skillet and heat over medium heat. Add garlic, thyme, and red pepper flakes and sauté for 1 minute. Add wine to the skillet and stir. Stir in clams and their juice. Add pasta to clam sauce. Toss and coat pasta in sauce and cook for 2–3 minutes. Remove from heat and season with salt and parsley and serve.

Curried Shrimp

The sweet coconut and warm curry offers a unique change of pace for a shrimp dish! Serve it alongside warm rice pilaf and a green vegetable.

2 tablespoons olive oil

½ large yellow onion, peeled and diced

2 tablespoons jarred minced garlic

2 tablespoons jarred minced ginger

1 (15-ounce) can unsweetened coconut milk

2 tablespoons curry powder

½ teaspoon ground cumin

⅛ teaspoon ground cinnamon

¼ cup lime juice

¼ teaspoon salt

⅛ teaspoon ground black pepper

1½ pounds raw shrimp, peeled and deveined

½ cup chopped fresh cilantro

SERVES 4

Per Serving:

Calories	250
Fat	12g
Protein	24g
Sodium	1,180mg
Fiber	1g
Carbohydrates	6g
Sugar	2g

1 In a large skillet, heat olive oil over medium-high heat. Add onions, garlic, and ginger to the skillet and sauté for 2–4 minutes. Add in milk, curry powder, cumin, cinnamon, lime juice, salt, and pepper and stir to combine. Bring to a boil, then reduce heat to medium-low and let simmer for 7–10 minutes.

2 Add in shrimp and let simmer for an additional 5–7 minutes until shrimp is cooked through. Top with cilantro.

Crispy Baked Fish Sticks

SERVES 4

Per Serving:

Calories	516
Fat	15g
Protein	26g
Sodium	760mg
Fiber	8g
Carbohydrates	65g
Sugar	2g

PANKO VERSUS BREAD CRUMBS

The biggest difference between panko and standard bread crumbs is that panko is made from bread without crusts. Panko is a type of flaky bread crumb that is commonly used in Asian cuisine. The panko bread is processed into large flakes, rather than crumbs, and then dried. It is ground into large flakes that give fried foods a light, crunchy coating.

This crispy, crunchy, and healthier version of traditional fish sticks will give your kids the flavor they like that is both gluten-free and dairy-free. Serve with Homemade Tartar Sauce (see recipe in Chapter 7) for dipping.

1 pound cod fillets, cut into 1" strips
2 teaspoons seasoned salt
1 cup gluten-free all-purpose flour with xanthan gum
2 large eggs
1 tablespoon Dijon mustard
1 cup gluten-free panko bread crumbs
1 cup gluten-free bread crumbs
½ teaspoon garlic powder
½ teaspoon onion powder

1 Preheat oven to 400°F and line a baking sheet with aluminum foil and spray with gluten-free nonstick cooking spray.

2 Season fish with seasoned salt. Add flour to a pie pan or shallow dish. In a second pie pan, whisk together eggs and mustard. In a third pie pan, combine panko, bread crumbs, garlic powder, and onion powder.

3 Press a fish stick in flour, making sure to cover all sides. Next dredge fish stick in the egg mixture. Then press fish stick in the bread-crumb mixture, patting to help coating adhere. Place coated fish stick on prepared baking sheet and repeat the process with remaining fish sticks. Spray fish with olive oil gluten-free nonstick cooking spray.

4 Bake for 6 minutes, then turn over fish sticks and spray with cooking spray again. Bake another 6–10 minutes until fish begins to flake easily with a fork.

CHAPTER 7

Sides, Sauces, and Dressings

Roasted Garlic Potatoes

SERVES 6

Per Serving:

Calories	250
Fat	10g
Protein	4g
Sodium	820mg
Fiber	4g
Carbohydrates	36g
Sugar	3g

This super simple side dish will perfectly complement just about any entrée. It's a classic, and it's gluten- and dairy-free naturally!

¼ cup olive oil
2 teaspoons salt
¼ teaspoon ground black pepper
2 tablespoons jarred minced garlic
3 pounds small red potatoes, cut in half

1 Preheat oven to 400°F. Line a baking sheet with aluminum foil and spray with gluten-free nonstick cooking spray.

2 Add olive oil, salt, pepper, and garlic in a large bowl and whisk together. Add potatoes and toss until potatoes are well coated.

3 Place potatoes on prepared sheet and spread out into one layer. Roast in the oven for 45 minutes to 1 hour until browned and crisp.

Easy Rice Pilaf

SERVES 4

Per Serving:

Calories	260
Fat	4g
Protein	8g
Sodium	410mg
Fiber	2g
Carbohydrates	49g
Sugar	2g

This recipe makes fluffy and flavorful rice every time. This dish is completely customizable; you can use your favorite frozen or fresh vegetables and even dried fruits and nuts.

2 teaspoons olive oil
½ cup peeled and chopped sweet onion
1 cup uncooked long-grain white rice
2 cups gluten-free chicken broth
2 teaspoons seasoned salt
⅛ teaspoon ground black pepper
1 cup frozen peas and carrots

1 Heat olive oil in a large skillet over medium heat. Add onions and cook for 3 minutes until translucent. Add rice and stir until rice is lightly toasted.

2 Stir in broth, salt, and pepper and bring to a boil. Reduce heat to a simmer, cover, and cook for 10 minutes.

3 Stir in peas and carrots, cover, and cook for an additional 10 minutes. Fluff with a fork and serve.

Baked Sweet Potato Fries

These light, crispy, and perfectly seasoned Baked Sweet Potato Fries are a nutrient-packed twist on fast-food fries. Not only are they scrumptious as a side with just about any entrée, but they are also a healthy choice! Sweet potatoes are packed with vitamin C, iron, potassium, vitamin B$_6$, and fiber.

1 pound sweet potatoes, peeled and cut into ¼" strips
2 tablespoons olive oil
2 tablespoons cornstarch
¼ teaspoon garlic powder
½ teaspoon paprika
¼ teaspoon ground black pepper
1 teaspoon salt

SERVES 4

Per Serving:

Calories	180
Fat	7g
Protein	2g
Sodium	645mg
Fiber	3g
Carbohydrates	26g
Sugar	5g

1 Add cut potatoes to a large bowl of water and soak for 30 minutes.

2 Preheat oven to 425°F. Line a large baking sheet with parchment paper and spray with gluten-free nonstick cooking spray.

3 Drain potatoes and blot dry with a paper towel. Add potatoes in a separate large bowl. Drizzle evenly with olive oil and toss until potatoes are evenly coated.

4 In a small bowl, whisk together cornstarch, garlic powder, paprika, and pepper until combined. Sprinkle the mixture evenly over potatoes and toss until they are evenly coated and cornstarch has soaked into oil.

5 Spread potatoes out in an even layer on prepared baking sheet, making sure not to overlap. Bake for 25 minutes. Then remove pan from oven and take the time to flip each fry with a spatula. Rearrange so that fries are evenly spaced and not overlapping again. Put back in the oven and bake for 20 minutes. Sprinkle with salt, then allow fries cool for 5 minutes. Serve warm.

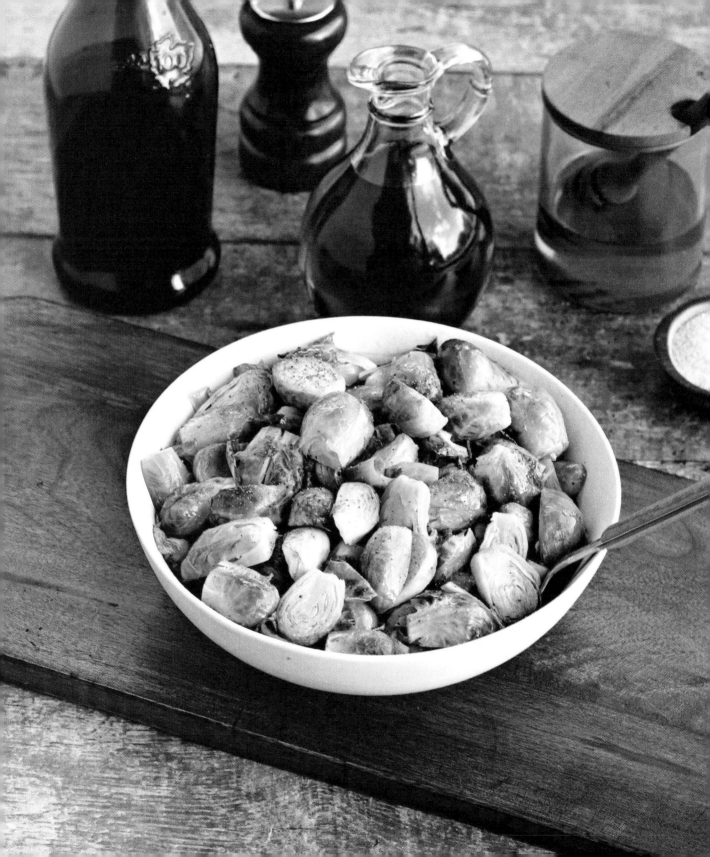

Balsamic-Roasted Brussels Sprouts

These flavor-packed Brussels sprouts are roasted in the oven. You can take them out just as they begin to brown, or leave them in longer until they are crisp and caramelized. Brussels sprouts are low in calories but high in fiber, vitamins, antioxidants, and minerals.

¼ cup olive oil
1 teaspoon salt
¼ teaspoon ground black pepper
1½ pounds Brussels sprouts, trimmed and cut in half through the core
1 tablespoon balsamic vinegar
2 tablespoons honey

1. Preheat oven to 400°F. Line a baking sheet with aluminum foil and spray with gluten-free nonstick cooking spray.

2. Add olive oil, salt, and pepper to a large bowl and stir to combine. Add Brussels sprouts to the bowl and toss to coat with the oil mixture.

3. Place Brussels sprouts on the baking sheet and roast for 20–30 minutes until tender and browned. Remove from the oven.

4. Add vinegar and honey to the large bowl and whisk to combine. Add the roasted sprouts to the bowl and toss to cover in the vinegar mixture. Serve warm.

SERVES 4

Per Serving:

Calories	180
Fat	14g
Protein	1g
Sodium	590mg
Fiber	1g
Carbohydrates	12g
Sugar	9g

Ratatouille

THE HEALTHY SIDE OF TOMATOES

Tomatoes are full of vitamin C, and they are also a powerful antioxidant. They can lower the risk of hypertension, coronary heart disease, and even stroke. Grow them in your garden for full-bodied, vine-ripened flavor!

This recipe will make heads turn as you walk it out from the kitchen to the dinner table thanks to the beautiful colors and fragrant aroma of the vegetables and herbs. Ratatouille is a very elegant dish that also tastes really good reheated the next day.

6 tablespoons olive oil, divided
1 large eggplant, cut into ⅓" cubes
1 teaspoon salt, divided
2 medium zucchini, cut into cubes
1 medium yellow onion, peeled and finely chopped
1 large red bell pepper, seeded and chopped
2 tablespoons jarred minced garlic
5 Roma tomatoes, chopped
1 tablespoon tomato paste
1 tablespoon dried thyme
3 tablespoons dried basil
1 teaspoon granulated sugar

1. In a large skillet, heat 3 tablespoons olive oil over medium heat. Add eggplant and sprinkle with ¼ teaspoon salt. Cook for 10–12 minutes, stirring frequently, until soft and starting to brown. Transfer to a plate.

2. Add 1 more tablespoon olive oil to the skillet and add the zucchini. Cook for 3–4 minutes, stirring frequently, until soft. Season with ¼ teaspoon salt and transfer to a plate.

3. Add remaining 2 tablespoons olive oil to the skillet and add onions, bell peppers, and garlic. Cook for 5 minutes, stirring frequently. Add tomatoes and their juices, tomato paste, thyme, basil, sugar, and remaining ½ teaspoon salt. Cook for 10 minutes, stirring occasionally, until tomatoes are broken down into a sauce.

4. Add eggplant back to the skillet; bring to a gentle boil, then reduce the heat to low and simmer uncovered for about 10 minutes until eggplant is soft. Add zucchini back and cook for 1–2 minutes. Serve warm or chilled.

Creamy Scalloped Potatoes

You don't have to skip scalloped potatoes when you avoid gluten and dairy! This rich recipe will go quickly at any get-together.

6 large russet potatoes, peeled and thinly sliced
6 tablespoons dairy-free buttery spread
4 tablespoons gluten-free flour with xanthan gum
1 tablespoon onion powder
1 tablespoon garlic powder
1 cup gluten-free chicken broth
2 cups unsweetened almond milk
2 teaspoons salt
¼ teaspoon ground black pepper
1 teaspoon tarragon

1 Preheat oven to 425°F. Lightly grease a 9" × 13" baking pan with gluten-free nonstick cooking spray. Place potato slices in a large bowl of cold water.

2 Melt buttery spread in a medium skillet over medium heat. Whisk in flour. Add onion powder and garlic powder. Pour in broth and whisk until combined. Add in milk, salt, pepper, and tarragon and whisk until combined. Cook for 2 minutes until sauce begins to simmer and thicken. Remove from heat.

3 Drain potato slices. Spread one-third of potato slices into the bottom of prepared baking dish. Top evenly with one-third of cream sauce. Add another layer of potatoes and sauce, and repeat once more for a total of three layers.

4 Bake for 45 minutes until potatoes are cooked through. The sauce should be bubbly around the edges. For a crisp topping, change the oven setting to broil for 5 minutes before removing the dish.

SERVES 6

Per Serving:

Calories	175
Fat	4g
Protein	4g
Sodium	960mg
Fiber	2g
Carbohydrates	31g
Sugar	1g

Potato Pancakes

SERVES 6

Per Serving:

Calories	195
Fat	12g
Protein	3g
Sodium	380mg
Fiber	1g
Carbohydrates	18g
Sugar	1g

If you have leftover mashed potatoes, use them in these glorious pancakes. There are dozens of ways to adapt this classic recipe. For example, adding vegetables like diced sweet onion, leeks, or scallions will amplify the flavor.

1 large egg
¼ cup gluten-free all-purpose flour with xanthan gum
2 teaspoons onion powder
¼ teaspoon salt
⅛ teaspoon ground black pepper
2 cups cooked mashed potatoes
3 tablespoons vegetable oil

1 In a large bowl, whisk together egg, flour, and seasonings. Add the mashed potatoes and stir to combine.

2 Heat oil in a large skillet over medium-high heat. Use an ice cream scoop to drop batter on the skillet. Cook for 5–6 minutes until pancakes start to turn golden brown. Turn pancakes over and press patties down, cooking for another 5–6 minutes, until golden brown.

Honey-Glazed Carrots

SERVES 4

Per Serving:

Calories	85
Fat	2g
Protein	1g
Sodium	290mg
Fiber	3g
Carbohydrates	18g
Sugar	13g

These sweet carrots are a tasty way to add vegetables to your plate. The honey and dill complement each other to create a sauce that's flavorful and popular.

1 pound baby carrots
2 tablespoons dairy-free buttery spread
2 tablespoons honey
1 tablespoon lemon juice
¼ teaspoon salt
2 teaspoons dried dill

1 In a medium saucepan, bring water to a boil over medium-high heat. Add carrots and cook 10–15 minutes until tender. Drain carrots and add back to the pan with buttery spread, honey, and lemon juice and stir to combine ingredients.

2 Cook for 5 minutes until glaze coats carrots. Season with salt and dill.

Southwestern Black Bean and Corn Salad

The deep and rich flavors of the Southwest are captured in this Southwestern Black Bean and Corn Salad. If you have leftover corn on the cob, remove the corn from the cob and use it in this dish. Serve with gluten-free tortilla chips or just eat it straight!

1 tablespoon olive oil
½ cup lime juice
¼ teaspoon gluten-free and dairy-free hot sauce
½ teaspoon salt
1 (15-ounce) can black beans, rinsed and drained
1 (15-ounce) can corn, drained
1 large tomato, chopped
⅓ cup peeled and chopped red onion
1 cup chopped fresh cilantro

SERVES 6	
Per Serving:	
Calories	142
Fat	3g
Protein	5g
Sodium	400mg
Fiber	3g
Carbohydrates	23g
Sugar	4g

1   Whisk together olive oil, lime juice, hot sauce, and salt in a small bowl.

2   In a large bowl, combine beans, corn, tomatoes, onions, and cilantro. Pour lime dressing over salad ingredients to coat. Cover and refrigerate for 30 minutes before serving.

Cheesy Green Bean Casserole

This is a new twist on the classic green bean casserole. It combines French-style green beans, a creamy yet dairy-free cheese sauce, and a crunchy potato stick topping. Store leftovers for 3 days in an airtight container in the refrigerator and eat for lunch!

2 (14-ounce) cans French-style green beans, drained
1 teaspoon onion powder
1 cup gluten-free and dairy-free Cream of Mushroom Soup (see recipe in Chapter 9)
1½ cups shredded dairy-free Cheddar cheese
1 cup crushed gluten-free potato sticks

SERVES 8	
Per Serving:	
Calories	120
Fat	6g
Protein	2g
Sodium	590mg
Fiber	2g
Carbohydrates	13g
Sugar	2g

1   Preheat oven to 350°F. Spray a 2-quart casserole dish with gluten-free nonstick cooking spray.

2   Add beans to prepared dish. Sprinkle onion powder over beans. Pour soup over the bean mixture and stir to combine. Add cheese and stir to combine.

3   Bake on the middle rack for 15 minutes. Add potato sticks and bake for an additional 15–25 minutes or until sides are bubbly and potato sticks are golden brown.

Italian Roasted Vegetables

SERVES 4

Per Serving:

Calories	85
Fat	0g
Protein	4g
Sodium	600mg
Fiber	3g
Carbohydrates	21g
Sugar	4g

This recipe is a fantastic combination of fresh and healthy vegetables and the rich Italian flavor of olive oil and basil. These vegetables are easily found no matter what season it is.

1 large zucchini, sliced
1 large yellow squash, sliced
2 large russet potatoes, diced
1 cup halved grape tomatoes
2 tablespoons olive oil
1 teaspoon salt
2 tablespoons dried basil

1 Preheat oven to 425°F. Line a baking sheet with aluminum foil and spray with gluten-free nonstick cooking spray.

2 In a large bowl, toss all vegetables together with olive oil, salt, and basil.

3 Place vegetables on prepared baking sheet. Bake for 35–40 minutes.

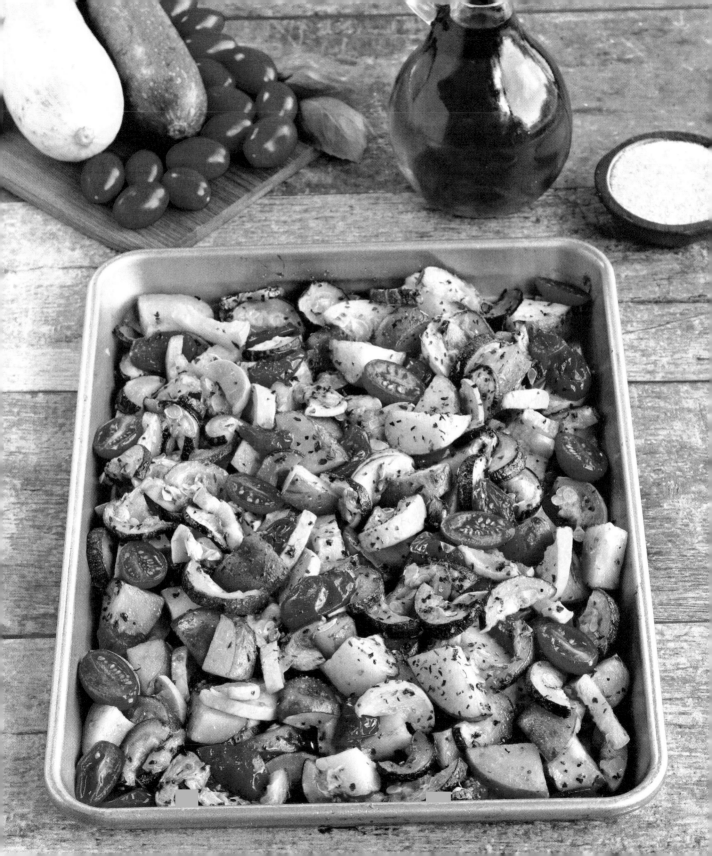

Roasted Butternut Squash

SERVES 4

Per Serving:

Calories	160
Fat	11g
Protein	1g
Sodium	300mg
Fiber	5g
Carbohydrates	16g
Sugar	3g

Roasted squash is a tender, easy way to eat squash. Eat it alongside Pecan-Crusted Honey Mustard Salmon (see recipe in Chapter 6).

3 tablespoons olive oil
½ teaspoon salt
⅛ teaspoon ground black pepper
1 large butternut squash, peeled, seeded, and cut into 1" cubes

1 Preheat oven to 400°F. Line a baking sheet with aluminum foil and spray with gluten-free nonstick cooking spray.

2 Add olive oil, salt, and pepper to a large bowl and stir to combine. Add squash and toss.

3 Place squash on prepared sheet and arrange squash in one layer. Bake for 25–30 minutes until the squash is tender and starting to brown on the edges.

Sautéed Garlic Green Beans

SERVES 4

Per Serving:

Calories	110
Fat	8g
Protein	2g
Sodium	560mg
Fiber	3g
Carbohydrates	8g
Sugar	4g

Try this simple recipe as a great side dish for chicken, beef, or seafood that can be whipped up in under 10 minutes. Resist the urge to overcook the green beans. Green beans are best when cooked to a lightly crunchy texture and with a bright green color. Overcooked green beans will be an olive-green color, and their texture will be more mushy. Overcooking can also cause nutrient loss.

1 pound green beans, trimmed
1 teaspoon salt, divided
2 tablespoons olive oil
1 tablespoon jarred minced garlic

1 Bring a large pot of water to a boil over medium-high heat. Add beans and ½ teaspoon salt and cook for 4 minutes. Drain beans in a colander.

2 Heat olive oil in a large skillet over medium-high heat. Add garlic and sauté for 30 seconds until fragrant. Add green beans and toss to coat with the oil mixture. Sauté beans for 2–4 minutes until they get a little caramelization. Add remaining salt and serve warm.

Zucchini Noodles

A perfectly gluten-free and dairy-free innovation for traditional pasta are zucchini noodles, aka zoodles. Zucchini Noodles are a great substitute for pasta dishes—they are nutritious and hold sauces well. There are several different spiraling machines on the market, from inexpensive handheld versions to large tabletop models.

4 medium zucchini, spiralized
½ teaspoon salt
1 tablespoon olive oil

1. Place zoodles in a colander, toss them with salt, and let sit for 20 minutes. Squeeze out excess water from zoodles with a paper towel.

2. Add olive oil to a large skillet and heat over medium-high heat. Add zucchini to the skillet and sauté for 3–5 minutes.

SERVES 4

Per Serving:

Calories	65
Fat	4g
Protein	2g
Sodium	310mg
Fiber	2g
Carbohydrates	6g
Sugar	5g

Easy Oven-Roasted Corn on the Cob

This corn on the cob is an easy way to make dinner extra special. Boiling corn might be the traditional method, but roasting cooks in a complex, sweet flavor and gives you the most tender corn!

6 ears of corn, in husks
½ teaspoon salt
¼ cup dairy-free buttery spread, melted

1. Preheat oven to 375°F.

2. Place ears of corn with the husks still on them on an ungreased baking sheet. Bake for 40 minutes.

3. Remove from the oven and allow to cool for several minutes. Peel back corn husks and snap the ends off. Serve with salt and buttery spread.

SERVES 6

Per Serving:

Calories	95
Fat	3g
Protein	3g
Sodium	280mg
Fiber	2g
Carbohydrates	17g
Sugar	3g

Southern-Style Sweet Potato Casserole

SERVES 10

Per Serving:

Calories	130
Fat	3g
Protein	3g
Sodium	95mg
Fiber	1g
Carbohydrates	25g
Sugar	14g

This traditional sweet potato casserole topped with roasted marshmallows is a crowd-pleaser at every holiday meal. It reheats well the next day, so save those leftovers.

3 cups cooked sweet potatoes
⅓ cup dairy-free buttery spread, melted
1 cup granulated sugar
⅛ teaspoon ground ginger
2 teaspoons ground cinnamon
¼ teaspoon ground nutmeg
2 large eggs
1 teaspoon pure vanilla extract
¼ cup unsweetened almond milk
3 cups gluten-free mini marshmallows

1 Preheat oven to 350°F and spray a 2-quart casserole dish with gluten-free nonstick cooking spray.

2 In a large bowl, beat mashed sweet potatoes, buttery spread, sugar, ginger, cinnamon, nutmeg, eggs, vanilla, and milk with an electric mixer until smooth. Pour the sweet potato mixture into prepared dish.

3 Bake for 30 minutes. Remove from the oven and top with mini marshmallows and bake for an additional 5–10 minutes. Watch the marshmallows carefully because all ovens are different—be sure they do not burn.

Bacon and Tomato Macaroni Salad

SERVES 12

Per Serving:

Calories	290
Fat	16g
Protein	4g
Sodium	200mg
Fiber	1g
Carbohydrates	33g
Sugar	11g

This gluten-free macaroni salad is perfect for potlucks, backyard barbecues, and everyday meals! Get-togethers and potlucks can be challenging for those on a specific diet, so bring dishes you know you can eat for peace of mind.

1 (12-ounce) box gluten-free elbow macaroni noodles, cooked
1 cup mayonnaise
2 tablespoons white vinegar
1 tablespoon yellow mustard
⅔ cup sugar
1½ teaspoons salt
½ teaspoon ground black pepper
1 teaspoon onion powder
1 cup chopped cooked gluten-free bacon
1 cup quartered grape tomatoes

1 Cook macaroni according to the package directions for al dente. After draining the pasta, rinse pasta with cold water. Add pasta to a large bowl.

2 In a small bowl, add mayonnaise, vinegar, mustard, sugar, salt, pepper, and onion powder and stir until fully combined. Add to pasta and stir until fully coated.

3 Add bacon and tomatoes to pasta and stir until fully combined. Cover and refrigerate for 30 minutes before serving.

Loaded Bacon Ranch Potato Salad

This recipe transfers all of your favorite flavors from a loaded baked potato into a potato salad format. It's a summer classic that everyone will love!

4 cups diced russet potatoes

1 tablespoon dried dill

1½ teaspoons garlic powder

1½ teaspoons onion powder

2 teaspoons dried parsley

1½ teaspoons salt

½ teaspoon ground black pepper

1 tablespoon granulated sugar

1 cup mayonnaise

1¼ cups chopped cooked gluten-free bacon, divided

½ cup sliced green onion, divided

2 large hard-boiled eggs, chopped

SERVES 8

Per Serving:

Calories	310
Fat	25g
Protein	7g
Sodium	790mg
Fiber	1g
Carbohydrates	15g
Sugar	3g

1 Add potatoes to a large pot and cover with water. Cook over high heat and bring to a boil. Once boiling, reduce the heat to medium and boil for 12–15 minutes or until potatoes are tender. Check with a fork to see if potatoes are cooked to your liking.

2 Drain potatoes and rinse with cold water. Add potatoes to a large bowl and place in the refrigerator to cool while you are making the dressing.

3 In a small bowl, add all seasonings and sugar together and stir to combine. Add mayonnaise and mix until fully combined.

4 Add dressing to chilled potatoes. Carefully stir to fully cover potatoes with dressing.

5 Add 1 cup bacon, ¼ cup green onions, and eggs to potato salad. Stir gently. Cover and chill for 2 hours. Sprinkle remaining ¼ cup of the bacon and remaining ¼ cup green onions on top of potato salad before serving.

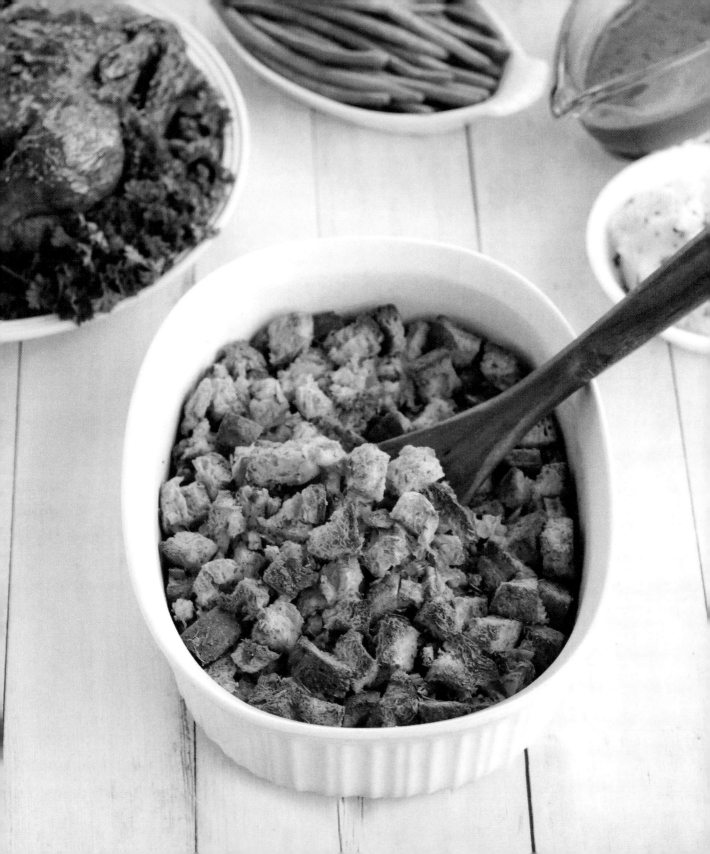

Savory Stuffing

Make the holidays easy and delicious for your gluten-free and dairy-free family members with this savory gluten-free stuffing. It is perfect for Thanksgiving or any holiday meal!

1 tablespoon olive oil

1 cup diced celery

½ teaspoon jarred minced garlic

1 teaspoon salt

1 tablespoon onion powder

1 tablespoon dried thyme

1 tablespoon dried sage

1 teaspoon dried rosemary

1 loaf gluten-free and dairy-free sandwich bread, cut into 1" cubes

2 large eggs, whisked

2 cups gluten-free chicken broth

SERVES 8

Per Serving:

Calories	170
Fat	7g
Protein	6g
Sodium	575mg
Fiber	1g
Carbohydrates	20g
Sugar	3g

1 Preheat oven to 350°F and spray a 2½-quart casserole dish with gluten-free nonstick cooking spray.

2 Add olive oil, celery, and jarred minced garlic to a small skillet and sauté over medium-high heat until soft, about 8–10 minutes.

3 Add spices to a small bowl and stir to combine.

4 Add bread pieces to a large bowl. Pour seasoning blend and whisked eggs over bread and stir. Add the celery mixture and stir. Add chicken broth and gently mix until bread is evenly moistened.

5 Pour the stuffing mixture into prepared dish.

6 Bake for 40–50 minutes until the top of stuffing is golden brown and lightly crisp.

Easy Homemade Gravy

SERVES 6

Per Serving:

Calories	240
Fat	10g
Protein	8g
Sodium	790mg
Fiber	2g
Carbohydrates	29g
Sugar	4g

No holiday meal is complete without gravy, but most store-bought options have gluten-based or dairy ingredients. This Easy Homemade Gravy is creamy, rich, and bursting with meaty flavor—and safe for you to eat!

2 cups gluten-free chicken broth
3 tablespoons water
3 tablespoons cornstarch
¼ teaspoon salt
⅛ teaspoon pepper

1 Add broth to a small saucepan over medium heat. Whisk water and cornstarch in a small bowl until smooth and add to broth, stirring constantly with a whisk, bringing to a boil.

2 Boil for 1 minute and season with salt and pepper. Serve warm.

Creamy Dill Sauce

SERVES 8

Per Serving:

Calories	98
Fat	11g
Protein	0g
Sodium	155mg
Fiber	0g
Carbohydrates	0g
Sugar	0g

If you are searching for the perfect topper for your salmon or other protein, this rich and creamy sauce is just the trick to make it a flawless dish. It is simple to make and uses ingredients you probably already have on hand.

½ cup mayonnaise
1 tablespoon dried dill
1 teaspoon horseradish sauce
1 teaspoon lemon juice
¼ teaspoon garlic salt

Combine all ingredients in a small bowl. Cover and chill in the refrigerator for 30 minutes before serving. Store in an airtight container in the refrigerator for up to 1 week.

Homemade Buttermilk Ranch Dressing

Finding a rich and creamy gluten-free and dairy-free salad dressing in a store or restaurant can be a challenge. This Homemade Buttermilk Ranch Dressing will quickly become a mainstay in your refrigerator. It will stay fresh in an airtight container in the refrigerator for up to 1 week.

1 cup unsweetened almond milk
1 tablespoon white vinegar
½ cup mayonnaise
1 tablespoon dried dill
1½ teaspoons garlic powder

1½ teaspoons onion powder
2 teaspoons dried parsley
1½ teaspoons salt
½ teaspoon ground black pepper
1 tablespoon granulated sugar

SERVES 12

Per Serving:

Calories	70
Fat	7g
Protein	0g
Sodium	365mg
Fiber	0g
Carbohydrates	1g
Sugar	1g

1 Add milk and vinegar to a small bowl and place in the refrigerator for 5–10 minutes to make buttermilk.

2 In a separate small bowl, add mayonnaise, seasonings, and sugar and whisk together. Pour in buttermilk and whisk. Cover and refrigerate for 30 minutes before stirring again and serving.

Homemade Honey Mustard Dressing

This recipe for Homemade Honey Mustard Dressing has all the flavors of your favorite store-bought dressing in a gluten- and dairy-free format. It also makes a perfect dipping sauce for chicken nuggets. It will stay fresh in an airtight container for up to 1 week in the refrigerator.

½ cup mayonnaise
2 tablespoons Dijon mustard
2 tablespoons honey
4 teaspoons lemon juice

SERVES 8

Per Serving:

Calories	115
Fat	10g
Protein	0g
Sodium	180mg
Fiber	0g
Carbohydrates	5g
Sugar	4g

In a small bowl, whisk together all ingredients. Cover and refrigerate for 30 minutes before serving. Stir well before serving.

Balsamic Vinaigrette Salad Dressing

SERVES 24

Per Serving:

Calories	70
Fat	7g
Protein	0g
Sodium	365mg
Fiber	0g
Carbohydrates	1g
Sugar	1g

This is the perfect Balsamic Vinaigrette Salad Dressing that is gluten-free and dairy-free and also safe for paleo and AIP diets. It will stay fresh in the refrigerator in an airtight container for up to 1 week.

½ teaspoon dried basil
½ teaspoon garlic powder
½ teaspoon onion powder
½ teaspoon dried oregano
1 teaspoon salt
2 tablespoons honey

2 tablespoons water
⅓ cup vinegar blend (made up of half apple cider vinegar, and half balsamic vinegar)
⅔ cup olive oil

1. In a small bowl, mix seasonings together.
2. Add honey, water, vinegar blend, and olive oil to dry ingredients and whisk until all ingredients are fully combined.
3. Cover and refrigerate for 30 minutes before serving. Stir well before serving.

Homemade Tartar Sauce

SERVES 8

Per Serving:

Calories	195
Fat	21g
Protein	0g
Sodium	320mg
Fiber	0g
Carbohydrates	1g
Sugar	1g

You can stop buying tartar sauce from the supermarket because this homemade version of the traditional will be everyone's choice from now on! And you know the ingredients fit your lifestyle. It will stay fresh in an airtight container in the refrigerator for up to 1 week.

1 cup mayonnaise
1 cup finely chopped dill pickles
2 tablespoons peeled and finely chopped sweet onion
1 tablespoon dried dill
1 tablespoon lemon juice
1 teaspoon granulated sugar
⅛ teaspoon freshly ground black pepper

In a small bowl, whisk together all ingredients. Cover and refrigerate for 30 minutes before serving. Stir before serving.

CHAPTER 8

Breads

Bread Machine Bread

SERVES 12

Per Serving:

Calories	170
Fat	2g
Protein	3g
Sodium	280mg
Fiber	0g
Carbohydrates	35g
Sugar	11g

GLUTEN-FREE SETTINGS ON BREAD MACHINES

Gluten-free flour does not bake the same as regular wheat flour. Bread machine settings for traditional wheat bread won't work for gluten-free dough. If you have a bread machine without a gluten-free setting, you will need to manually adjust the settings of your bread machine to a 20-minute mix cycle, a 1-hour rise cycle, and a 1-hour bake cycle. Also, do not allow the machine to do a punch down or second rise.

Looking for that perfect loaf of homemade gluten-free and dairy-free bread? Try this easy bread machine recipe that will satisfy cravings for soft and tasty bread.

1½ cups unsweetened almond milk, warm
¼ cup dairy-free buttery spread, melted
½ cup honey
2 large eggs, room temperature and whisked
1 teaspoon apple cider vinegar
3 cups gluten-free all-purpose flour with xanthan gum
1 teaspoon salt
1¾ teaspoons instant yeast

1   Grease a bread pan with gluten-free nonstick cooking spray.

2   Pour warm milk, buttery spread, honey, eggs, and vinegar into the bread pan.

3   Add flour and salt to the bread pan. Make a small hole with your finger in the flour. Pour yeast into the hole.

4   Start the bread machine and set to the gluten-free setting. As bread machine is mixing, you may need to go in and scrape the sides down into the batter with a spatula.

5   Once the bread machine has finished the baking cycle, allow bread to cool 5–10 minutes before removing from the pan and slicing. Store in an airtight container at room temperature for up to 3 days.

Easy One-Bowl Banana Bread

This is the only gluten-free banana bread recipe you'll ever need—it's a one-bowl wonder with great banana flavor and texture! Plus, you don't need a mixer for this super moist banana bread.

2 large ripe bananas, peeled
1 teaspoon baking soda
⅓ cup dairy-free buttery spread, melted
⅛ teaspoon salt
¾ cup granulated sugar

2 large eggs, whisked
1 teaspoon pure vanilla extract
1½ cups gluten-free all-purpose flour with xanthan gum

1 Preheat oven to 350°F. Spray a 4" × 8" loaf pan with gluten-free non-stick cooking spray.

2 In a large bowl, mash bananas until smooth, add baking soda, and stir to combine. Add buttery spread. Stir in salt, sugar, eggs, and vanilla extract. Mix in flour. Pour batter into prepared loaf pan.

3 Bake on the center rack for 50 minutes to 1 hour or until a toothpick inserted in the center comes out clean. Allow bread to cool for 3–5 minutes before removing from the pan for further cooling and slicing.

SERVES 8	
Per Serving:	
Calories	190
Fat	3g
Protein	3g
Sodium	260mg
Fiber	1g
Carbohydrates	37g
Sugar	19g

Double Chocolate Banana Bread

The comforting and rich taste of this chocolate and banana bread is a favorite for people of all ages. It's a perfect way to use up bananas that are past their prime.

2 ripe large bananas, peeled and mashed
1 teaspoon baking soda
⅓ cup dairy-free buttery spread, melted
¾ cup sugar
¼ cup cocoa powder
⅛ teaspoon salt

2 large eggs, whisked
1 teaspoon pure vanilla extract
1½ cups gluten-free all-purpose flour with xanthan gum
½ cup gluten-free and dairy-free mini chocolate chips

1 Preheat oven to 350°F. Spray a 4" × 8" loaf pan with gluten-free non-stick cooking spray.

2 In a large bowl, combine bananas and baking soda. Stir in buttery spread, sugar, cocoa powder, salt, eggs, and vanilla. Mix in flour. Stir in chocolate chips. Pour batter into prepared loaf pan.

3 Bake on the center rack for 50 minutes to 1 hour or until a toothpick inserted in the center comes out clean. Allow bread to cool for 3–5 minutes before removing from the pan and slicing. Store leftovers in an airtight container at room temperature for up to 3 days.

SERVES 8	
Per Serving:	
Calories	275
Fat	10g
Protein	4g
Sodium	300mg
Fiber	2g
Carbohydrates	41g
Sugar	19g

Soft Homemade Dinner Rolls

MAKES 18 ROLLS

**Per Serving
(Serving Size: 2 rolls):**

Calories	115
Fat	2g
Protein	2g
Sodium	195mg
Fiber	0g
Carbohydrates	23g
Sugar	7g

WARM THEM UP!

Recipes often call for room-temperature eggs because room-temperature ingredients mix together better than cold ingredients. Add very warm, but not hot, water into a bowl. Place your cold eggs into the water gently for 5–7 minutes.

These easy homemade yeast dinner rolls will satisfy your cravings for soft and tasty bread. These rolls are made with instant quick-rise yeast, so you don't have to proof your yeast. Using instant quick-rise yeast also cuts the dough's rising time in half!

3 cups gluten-free all-purpose flour with xanthan gum
1 teaspoon salt
1¾ teaspoons instant yeast
1¼ cups unsweetened almond milk, warmed to 110°F–115°F
¼ cup dairy-free buttery spread, softened
2 large eggs, room temperature
1 teaspoon apple cider vinegar
½ cup honey
2 tablespoons dairy-free buttery spread, melted

1 Preheat oven to 200°F. Once it gets to 100°F, turn off oven. Spray two 9" metal cake pans with gluten-free nonstick cooking spray.

2 In a large bowl, add flour and salt. Make a small hole in the center and pour yeast into the hole.

3 Check the temperature of warm milk with a thermometer. (If your milk is too hot it will kill the yeast.) Pour milk over yeast.

4 Add softened buttery spread, eggs, vinegar, and honey to the flour mixture and mix for 2–3 minutes until fully combined. The dough will be sticky.

5 Using a greased ice cream scoop, scoop dough balls and place into prepared pans. Take a small spatula and smooth out the tops of dough. There will be eight dough balls around each pan and one dough ball in the center. Cover the pans with a kitchen towel and allow to rise in the warm oven for 1 hour. Take the pans out and keep covered while preheating the oven.

6 Preheat oven to 400°F. Bake rolls on the middle rack for 14–16 minutes until light golden brown. The temperature of the rolls should measure 200°F internally. Melt 2 tablespoons buttery spread in a small microwave-safe bowl and brush the tops of rolls before serving warm.

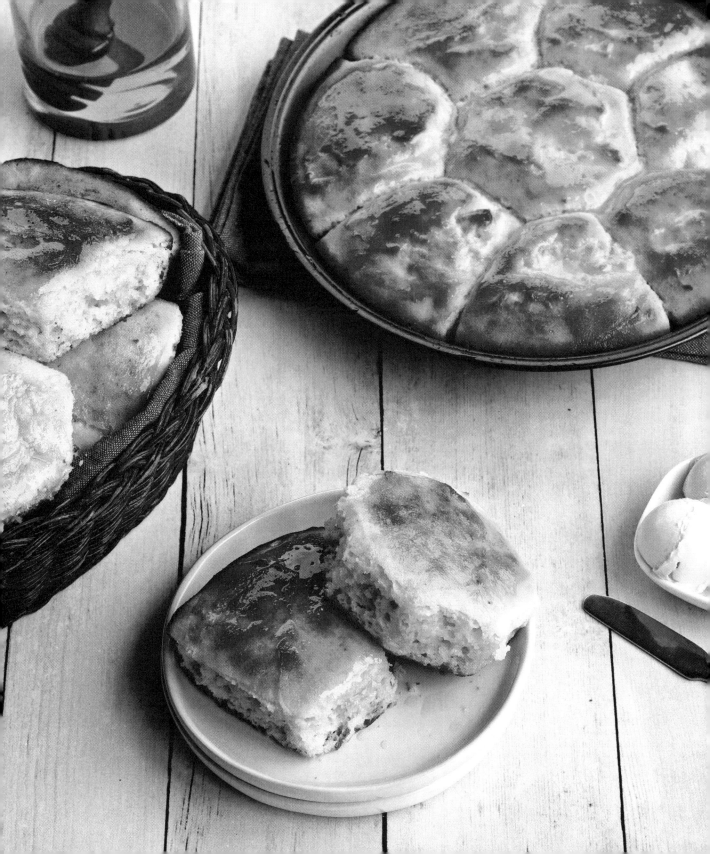

Easy Thick-Crust Pizza Dough

COOKING THE PIZZA

To cook your pizza, place parchment paper on a pizza pan or baking sheet. Bake for 15 minutes. Remove the pizza crust from the oven and top with your favorite toppings. Bake for another 5 minutes until the crust is golden brown. Allow the pizza to cool for 3–5 minutes before slicing.

Make your own Easy Thick-Crust Pizza Dough with only a few simple ingredients. This thick and chewy pizza crust is ready for your favorite gluten- and dairy-free toppings!

2½ cups plus 2 tablespoons gluten-free all-purpose flour with xanthan gum, divided
1 packet (2¼ teaspoons) instant yeast
1 tablespoon gluten-free baking powder
1 teaspoon salt
1 tablespoon honey
1½ cups warm water (110°F–115°F)
½ cup olive oil
1 teaspoon apple cider vinegar

1. Preheat oven to 200°F. Once it gets to 100°F, turn off oven.
2. In a large bowl, combine 2½ cups flour, yeast, baking powder, and salt.
3. In a small bowl, add honey and warm water and stir until honey is dissolved.
4. Pour the honey mixture into the flour mixture and mix with your mixer with a dough hook or paddle attachment on low.
5. Pour olive oil and vinegar into the dough mixture and mix on medium speed for 3 minutes. The dough will be very sticky.
6. Place dough in a large ovenproof bowl sprayed with gluten-free non-stick cooking spray. Cover with plastic wrap and then with a kitchen towel and place in warm oven for 30 minutes to rise.
7. Remove dough from the oven and preheat oven to 425°F.
8. Pour remaining 2 tablespoons flour onto a sheet of parchment paper and spread into a large 15" circle.
9. Turn the bowl over on top of floured parchment paper. Gently pat dough into a circle in an outward motion. Work from the middle and push to spread the dough out to the edge to make a 15" circle. Use your fingertips to press down into the dough to form the crust edge. Use your hands to finish shaping and rounding the edges.
10. Place the parchment paper on a pizza pan or baking sheet. Bake for 15 minutes. Remove the pizza crust from the oven and top with your favorite toppings. Bake for another 5 minutes, until the crust is golden brown. Allow the pizza to cool for 2–3 minutes before slicing.

Chocolate Chip Quick Bread

This soft, chocolaty quick bread will take only a few minutes to prepare, but it will make your guests think it took all day! Carefully cut your loaf in 2"-thick slices for a delicious take-along breakfast or snack all week!

⅓ cup dairy-free buttery spread, melted

2 large eggs, whisked

1 tablespoon pure vanilla extract

1½ cups gluten-free all-purpose flour with xanthan gum

½ cup sugar

1 teaspoon baking soda

½ teaspoon gluten-free baking powder

¼ teaspoon salt

1 cup unsweetened almond milk

1 cup gluten-free and dairy-free chocolate chips

1 Preheat oven to 350°F. Spray a 4" × 8" loaf pan with gluten-free non-stick cooking spray.

2 In a large bowl, add buttery spread, eggs, and vanilla and stir to combine. Add flour, sugar, baking soda, baking powder, and salt and mix until fully combined. Add milk and mix until smooth. Stir in chocolate chips.

3 Pour batter into a prepared loaf pan. Bake on the center rack for 50 minutes to 1 hour or until a toothpick inserted in the center comes out clean. Allow bread to cool for 3–5 minutes before removing from the pan and slicing. Store leftovers in an airtight container at room temperature for up to 3 days.

SERVES 8

Per Serving:

Calories	170
Fat	4g
Protein	3g
Sodium	355mg
Fiber	0g
Carbohydrates	30g
Sugar	13g

MILKING THE CASHEW

You can also use cashew milk in this recipe. Making cashew milk is not as complicated as it sounds. The preferred method is to soak 1 cup of cashews overnight, then rinse and drain them thoroughly. The next step is to take the cashews and add 4 cups of water and place into a powerful blender for a minute or two. Add your choice of sweetener to the blend and refrigerate. It's that easy!

Southern Sweet Corn Bread

SERVES 12

Per Serving:

Calories	112
Fat	3g
Protein	2g
Sodium	360mg
Fiber	0g
Carbohydrates	19g
Sugar	10g

THE BENEFITS OF HONEY

Raw honey is considered the best quality and is full of flavonoids that are scientifically proven to fight many diseases. High-quality honey is rich in antioxidants. Raw honey also contains bee pollen, which provides natural allergy relief and boosts immunity.

Welcome everyone to your table with fresh, soft corn bread! It goes perfectly with beef stew or chili or all by itself smothered with dairy-free buttery spread and strawberry preserves.

1½ cups unsweetened almond milk
1½ tablespoons white vinegar
1½ cups gluten-free cornmeal
1 cup gluten-free all-purpose flour with xanthan gum
½ cup sugar
½ teaspoon baking soda
2 teaspoons gluten-free baking powder
1 teaspoon salt
½ cup dairy-free buttery spread, melted
1 tablespoon honey
2 large eggs, whisked

1 Preheat oven to 400°F. Spray the bottom and sides of an 8" square pan or 8" cast-iron pan with gluten-free nonstick cooking spray.

2 In a small bowl, add milk and vinegar together and allow to sit for 2 minutes to make buttermilk.

3 In a large bowl, mix together cornmeal, flour, sugar, baking soda, baking powder, and salt.

4 Stir in buttery spread, honey, eggs, and the milk mixture and mix until fully combined.

5 Pour batter into prepared pan and smooth top of batter. Bake 20–25 minutes or until golden brown and a toothpick inserted in the center comes out clean. Cool for 5 minutes before cutting. Serve warm.

Apple Cinnamon Quick Bread

This soft and sweet Apple Cinnamon Quick Bread is an excellent pick at any time of the year. If you've just been apple picking, you can make your own applesauce to use.

1½ cups applesauce

⅓ cup dairy-free buttery spread, melted

½ cup sugar

2 large eggs, whisked

1 teaspoon pure vanilla extract

1½ cups gluten-free all-purpose flour with xanthan gum

1 teaspoon baking soda

½ teaspoon gluten-free baking powder

1 tablespoon ground cinnamon

⅛ teaspoon salt

1 cup unsweetened almond milk

1 Preheat oven to 350°F. Spray a 4" × 8" loaf pan with gluten-free non-stick cooking spray.

2 Add applesauce to a large bowl. Stir in buttery spread, sugar, eggs, and vanilla extract. Mix in flour, baking soda, baking powder, cinnamon, and salt and mix until all ingredients are fully combined. Add milk and mix until smooth. Pour batter into prepared loaf pan.

3 Bake on the center rack for 50 minutes to 1 hour or until a toothpick inserted in the center comes out clean. Allow the bread to cool for 3–5 minutes before removing from the pan and slicing. Store leftovers in an airtight container at room temperature for up to 3 days.

SERVES 8

Per Serving:

Calories	200
Fat	4g
Protein	3g
Sodium	320mg
Fiber	1g
Carbohydrates	39g
Sugar	20g

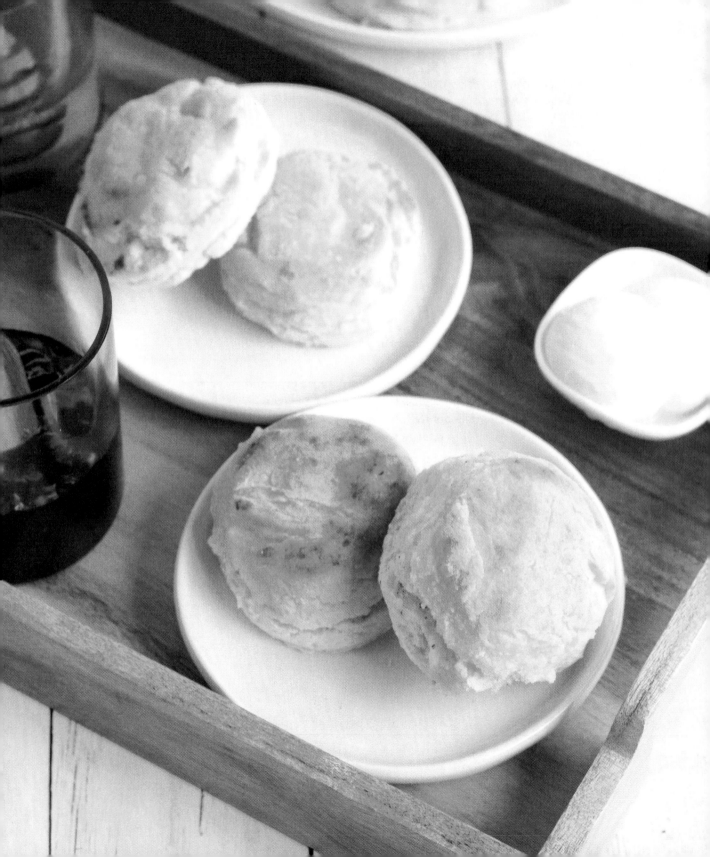

Southern Buttermilk Biscuits

Southern Buttermilk Biscuits hold an honored place at your table, no matter which meal is being served. These tender and flaky biscuits can be eaten at breakfast, lunch, and dinner.

8 tablespoons dairy-free buttery spread, divided

1 cup unsweetened almond milk

1 tablespoon white vinegar

2 cups plus 2 tablespoons gluten-free all-purpose flour with xanthan gum, divided

1 tablespoon gluten-free baking powder

1 teaspoon salt

2 tablespoons granulated sugar

1 large egg, whisked

MAKES 12 BISCUITS

**Per Serving
(Serving Size: 1 biscuit):**

Calories	105
Fat	3g
Protein	4g
Sodium	500mg
Fiber	1g
Carbohydrates	18g
Sugar	3g

1. Preheat oven to 450°F and grease a large cast-iron pan with vegetable oil or line a baking sheet with parchment paper.

2. Add 6 tablespoons buttery spread in a small bowl and place in the freezer for 5 minutes. In a separate small bowl, add milk and vinegar, then let stand 5 minutes in the refrigerator to keep cold.

3. In a large bowl, stir together 2 cups flour, baking powder, salt, and sugar.

4. Cut in chilled buttery spread into flour with a pastry cutter or fork until it looks like small peas.

5. Add in the milk mixture and whisked egg and stir until a soft dough forms. The key is to not overmix because that will create tough biscuits. The dough will be sticky.

6. Add 1 tablespoon flour to a large piece of parchment paper. Place dough on top of floured parchment paper. Dust the top of dough with remaining 1 tablespoon flour and gently fold dough in half on top of itself and then repeat.

7. With your hands, form a dough round that is about 7" in diameter and 1" thick. (If you make it any larger or flatter you will end up with hard, flat biscuits.)

8. Cut out 2" biscuits using a biscuit cutter, the mouth of a glass, or the lid of a Mason jar. Do not twist cutter when cutting; this will crimp the edges of biscuits, causing them not to rise well. Re-form dough scraps into a dough round and cut out more biscuits. Put biscuits on prepared pan or baking sheet.

9. Bake biscuits for 15–20 minutes. At the 15-minute point, check to see if biscuits are golden brown. In a small bowl, melt remaining 2 tablespoons buttery spread and brush on top of warm biscuits. Serve warm. Store leftovers in an airtight container for up to 3 days.

BUTTERMILK IS THE TRICK

Buttermilk can improve many baked goods. It adds a slight tangy flavor helps the bread rise nicely, and makes items less likely to become overly brown. Buttermilk is easily made dairy-free by adding either 1 tablespoon white vinegar or lemon juice to 1 cup dairy-free milk and allowing it to sit for 3–5 minutes.

Lemon Blueberry Scones

MAKES 8 SCONES

**Per Serving
(Serving Size: 1 scone):**

Calories	315
Fat	5g
Protein	3g
Sodium	310mg
Fiber	1g
Carbohydrates	63g
Sugar	25g

WHAT IS A SCONE?

The scone is best known as a single-serving sweet bread alongside British afternoon tea, which is usually served at 4:00 p.m. In the United States, you can find premade scones at coffee shops and grocery stores, but keep a close eye on the ingredients because traditional scones are made with both gluten and dairy.

These flaky, sweet morning treats are an excellent choice for a quick, on-the-go breakfast. They are crispy and buttery, and they go perfectly with your fresh-brewed coffee or tea.

SCONES

½ cup dairy-free buttery spread
1 tablespoon white vinegar
¾ cup plus 2 tablespoons unsweetened almond milk, divided
3 cups plus 2 tablespoons gluten-free all-purpose flour with xanthan gum
⅓ cup sugar
2 tablespoons gluten-free baking powder
½ teaspoon salt
1 tablespoon dried lemon peel
2 large eggs, whisked
1 cup frozen blueberries

LEMON GLAZE

1 cup confectioners' sugar
1 tablespoon lemon juice
½ teaspoon pure vanilla extract
1 tablespoon water

1 Preheat oven to 425°F. Line a baking sheet with parchment paper.

2 Cut buttery spread into small pieces and freeze for 10 minutes. Combine vinegar and ¾ cup milk in a small bowl and set aside 2–5 minutes in the refrigerator.

3 In a large bowl, add flour, sugar, baking powder, salt, and lemon peel and stir to combine.

4 Cut buttery spread into flour mixture with a pastry cutter or fork until it looks like small peas. Add milk mixture and eggs and stir until a soft, sticky dough forms. Carefully stir in blueberries.

5 Add 1 tablespoon flour to a piece of parchment paper. Place dough on top of the floured parchment paper. Dust the top of dough with remaining 1 tablespoon flour and fold dough over on itself two times.

6 With your hands, form a dough round that is about 7" in diameter and 2" thick. If you make it any larger or flatter you will end up with flat scones.

7 Run a sharp knife under warm water and cut dough round in half. Then cut each half into four slices. You will now have eight dough triangles. Carefully place dough on prepared baking sheet. Brush the tops of dough with remaining 2 tablespoons milk. Bake for 15–20 minutes until the tops are golden brown.

8 Add the glaze ingredients to a small bowl and stir together until smooth. Drizzle over warm scones. Store in an airtight container for up to 3 days.

Jam-Filled Danish

Everyone at the next office meeting will be amazed that these delicious treats are gluten-free and dairy-free!

1/4 cup warm water (110°F to 115°F) plus 5 tablespoons water, divided

1/2 cup plus 1 tablespoon granulated sugar, divided

1 packet (2 1/4 teaspoons) instant yeast

2 cups plus 2 tablespoons gluten-free all-purpose flour with xanthan gum, divided

1 teaspoon salt

1/2 cup dairy-free buttery spread

2 large eggs, yolks and whites divided

1/2 cup unsweetened almond milk

1/4 teaspoon plus 1/8 teaspoon pure vanilla extract, divided

1/4 teaspoon plus 1/8 teaspoon pure almond extract, divided

8 teaspoons gluten-free raspberry jam

1 cup confectioners' sugar

MAKES 8 DANISH

Per Serving (Serving Size: 1 Danish):

Calories	300
Fat	4g
Protein	3g
Sodium	440mg
Fiber	0g
Carbohydrates	62g
Sugar	33g

1. Add 1/4 cup warm water and 1 tablespoon granulated sugar to a small bowl. Pour in the yeast and allow to sit for 2–3 minutes until foamy.

2. In a large bowl, add 2 cups flour, 1/2 cup sugar, and salt. Cut in buttery spread with a pastry cutter or fork until it looks like small peas.

3. Separate eggs and place whites in a small bowl, cover, and place in the refrigerator.

4. Add yeast mixture, yolks, milk, 1/4 teaspoon vanilla, and 1/4 teaspoon almond extract to flour mixture and mix until smooth. Cover the bowl and place in the freezer for 30 minutes.

5. Add 1 tablespoon flour to a large piece of parchment paper. Place dough on the floured parchment paper. Dust the top of dough with 1 tablespoon flour and fold dough in half on top of itself and then in half on itself again.

6. Form the dough into a round 7" in diameter and 1" thick. Cut out dough using a greased 3" biscuit cutter. Do not twist cutter when cutting; this will crimp the edges of the dough, causing it not to rise well. Put dough rounds on a baking sheet lined with parchment paper, cover with a kitchen towel, and let rise in a warm place for 30 minutes.

7. Use the back of a rounded tablespoon to press down on the center of each dough round. Place 1 teaspoon of jam in the center of each. Add 1 tablespoon water to the egg whites and whisk. Brush the tops of dough with the egg white mixture.

8. Bake for 18–20 minutes until the tops start to turn golden brown. In a small bowl, whisk together confectioners' sugar, 1/8 teaspoon vanilla extract, 1/8 teaspoon pure almond extract, and remaining 4 tablespoons water. Drizzle glaze on top. Allow Danish to cool for 5–10 minutes until jam is no longer hot before serving.

Cinnamon Biscuits

MAKES 12 BISCUITS

Per Serving
(Serving Size: 1 biscuit):

Calories	170
Fat	2g
Protein	1g
Sodium	270mg
Fiber	0g
Carbohydrates	36g
Sugar	16g

These tender and flaky gluten-free buttermilk biscuits are layered with cinnamon and sugar and topped with a sweet vanilla glaze.

BISCUITS
6 tablespoons dairy-free buttery spread
1 tablespoon white vinegar
1 cup unsweetened almond milk
2 cups plus 2 tablespoons gluten-free all-purpose flour with xanthan gum
1 tablespoon gluten-free baking powder
1 teaspoon salt
2 tablespoons granulated sugar
1 large egg, whisked
¼ cup light brown sugar, packed
1 tablespoon ground cinnamon

GLAZE
1 cup confectioners' sugar
1 teaspoon pure vanilla extract
2 teaspoons unsweetened almond milk

1. Preheat oven to 450°F.

2. Cut buttery spread into small pieces and put in the freezer for 10 minutes. In a small bowl, add vinegar and milk and let stand 2–5 minutes in the refrigerator to keep cold.

3. In a large bowl, add 2 cups flour, baking powder, salt, and sugar and stir. Cut in buttery spread into the flour mixture with a pastry cutter or fork until it looks like small peas.

4. Add in the milk mixture and egg and stir until a soft dough forms. Do not overmix. The dough will be sticky. Do not roll out dough.

5. Add 1 tablespoon flour to a large piece of parchment paper. Place dough on top of floured parchment paper. Form a dough round that is 7" in diameter and 1" thick.

6. In a small bowl, add brown sugar and cinnamon and stir to combine. Sprinkle 2 tablespoons sugar mixture all over the top of dough round.

7. Gently fold dough over on itself. Sprinkle another 2 tablespoons sugar mixture over dough. Fold dough in half on top of itself again.

8. With your hands form a dough round 7" in diameter and 1" thick. Sprinkle remaining sugar mixture over dough round.

9. Grease a large cast-iron pan with vegetable oil or line a baking sheet with parchment paper. Cut out twelve 2" biscuits using a biscuit cutter or the mouth of a glass. Do not twist cutter when cutting. Put biscuits on prepared pan or baking sheet.

10. Bake biscuits for 15–20 minutes. At the 15-minute point, check to see if they are golden brown.

11. In a small bowl, stir glaze ingredients until smooth. Spread over biscuits and serve warm. Store in an airtight container for up to 3 days.

Homemade Bagels

These big, soft, and chewy bagels are just like the $5 bagels at your favorite coffee shop! Add mix-ins like cinnamon and raisins or sprinkle everything bagel seasoning on top.

2¼ cups plus 1 tablespoon water, warmed to 100°F–110°F

1 tablespoon instant yeast

1 tablespoon granulated sugar

3½ cups gluten-free all-purpose flour with xanthan gum

3 tablespoons psyllium husk powder

2 teaspoons gluten-free baking powder

1½ teaspoons salt

1 tablespoon light brown sugar, packed

1 cup dairy-free buttery spread, melted

1 teaspoon apple cider vinegar

¼ cup honey

1 large egg white, whisked

MAKES 8 BAGELS

Per Serving (Serving Size: 1 bagel):

Calories	300
Fat	7g
Protein	3g
Sodium	685mg
Fiber	2g
Carbohydrates	55g
Sugar	11g

1 Preheat oven to 200°F. Once it gets to 100°F, turn off the oven.

2 Combine water, yeast, and granulated sugar in the bowl of a stand-up mixer fitted with a dough hook. Stir; let stand 5 minutes until foamy.

3 Add flour, psyllium husk powder, baking powder, salt, and brown sugar and mix until fully combined. Add buttery spread and vinegar and beat on low speed for 2 minutes. Raise the mixer speed to medium and knead for 5 minutes.

4 Place dough in an ovenproof bowl sprayed with gluten-free nonstick cooking spray. Cover the bowl with plastic wrap and then a kitchen towel. Allow dough to rise for 20 minutes in the warm oven.

5 Line a baking sheet with parchment paper. Turn dough out onto parchment paper and cut into eight pieces. Roll each piece into a ball. Press your finger through the center of each ball to make a hole about 1" in diameter. Cover the shaped bagels with a kitchen towel and let rise on the counter for 10 minutes.

6 Preheat oven to 425°F.

7 Fill a large pot with 2 quarts water. Whisk in honey. Bring water to a boil, then reduce heat to medium-high. Drop bagels in one at a time. Cook bagels for 30 seconds on each side. Remove with a slotted spoon and return boiled bagels to the sheet, right side up, with flat bottoms against pan.

8 Whisk the egg white and 1 tablespoon water together in a small bowl. Brush the tops of bagels with egg wash on top and around the sides. Bake for 7 minutes and then rotate the pan and cook for another 8 minutes until golden brown and internal temperature reaches 180°F. Remove from the oven and allow bagels to cool on the baking sheet for 10 minutes before serving. Store in an airtight container for up to 3 days.

Rosemary Focaccia Bread

SERVES 12

Per Serving:

Calories	270
Fat	19g
Protein	1g
Sodium	400mg
Fiber	0g
Carbohydrates	22g
Sugar	1g

HEALTH BENEFITS OF ROSEMARY

Not only does rosemary taste and smell great, but it is also a great source of vitamin B_6, calcium, and iron. For thousands of years, the rosemary plant has been thought to have various medicinal qualities, such as treating indigestion, enhancing memory and concentration, boosting the immune system, and improving blood circulation.

This savory bread is crispy on the outside crust and soft and fluffy inside! If you have any fresh rosemary from an herb garden, use 1 tablespoon chopped fresh rosemary instead of the 1½ teaspoons dried.

2½ cups plus 1 tablespoon gluten-free all-purpose flour with xanthan gum
1 packet (2¼ teaspoons) instant yeast
1 tablespoon gluten-free baking powder
2 teaspoons salt, divided
1½ teaspoons dried rosemary, divided
1 tablespoon honey
1½ cups warm water (110°F–115°F)
1 teaspoon apple cider vinegar
1 cup olive oil, divided

1 Preheat oven to 200°F. Once it gets to 100°F, turn off oven.

2 In a large bowl, combine flour, yeast, baking powder, ½ teaspoon salt, and 1 teaspoon rosemary. Stir to combine ingredients.

3 Add honey to warm water and stir until honey is dissolved.

4 Pour the warm water mixture into the flour mixture and mix with your mixer with a dough hook or paddle attachment on low.

5 Pour vinegar and ½ cup olive oil into the dough mixture and mix on medium speed for 3 minutes. The dough will be very sticky.

6 Place dough in an ovenproof bowl sprayed with gluten-free nonstick cooking spray. Cover the bowl with plastic wrap and then with a kitchen towel and place in warm oven for 30 minutes to rise.

7 Remove dough from the oven and preheat oven to 425°F. Coat a jelly pan with ¼ cup olive oil. Put dough onto the pan and begin pressing it out to fit the size of the pan. Using your fingers make impressions throughout the dough, but do not poke holes. Spread the remaining ¼ cup olive on top of the dough. Sprinkle with remaining 1 teaspoon salt and ½ teaspoon rosemary. Bake for 20 minutes until golden brown. Allow to cool for 3–5 minutes before slicing the bread. Store in an airtight container for up to 3 days.

Soft Pretzels

If you are tired of walking by the famous pretzel shop in the mall and wishing it had gluten-free and dairy-free pretzels, look no further. These pretzels are as good as any freshly baked pretzel from a pretzel shop, and they are much easier to make at home than you might imagine!

½ cup unsweetened almond milk, warm (100°F–110°F)

1 teaspoon granulated sugar

1 packet (2¼ teaspoons) instant yeast

3⅓ cups plus 1 tablespoon gluten-free all-purpose flour with xanthan gum, divided

1½ teaspoons gluten-free baking powder

1½ teaspoons salt

1 cup dairy-free plain coconut yogurt

2 large eggs, divided

6 tablespoons baking soda

1 tablespoon coarse sea salt

1. Preheat oven to 200°F. Once it gets to 100°F turn off oven.

2. In a small bowl, stir together milk, sugar, and yeast. Let stand for 5–10 minutes until foamy. In a large bowl, combine flour, baking powder, and salt. In a separate small bowl, whisk together yogurt and one egg.

3. Add the yeast mixture and yogurt mixture to the flour mixture. Mix together until it forms a sticky dough.

4. Add dough to an ovenproof bowl sprayed with gluten-free nonstick cooking spray. Cover the bowl with plastic wrap and a kitchen towel, and place in the warm oven for 30 minutes.

5. Add 1 tablespoon flour to a piece of parchment paper. Turn out dough onto the parchment paper and divide into eight balls.

6. Take each piece of dough and begin rolling them into a long rope, about the length of the parchment paper (11"). Take the ends of the dough rope and bring them together so the dough forms a circle. Twist the ends over each other twice, then bring them toward yourself and press them down into a pretzel shape.

7. Preheat oven to 450°F and line a baking sheet with parchment paper. Add 2 quarts water in a large pot and stir in baking soda. Bring water to a boil, then reduce heat to medium-high. Drop pretzels in the boiling water one at a time and boil for 30 seconds. Using a wire skimmer or slotted spoon, return pretzels to the sheet, right side up, with flat bottoms against the sheet. Repeat until all pretzels have been boiled.

8. In a small bowl, whisk remaining egg. Brush pretzels with egg and sprinkle with salt. Bake for 15 minutes or until golden brown. Allow to cool for 2–3 minutes and serve warm.

MAKES 8 PRETZELS

Per Serving (Serving Size: 1 pretzel):

Calories	220
Fat	2g
Protein	4g
Sodium	4,200mg
Fiber	0g
Carbohydrates	1g
Sugar	0g

EXPLORE DAIRY-FREE YOGURT

There are several different options for dairy-free yogurt. Dairy-free yogurts are made from either coconut, almond, or soy milk. Dairy-free yogurt can be used in a variety of ways. It can be used in baking, to make sauces, and to make dairy-free sour cream. There are also lots of fun flavors to enjoy eating on their own as well.

Flatbread

From gyros to lunch wraps, this wonderful Flatbread is versatile and helps you enjoy some of your favorite foods in a gluten-free and dairy-free way. It is best served fresh and hot with your choice of marinated meat, vegetables, and sauce.

INVEST IN PARCHMENT PAPER

If you do not regularly use parchment paper, try it out. Lining your baking sheets with parchment paper prevents the hard-to-clean, burnt-on batter of cookies, pies, and tons of other baked goods from covering your favorite baking sheets. It also allows the food to slide right off the pan when it's done.

1 packet (2¼ teaspoons) instant yeast
1 tablespoon honey
1½ cups warm water (100°F–110°F)
1 tablespoon gluten-free baking powder
1 teaspoon salt
1 teaspoon apple cider vinegar
¼ cup plus 2 tablespoons olive oil, divided
3 cups plus 1 tablespoon gluten-free all-purpose flour with xanthan gum, divided

1 Preheat oven to 200°F. Once it gets to 100°F, turn off oven.

2 In the bowl of a stand-up mixer fitted with a dough hook, combine the yeast, honey, and water; mix until combined. Let yeast sit for 5 minutes until foamy.

3 Add baking powder, salt, vinegar, and ¼ cup olive oil and mix. Add 3 cups flour, 1 cup at a time, mixing at the lowest speed until all the flour has been incorporated and dough pulls away from the side of the bowl, about 4 minutes.

4 Place dough in a greased ovenproof bowl covered with plastic wrap and then a kitchen towel and let rise in a warm oven for 30 minutes.

5 Flour a piece of parchment paper with remaining 1 tablespoon flour. Divide dough into eight pieces and flatten them out with the palms of your hands, then use a rolling pin to roll each piece into a thin circle.

6 Heat remaining 2 tablespoons olive oil in a large skillet over medium-high heat. Once the skillet is hot, place dough into the skillet. Cook for 1 minute. When the edges are starting to look golden, flip the bread carefully with a spatula and cook for another minute. Remove to a plate and cover with aluminum foil to keep warm. Store in an airtight container for up to 3 days.

Homemade Popovers

Popovers are unique, light, air-filled rolls. Try serving these popovers with dairy-free buttery spread and your choice of gluten-free sweet jam for a great late-afternoon snack! Popover pans are different from regular muffin tins by their deep, steep-sided wells. This forces the batter upward and results in a popover with a puffy dome and crispy sides. If you don't have one, muffin tins will work, but the popovers won't rise as high.

2 large eggs
1 cup gluten-free all-purpose flour
 with xanthan gum

½ teaspoon salt
1 cup unsweetened almond milk

1 Preheat oven to 450°F and grease a twelve-cup popover pan with gluten-free nonstick cooking spray.

2 In a large bowl, beat eggs. Beat in flour, salt, and milk until smooth.

3 Fill baking cups three-quarters full and bake for 20 minutes. Decrease the oven temperature to 350°F and bake for 20 minutes longer until golden brown. Do not open the oven during the baking process. Remove popovers immediately from the baking cups and serve immediately while hot. Store in an airtight container for up to 3 days.

MAKES 12 POPOVERS

Per Serving
(Serving Size: 1 popover):

Calories	50
Fat	1g
Protein	2g
Sodium	130mg
Fiber	0g
Carbohydrates	8g
Sugar	0g

Herbed Crusty Bread

Serve this bread with your favorite flavored olive oil.

3 cups gluten-free all-purpose flour
 with xanthan gum, divided
1 tablespoon granulated sugar
1 teaspoon salt
1 packet (2¼ teaspoons) instant yeast
1½ cups warm water (110°F)
¼ cup dairy-free buttery spread

2 large eggs, room temperature and
 beaten
1 teaspoon apple cider vinegar
½ teaspoon dried rosemary
¼ teaspoon dried thyme
¼ teaspoon garlic powder

1 Preheat oven to 200°F. Once it gets to 100°F, turn off your oven.

2 In a large bowl, combine 2 cups flour, sugar, salt, and yeast. Add water, buttery spread, eggs, vinegar, rosemary, thyme, and garlic powder and beat on low 1 minute. Stir in remaining 1 cup flour; beat 2 minutes on medium.

3 Transfer dough to a greased 9" × 5" pan. Cover with plastic wrap and then a kitchen towel and place in the warm oven for 30 minutes to rise. Remove from the oven and keep covered. Preheat oven to 375°F. Bake for 40–45 minutes. Remove from pan and cool on a wire rack for 20 minutes before slicing and serving warm.

SERVES 8

Per Serving:

Calories	190
Fat	3g
Protein	4g
Sodium	385mg
Fiber	0g
Carbohydrates	36g
Sugar	1g

Lemon Blueberry Quick Bread

SERVES 8

Per Serving:

Calories	185
Fat	4g
Protein	3g
Sodium	280mg
Fiber	1g
Carbohydrates	32g
Sugar	14g

This bread combines the distinctive tart flavor of lemon with sweet blueberries into a rich and unique bread loaf that tastes so much better than anything you can buy from the store! Slice and serve it to guests or give loaves as gifts at the holidays.

⅓ cup dairy-free buttery spread, melted

2 large eggs, whisked

1 teaspoon pure vanilla extract

1 tablespoon gluten-free lemon extract

1½ cups gluten-free all-purpose flour with xanthan gum

½ cup sugar

1 teaspoon baking soda

½ teaspoon gluten-free baking powder

¼ teaspoon salt

1 cup unsweetened almond milk

1 cup frozen blueberries

1. Preheat oven to 350°F. Spray a 4" × 8" loaf pan with gluten-free non-stick cooking spray.

2. In a large bowl, add buttery spread, eggs, vanilla extract, and lemon extract and stir to combine ingredients. Add flour, sugar, baking soda, baking powder, and salt to the mixture and mix until fully combined. Add milk and mix until smooth. Fold in blueberries. Pour batter into prepared loaf pan.

3. Bake on the center rack for 50 minutes to 1 hour or until a toothpick inserted in the center comes out clean. Allow the bread to cool for 3–5 minutes before removing from the pan and slicing. Store leftovers in an airtight container at room temperature for up to 3 days.

Garlic Breadsticks

You can stop bypassing the breadsticks because you can't find a gluten- and dairy-free version! These Garlic Breadsticks are soft on the inside and golden brown on the outside.

2½ cups plus 1 tablespoon gluten-free all-purpose flour with xanthan gum

1 packet (2¼ teaspoons) instant yeast

1 tablespoon gluten-free baking powder

¼ teaspoon garlic powder

1 teaspoon salt

1 tablespoon honey

1½ cups warm water (110°F–115°F)

½ cup plus 1 teaspoon olive oil, divided

1 teaspoon apple cider vinegar

2 tablespoons dairy-free buttery spread, melted

MAKES 16 BREADSTICKS

Per Serving
(Serving Size: 1 breadstick):

Calories	145
Fat	8g
Protein	1g
Sodium	170mg
Fiber	0g
Carbohydrates	16g
Sugar	1g

1 Preheat oven to 200°F. Once it gets to 100°F turn off oven.

2 In a large bowl, combine flour, yeast, baking powder, garlic powder, and salt. Stir to combine ingredients.

3 Add honey to warm water and stir until it is dissolved.

4 Pour the warm water mixture into the flour mixture and mix with your mixer with a dough hook or paddle attachment on low.

5 Pour ½ cup olive oil and vinegar into the dough mixture and mix on medium speed for 3 minutes. The dough will be very sticky.

6 Line a baking sheet with parchment paper. Pour remaining 1 teaspoon oil into a sealable plastic bag and spread around so the bag is coated. Add dough to the bag toward one of the bottom corners. Cut 1" off of the corner of the bag. Squeeze the bag toward the cut corner so the dough comes out of the corner of the bag. Pipe dough down to make a length of breadstick, about 7", on the baking sheet. Repeat piping dough into breadstick shapes until all dough is used. Place in the warm oven and let rise for 30 minutes.

7 Remove dough from the oven and preheat oven to 425°F.

8 Bake for 15 minutes until golden brown. Brush tops with melted buttery spread. Allow to cool for 1–2 minutes, then serve warm. Store in an airtight container for up to 3 days.

Marbled Quick Bread

SERVES 8

Per Serving:

Calories	125
Fat	4g
Protein	3g
Sodium	360mg
Fiber	0g
Carbohydrates	18g
Sugar	0g

This sweetly delicious loaf is tender and flaky and will satisfy your sweet tooth for chocolaty goodness! Lightly dust it with confectioners' sugar for a nice finishing touch.

⅓ cup dairy-free buttery spread, melted
2 large eggs, whisked
1 tablespoon pure vanilla extract
1½ cups gluten-free all-purpose flour with xanthan gum
½ cup sugar
1 teaspoon baking soda
½ teaspoon gluten-free baking powder
¼ teaspoon salt
1 cup unsweetened almond milk
1 tablespoon cocoa powder

1 Preheat oven to 350°F. Spray a 4" × 8" loaf pan with gluten-free non-stick cooking spray.

2 In a large bowl, add buttery spread, eggs, and vanilla extract, and stir to combine. Add flour, sugar, baking soda, baking powder, and salt to the mixture and mix until fully combined. Add milk and stir until smooth.

3 Add 1 cup of batter to a small bowl. Stir in cocoa powder and mix until fully combined to make chocolate batter.

4 Pour vanilla batter into prepared loaf pan. Drizzle chocolate batter on top and use a knife to swirl through the vanilla batter.

5 Bake on the center rack for 50 minutes to 1 hour or until a toothpick inserted in the center comes out clean. Allow bread to cool for 3–5 minutes before removing from the pan and slicing. Store leftovers in an airtight at room temperature container for 3 days.

Potato Rolls

Homemade dinner rolls will make any meal even more special. These are soft, fluffy, and packed with homemade bread flavor!

⅓ cup plus ½ cup warm water (110°F to 115°F), divided

1 tablespoon honey

1 packet (2¼ teaspoons) instant yeast

½ cup mashed potatoes (1 large baked potato, peeled, cooked, and mashed)

⅓ cup sugar

⅓ cup dairy-free buttery spread

1 large egg, room temperature

1¼ teaspoons salt

1 teaspoon apple cider vinegar

3 cups gluten-free all-purpose flour with xanthan gum

1 Preheat oven to 200°F. Once it gets to 100°F, turn off oven.

2 In a large bowl, add ⅓ cup warm water, honey, and yeast. Stir to combine and allow to sit for 5 minutes until foamy.

3 Add potatoes, sugar, buttery spread, egg, salt, vinegar, flour, and remaining ½ cup water to the yeast mixture and mix until smooth. The dough will be sticky.

4 Spray two 9" metal cake pans with gluten-free nonstick cooking spray. Using a greased ice cream scoop, make sixteen dough balls; place eight into the first pan and eight into the second pan. Cover the pans with a kitchen towel and allow to rise in the warm oven for 30 minutes. Remove from the oven and keep covered while preheating oven to 375°F.

5 Bake rolls on the middle rack for 20 minutes until light golden brown. The temperature of the rolls should measure 200°F internally. Allow rolls to cool for 1–2 minutes. Serve warm. Store in an airtight container for up to 3 days.

MAKES 16 ROLLS

Per Serving
(Serving Size: 1 roll):

Calories	120
Fat	2g
Protein	2g
Sodium	260mg
Fiber	0g
Carbohydrates	24g
Sugar	5g

VEGETABLE PEELERS

If you haven't upgraded your vegetable peeler lately, there are several great and affordable options on the market nowadays. You will find peelers with dual blades, oversized hand grips, rust-resistant stainless steel, swiveling action, multiple uses, and even sleek colors to match your kitchen. Avoid using a dull peeler to make prepping easy and safe.

Cranberry Orange Quick Bread

SERVES 8

Per Serving:

Calories	180
Fat	3g
Protein	3g
Sodium	350mg
Fiber	1g
Carbohydrates	33g
Sugar	15g

DON'T CONFUSE FOLDING WITH MIXING

For the record, mixing refers to thoroughly stirring ingredients, while folding describes the practice of gently combining ingredients without stirring or agitating. Plump berries and other soft fruits often respond better to folding than mixing.

If you love the taste combination of cranberry and citrus, then this quick bread recipe is one for you! This bread loaf is not only delicious, but each slice is delightfully filled with cranberries and looks beautiful displayed on a platter.

⅓ cup dairy-free buttery spread, melted

2 large eggs, whisked

1 teaspoon pure vanilla extract

¼ teaspoon pure almond extract

½ teaspoon dried orange peel

1½ cups gluten-free all-purpose flour with xanthan gum

½ cup sugar

1 teaspoon baking soda

½ teaspoon gluten-free baking powder

¼ teaspoon salt

½ cup unsweetened almond milk

½ cup orange juice

1 cup frozen cranberries

1. Preheat oven to 350°F. Spray a 4" × 8" loaf pan with gluten-free non-stick cooking spray.

2. In a large bowl, add buttery spread, eggs, vanilla extract, almond extract, and orange peel and stir to combine. Add flour, sugar, baking soda, baking powder, and salt to the mixture and stir until fully combined. Add milk and orange juice and mix until smooth. Carefully fold in cranberries. Pour batter into prepared loaf pan.

3. Bake on the center rack for 50 minutes to 1 hour or until a toothpick inserted in the center comes out clean. Allow the bread to cool for 3–5 minutes before removing from the pan and slicing. Store leftovers in an airtight container at room temperature for up to 3 days.

CHAPTER 9

Soups

Cream of Mushroom Soup

SERVES 4

Per Serving:

Calories	85
Fat	3g
Protein	3g
Sodium	390mg
Fiber	0g
Carbohydrates	11g
Sugar	1g

This homemade Cream of Mushroom Soup is a filling and delicious meal on its own, and it can also be used in any recipe that calls for the canned version, such as green bean casserole.

2 tablespoons dairy-free buttery spread
1 cup finely chopped mushrooms
½ teaspoon jarred minced garlic
6 tablespoons gluten-free all-purpose flour with xanthan gum
1 teaspoon onion powder
2 cups gluten-free chicken broth
½ teaspoon salt
⅛ teaspoon ground black pepper
⅛ teaspoon ground nutmeg
1 cup unsweetened almond milk

1 Add buttery spread, mushrooms, and garlic to a large pot and sauté over medium-high heat for 1–2 minutes until mushrooms are tender.

2 Sprinkle flour and onion powder over mushrooms and stir to coat. Stir in broth, salt, pepper, and nutmeg until flour dissolves. Bring to a boil and stir until thickened, about 2 minutes.

3 Reduce the heat to low to simmer and stir in milk. Simmer, uncovered, for about 10–15 minutes, stirring occasionally. Remove soup from the heat when it reaches desired thickness.

Savory Chicken and Rice Soup

SERVES 6

Per Serving:

Calories	150
Fat	5g
Protein	19g
Sodium	320mg
Fiber	1g
Carbohydrates	6g
Sugar	2g

This classic soup is both filling and delicious. Pack leftovers in a storage container to reheat for lunch the next day.

1 tablespoon olive oil
3 large carrots, peeled and diced
1 stalk celery, diced
1 teaspoon jarred minced garlic
1 tablespoon onion powder
½ teaspoon dried thyme
5 cups gluten-free chicken broth
½ teaspoon seasoned salt
⅛ teaspoon ground black pepper
2 (5-ounce) boneless, skinless chicken breasts, diced
1 cup long-grain white rice

1 Heat olive oil in a large pot over medium heat. Add carrots and celery and sauté vegetables for 5–7 minutes until very tender, stirring occasionally. Add garlic, onion powder, and thyme and sauté for 30 seconds until fragrant.

2 Add broth, salt, and pepper and bring to a boil over medium-high heat. Add chicken and rice and stir to combine. Turn heat down to medium and simmer uncovered for 15–20 minutes until rice is tender. Remove from the heat and cover and let sit for 5 minutes. Serve warm.

Loaded Baked Potato Soup

If you've had this type of soup at your favorite restaurant, try making it at home in a gluten- and dairy-free way. It stores well for taking to lunch the next day.

1 (12-ounce) package gluten-free bacon
1 cup peeled and chopped sweet onion
6 cups gluten-free chicken broth
2 pounds baking potatoes, peeled and cubed
⅔ cup dairy-free buttery spread
¾ cup gluten-free all-purpose flour with xanthan gum
4 cups unsweetened almond milk, divided
1 teaspoon salt
¼ teaspoon ground black pepper
¼ cup sliced green onion

SERVES 6

Per Serving:

Calories	530
Fat	25g
Protein	31g
Sodium	1,820mg
Fiber	4g
Carbohydrates	42g
Sugar	3g

1 In a large skillet, cook bacon for 6–8 minutes over medium heat until crisp; set on a paper towel–lined plate. Allow to cool for 5 minutes and crumble bacon; set aside. Drain bacon grease, reserving 2 tablespoons in the skillet. Add onions and sauté over medium-high heat for 6 minutes until tender.

2 Add broth and potatoes to a large pot and bring to a boil over medium-high heat. Reduce heat to medium and simmer for 10 minutes until potatoes are fork-tender.

3 Melt buttery spread in the skillet with onions over low heat. Stir in flour and whisk until smooth. Stir in 2 cups milk and whisk until fully combined and flour is dissolved. Pour the milk mixture into the potato mixture. Add remaining 2 cups milk, salt, and pepper to the pot. Cook over medium heat for 5 minutes, stirring constantly, until the mixture has thickened.

4 Stir in the bacon and cook until thoroughly heated. Serve and garnish with green onions.

Creamy Chicken Corn Chowder

SERVES 6

Per Serving:

Calories	220
Fat	8g
Protein	16g
Sodium	335mg
Fiber	1g
Carbohydrates	20g
Sugar	0g

MORE ON CHOWDER

The term *chowder* refers to a type of soup that is prepared with milk or cream. There are many great varieties of chowder, from seafood to corn. Chowder recipes can be easily adapted to be gluten-free and dairy-free by using a roux of gluten-free flour and dairy-free milk.

This creamy soup is comforting and rich and will warm you up on even the coldest day. The soft potatoes and corn complete the chicken and sauce in a way that will make your mouth water! Top with a pinch of diced gluten-free bacon and spices, if desired.

2 tablespoons dairy-free buttery spread
1 teaspoon jarred minced garlic
⅔ cup gluten-free all-purpose flour with xanthan gum
1 tablespoon onion powder
1 teaspoon dried thyme
2 cups gluten-free chicken broth
½ teaspoon salt
⅛ teaspoon ground black pepper
2 cups peeled and diced russet potatoes
2 cups chopped cooked chicken
1 (15-ounce) can corn, drained
1 cup unsweetened almond milk

1 Add buttery spread and garlic to a large pot and sauté over medium-high heat for 30 seconds until garlic is tender.

2 Sprinkle flour, onion powder, and thyme over garlic. Stir in broth, salt, and pepper. Stir the mixture until flour dissolves. Add potatoes and bring the mixture to a boil, stirring frequently, then reduce heat to medium-low and cook uncovered for 10 minutes or just until potatoes are tender. Bring soup to a boil for 2 minutes, stirring until thickened.

3 Add chicken and corn and stir to combine. Reduce the heat to low and stir in milk. Simmer uncovered for about 10–15 minutes, stirring occasionally. Remove soup from the heat when it reaches desired thickness.

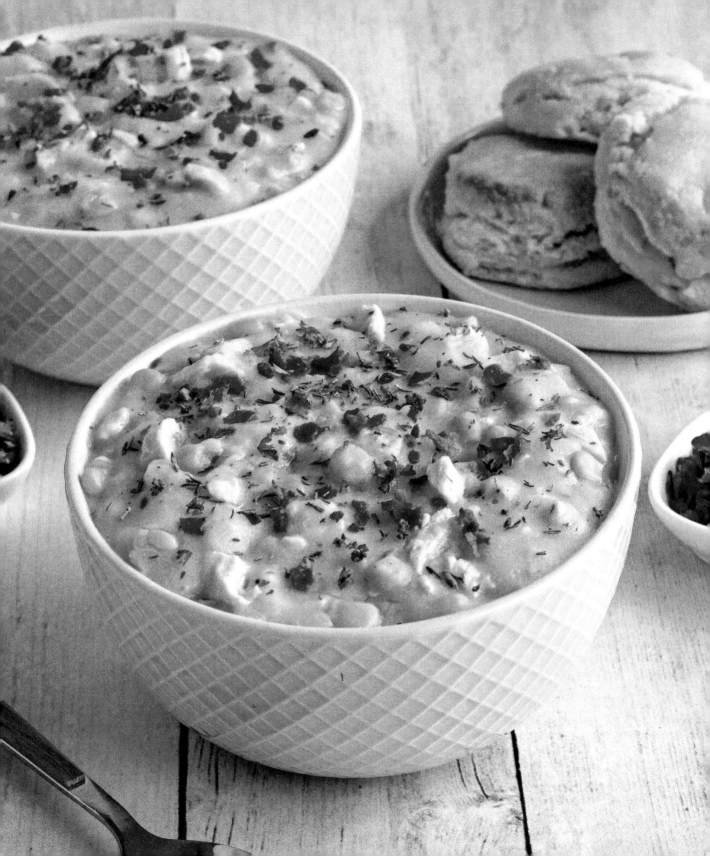

Zuppa Toscana

SERVES 6

Per Serving:

Calories	300
Fat	12g
Protein	21g
Sodium	805mg
Fiber	2g
Carbohydrates	25g
Sugar	2g

SLICING AND DICING

What's the difference between chopping, mincing, and dicing? When you chop, the pieces are not necessarily evenly cut. Dicing is smaller than a chop and are uniform in size. Mincing refers to cutting into very small parts.

Surprise your family tonight with the delicious soup they've only eaten at Italian restaurants. This version uses potatoes instead of beans for a slightly different twist. This soup goes great with fresh gluten-free and dairy-free breadsticks.

1 tablespoon olive oil
1 pound mild gluten-free Italian sausage, chopped
½ teaspoon crushed red pepper flakes
6 strips gluten-free bacon, diced
1 large sweet onion, peeled and chopped
3 tablespoons jarred minced garlic
4 cups gluten-free chicken broth
2 cups water
4 cups diced russet potatoes
½ teaspoon salt
¼ teaspoon ground black pepper
1 cup unsweetened almond milk
3 tablespoons gluten-free all-purpose flour with xanthan gum
2 cups chopped baby spinach leaves, stems removed

1 Add olive oil, sausage, and red pepper flakes to a large pot and cook for 10–15 minutes over medium-high heat until sausage is browned. Drain excess grease and set sausage aside.

2 Add bacon, onions, and garlic to the pot and sauté for 5 minutes until bacon is browned and onions are tender.

3 Add the chicken broth, water, potatoes, salt, and pepper. Boil for 20 minutes until potatoes are fork-tender.

4 In a small bowl, whisk together milk and flour. Reduce the heat to medium and stir in the milk mixture and cooked sausage and cook for 5 minutes. Stir spinach into soup just before serving.

Cream of Chicken Soup

This rich, creamy soup is loaded with flavor. It's used in a lot of casserole recipes, so it's good to have a gluten- and dairy-free version.

2 tablespoons dairy-free buttery spread
½ teaspoon jarred minced garlic
6 tablespoons gluten-free all-purpose flour with xanthan gum
1 teaspoon onion powder
1 teaspoon dried thyme
2 cups gluten-free chicken broth
½ teaspoon salt
⅛ teaspoon ground black pepper
⅛ teaspoon ground nutmeg
2 cups chopped cooked chicken
1 cup unsweetened almond milk

SERVES 4

Per Serving:

Calories	140
Fat	4g
Protein	16g
Sodium	460mg
Fiber	0g
Carbohydrates	11g
Sugar	0g

1 Add buttery spread and garlic to a large pot and sauté over medium-high heat for 30 seconds until garlic is tender.

2 Sprinkle in flour, onion powder, and thyme. Stir in broth, salt, pepper, and nutmeg until flour dissolves. Bring to a boil and stir until thickened, about 2 minutes.

3 Add chicken to soup and stir to combine. Reduce the heat to low to simmer and stir in milk. Simmer uncovered for about 10–15 minutes, stirring occasionally.

Hearty Hamburger Soup

This soup has all your favorite burger flavors without having to worry about the bun. It's a great choice to fill you up on a chilly day.

1 teaspoon olive oil
1 pound 90/10 ground beef
1 medium sweet onion, peeled and chopped
1 cup chopped celery
1½ teaspoons jarred minced garlic
6 cups gluten-free beef broth
1 (14-ounce) can diced tomatoes, including liquid
1 (8-ounce) can tomato sauce
1 teaspoon Italian seasoning
1½ teaspoons salt
¼ teaspoon ground black pepper
2 medium russet potatoes, peeled and cubed
3 cups frozen mixed vegetables

SERVES 6

Per Serving:

Calories	290
Fat	12g
Protein	22g
Sodium	1,380mg
Fiber	5g
Carbohydrates	24g
Sugar	6g

1 Add olive oil, beef, onions, celery, and garlic to a large pot and cook over medium-high heat for 5–7 minutes until meat is browned. Drain excess fat.

2 Add broth, tomatoes, tomato sauce, Italian seasoning, salt, pepper, potatoes, and mixed vegetables. Stir to combine, then bring to a boil. Reduce the heat, cover the pot, and simmer for 20–25 minutes until potatoes are fork-tender.

Italian Vegetable Soup

SERVES 6

Per Serving:

Calories	305
Fat	3g
Protein	18g
Sodium	1,750mg
Fiber	16g
Carbohydrates	52g
Sugar	10g

This zesty Italian Vegetable Soup is a crowd-pleaser with fresh aromas that will fill your home as you simmer it. It goes great with gluten-free and dairy-free breadsticks.

1 tablespoon olive oil

2 (14-ounce) cans petite-diced tomatoes, including liquid

1 tablespoon garlic powder

1 tablespoon onion powder

1 tablespoon dried basil

1 teaspoon salt

2 gluten-free beef bouillon cubes

1 (16-ounce) can kidney beans

1 (16-ounce) can cannellini beans

1 (16-ounce) can great northern beans

1 cup peeled and chopped carrots

1 cup chopped trimmed green beans

1 large zucchini, diced

1 large yellow squash, diced

1 (10-ounce) package baby spinach

1 cup water

Add olive oil into the bottom of a slow cooker. Add remaining ingredients and stir. Cook on high for 4 hours until vegetables are softened.

Southern Ham and Bean Soup

SERVES 6

Per Serving:

Calories	290
Fat	11g
Protein	23g
Sodium	410mg
Fiber	7g
Carbohydrates	24g
Sugar	1g

If you have never had a hot bowl of ham and bean soup, then pull up a chair and start enjoying! This easy-to-make soup has only a few simple ingredients, but the flavorful finished product will make you think differently.

1 tablespoon olive oil

1 small sweet onion, peeled and finely chopped

1 teaspoon jarred minced garlic

2 cups diced cooked ham

2 teaspoons dried thyme

2 (15-ounce) cans white beans, drained and rinsed

4 cups gluten-free chicken broth

1 teaspoon seasoned salt

⅛ teaspoon ground black pepper

1 Add olive oil, onions, garlic, ham, and thyme to a large pot over medium-high heat and cook for 4 minutes until onions are softened, stirring occasionally.

2 Add beans, broth, salt, and pepper and simmer uncovered for 20 minutes, stirring occasionally. Serve warm.

Chicken Fajita Soup

This delicious soup brings the flavors of sizzling chicken fajitas into a bowl of piping hot soup! Instead of sour cream, you can top the soup with a dollop of dairy-free plain yogurt.

1 teaspoon olive oil
1 large green bell pepper, seeded and chopped
1 large red bell pepper, seeded and chopped
1 cup peeled and chopped sweet onion
1 tablespoon jarred minced garlic
1 pound boneless, skinless chicken breasts
1 (15-ounce) can black beans, rinsed and drained
1 (15-ounce) can fire-roasted diced tomatoes, drained
5 cups gluten-free chicken broth
1 teaspoon chili powder
1 teaspoon paprika
1 teaspoon ground cumin
½ teaspoon dried oregano
1 teaspoon salt
¼ teaspoon ground black pepper
1 cup dry long-grain white rice
2 cups water
¼ cup chopped fresh cilantro

SERVES 6

Per Serving:

Calories	365
Fat	5g
Protein	29g
Sodium	740mg
Fiber	9g
Carbohydrates	50g
Sugar	3g

1 Add olive oil, bell peppers, onions, and garlic in a large pot and sauté over medium-high heat for 3–5 minutes until vegetables are softened.

2 Add chicken, black beans, tomatoes, broth, seasonings, rice, and water and stir to combine. Bring to a boil, then lower the heat and simmer for 20 minutes.

3 Use tongs to remove cooked chicken breasts to a plate, cool for 5 minutes, then shred with two forks. Continue simmering for 10–15 minutes until rice is tender. Add shredded chicken back to soup and stir to combine. Serve garnished with cilantro.

French Onion Soup

SERVES 6

Per Serving:

Calories	112
Fat	4g
Protein	4g
Sodium	860mg
Fiber	2g
Carbohydrates	13g
Sugar	5g

Finding gluten- and dairy-free French Onion Soup at a restaurant might be difficult, but you don't have to miss out on this classic soup forever!

½ cup dairy-free buttery spread
4 large sweet onions, peeled and thinly sliced
1 teaspoon jarred minced garlic
2 bay leaves
2 teaspoons dried thyme
½ teaspoon salt
¼ teaspoon ground black pepper
1 cup dry white wine
3 tablespoons gluten-free all-purpose flour with xanthan gum
8 cups gluten-free beef broth

1 Melt buttery spread in a large pot over medium heat. Add onions, garlic, bay leaves, thyme, salt, and pepper and cook for 20–25 minutes until onions are very soft and caramelized.

2 Add wine and bring to a boil, then reduce heat to medium and simmer 5 minutes. Remove bay leaves. Sprinkle mixture with flour and stir. Reduce heat to medium-low and cook 10 minutes.

3 Add beef broth and bring soup back to a simmer. Cook for 10 minutes.

Classic Tomato Soup

SERVES 6

Per Serving:

Calories	70
Fat	2g
Protein	2g
Sodium	300mg
Fiber	2g
Carbohydrates	10g
Sugar	6g

This Classic Tomato Soup is a go-to favorite on a cold day. It is often served with a grilled cheese sandwich, but it is also great served with Garlic Breadsticks (see recipe in Chapter 8).

4 tablespoons dairy-free buttery spread
½ large sweet onion, peeled and sliced
1½ cups gluten-free chicken stock
1 (28-ounce) can peeled tomatoes, including liquid
½ teaspoon salt
1 teaspoon granulated sugar

1 Melt buttery spread in a large pot over medium heat. Add onions, stock, tomatoes, salt, and sugar and stir to combine. Bring to a simmer and cook uncovered for 40 minutes, stirring occasionally.

2 Blend with an immersion blender or transfer to a blender and blend in batches until smooth and well combined. Serve warm.

Butternut Squash Soup

This rich Butternut Squash Soup is a healthy dinner that you can have on the table in about 30 minutes. It goes great with homemade gluten-free and dairy-free bread or rolls.

2 tablespoons dairy-free buttery spread

1 medium sweet onion, peeled and chopped

1 (3-pound) butternut squash, peeled, seeded, and diced

4 cups gluten-free chicken stock

1 tablespoon pure maple syrup

⅛ teaspoon ground nutmeg

½ teaspoon salt

¼ teaspoon ground black pepper

SERVES 6	
Per Serving:	
Calories	150
Fat	2g
Protein	6g
Sodium	300mg
Fiber	8g
Carbohydrates	32g
Sugar	10g

1 In a large pot, melt the buttery spread over medium heat. Add onions and cook for 6–8 minutes until translucent. Add squash and stock. Bring to a simmer and cook for 15–20 minutes until squash is tender.

2 Remove squash with a slotted spoon and place in a blender and purée. Return blended squash to the pot. Stir in maple syrup, nutmeg, salt, and pepper. Serve.

Ramen Soup with Eggs

Store-bought ramen has nothing on this classic ramen recipe that is packed with fresh, savory ingredients! This makes a great take-along lunch to school or work.

2 teaspoons sesame oil

1 tablespoon jarred minced ginger

1 tablespoon jarred minced garlic

½ cup sliced shitake mushrooms

3 tablespoons gluten-free soy sauce

1 tablespoon rice wine vinegar

6 cups gluten-free chicken stock

4 servings gluten-free ramen noodles (4 cubes dried ramen)

2 large soft-boiled eggs, halved

¼ cup sliced green onion

SERVES 4	
Per Serving:	
Calories	240
Fat	11g
Protein	14g
Sodium	1,290mg
Fiber	1g
Carbohydrates	20g
Sugar	2g

1 Heat oil in a large pot over medium heat. Add ginger and garlic and sauté for 30 seconds until fragrant. Add mushrooms and sauté for 2 minutes until tender. Add soy sauce and vinegar and stir to combine. Add stock, cover, and bring to a boil. Remove the lid and let simmer uncovered for 2 minutes.

2 Add ramen noodles to pot and cook according to the package directions until soft. Divide noodles into four bowls, pour in broth, and top with a half of a soft-boiled egg and green onions.

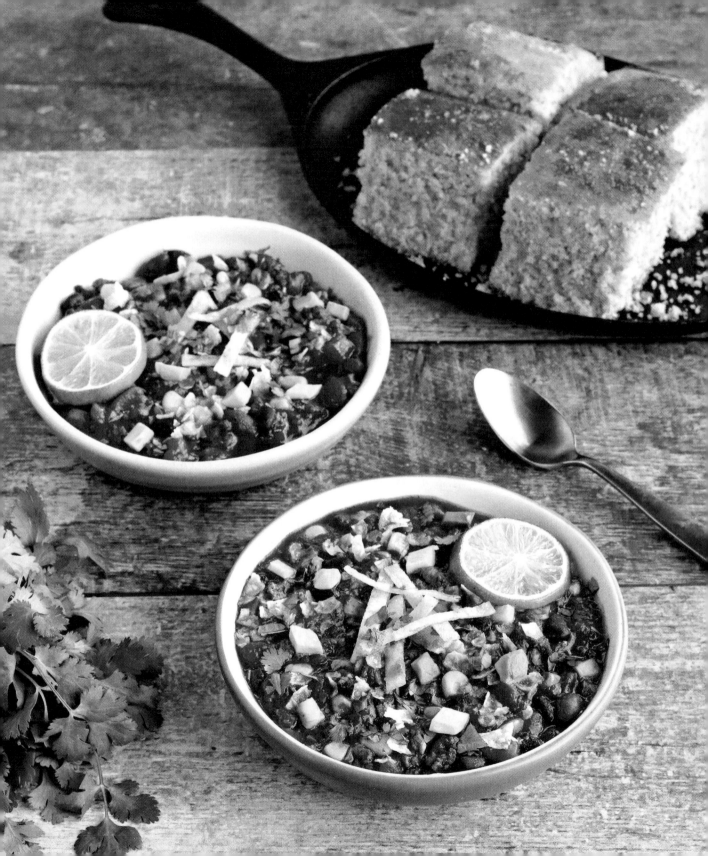

Taco Soup

If you have not tried your favorite taco flavors as a soup, you're missing out! When you've run out of gluten-free and dairy-free tortillas, this is a great way to satisfy a taco craving. Top with diced avocado and lime and serve with Southern Sweet Corn Bread (see recipe in Chapter 8), if desired.

1 teaspoon olive oil

1 tablespoon jarred minced garlic

1 pound 90/10 ground beef

1 tablespoon onion powder

2 teaspoons chili powder

½ teaspoon dried oregano

1 teaspoon ground cumin

½ teaspoon paprika

1 teaspoon salt

⅛ teaspoon ground black pepper

1 (28-ounce) can crushed tomatoes, including liquid

1 (4-ounce) can diced green chiles

1 (15-ounce) can kidney beans, drained and rinsed

1 (15-ounce) can black beans, drained and rinsed

1 (15-ounce) can corn, drained

2 cups gluten-free beef broth

1 cup crushed gluten-free corn chips

1   In a large pot, heat olive oil over medium heat. Add garlic and sauté for 30 seconds until tender. Add beef and cook for 5–7 minutes, stirring frequently, until beef is brown and crumbled; drain excess fat. Add remaining ingredients except corn chips and stir to combine. Bring to a boil, then reduce heat and simmer for 20 minutes.

2   Garnish with crushed corn chips to serve.

SERVES 6

Per Serving:

Calories	500
Fat	18g
Protein	30g
Sodium	1,290mg
Fiber	12g
Carbohydrates	55g
Sugar	6g

SPOTLIGHT ON VITAMIN A

Vitamin A is important for various processes in the body. It is most well known for promoting vision, lowering risks of cancer, and supporting a healthy immune system. It is found in many foods, including carrots, beans, eggs, and green leafy vegetables.

Maryland-Style Cream of Crab Soup

SERVES 6

Per Serving:

Calories	165
Fat	7g
Protein	14g
Sodium	800mg
Fiber	0g
Carbohydrates	10g
Sugar	1g

You won't believe this creamy, rich soup is dairy-free! Pair it with home-made gluten-free and dairy-free bread, and you've got a full meal.

½ cup dairy-free buttery spread
½ cup peeled and minced sweet onion
½ cup gluten-free all-purpose flour with xanthan gum
1 tablespoon Old Bay Seasoning
4 cups unsweetened almond milk
1 pound lump crabmeat, drained and picked over to remove any shells
3 tablespoons cooking sherry

1 Melt buttery spread in a medium saucepan over medium heat. Add onions; cook and stir 5 minutes until softened. Add flour and Old Bay Seasoning and whisk until well blended. Pour in milk and whisk constantly, bringing to a boil.

2 Stir in crabmeat. Reduce heat to low; simmer for 20 minutes, stirring occasionally. Stir in sherry and cook for 1 minute. Serve.

White Chicken Chili

SERVES 4

Per Serving:

Calories	480
Fat	10g
Protein	41g
Sodium	470mg
Fiber	13g
Carbohydrates	56g
Sugar	9g

If you like traditional tomato-based chili, try this White Chicken Chili for a delicious variation! It goes great with restaurant-quality gluten-free tortilla chips.

1 tablespoon olive oil
2 (6-ounce) boneless, skinless chicken breasts, cut into 1" pieces
1 large sweet onion, peeled and chopped
1 teaspoon jarred minced garlic
5 cups gluten-free chicken broth
3 (15-ounce) cans cannellini (white kidney) beans, rinsed and drained
2 (4-ounce) cans chopped green chiles
1 tablespoon dried oregano
2 teaspoons ground cumin
½ teaspoon salt
¼ cup chopped fresh cilantro

1 Heat olive oil in a large pot over medium heat. Add chicken, onions, and garlic. Cook for 5–8 minutes until chicken is browned.

2 Add the broth, beans, chiles, oregano, cumin, and salt. Bring the mixture to a simmer and cook for 20–30 minutes until chicken is no longer pink and is cooked through. Divide into four bowls and top with cilantro.

New England Clam Chowder

Everyone will go wild for this rich and creamy New England Clam Chowder! This chowder combines the flavors of clam, bacon, and garlic in a unique and sensational way.

6 strips thick-cut gluten-free bacon, diced
2 tablespoons dairy-free buttery spread
2 celery stalks, chopped
1 medium sweet onion, peeled and finely diced
1 teaspoon jarred minced garlic
2 cups gluten-free chicken broth
3 cups peeled and diced russet potatoes
1 (8-ounce) bottle clam juice
2 bay leaves
½ teaspoon dried parsley
¼ teaspoon dried thyme
½ cup gluten-free all-purpose flour with xanthan gum
1 cup unsweetened almond milk
2 (10-ounce) cans chopped clams in juice

1 In a large pot, cook bacon for 3–5 minutes over medium heat until crisp. Remove to paper towels to drain; set aside. Add buttery spread and sauté celery and onions for 3–5 minutes until tender. Add garlic; sauté for 1 minute.

2 Add broth, potatoes, clam juice, bay leaves, parsley, and thyme. Bring to a boil. Reduce heat to medium and simmer uncovered for 15–20 minutes until potatoes are fork-tender.

3 In a small bowl, whisk together flour and milk until smooth, and gradually stir the mixture into soup. Bring to a boil, stirring frequently, and cook for 1–2 minutes until thickened. Stir in clams and remove bay leaves. Crumble cooked bacon and sprinkle over each serving.

SERVES 6

Per Serving:

Calories	360
Fat	6g
Protein	41g
Sodium	460mg
Fiber	2g
Carbohydrates	33g
Sugar	2g

Mexican Pork Posole

Posole a traditional Mexican pork stew made with hominy, a type of dried corn. The ingredients and spices used create an intricate flavor sensation.

SERVES 8

Per Serving:

Calories	260
Fat	8g
Protein	14g
Sodium	960mg
Fiber	1g
Carbohydrates	35g
Sugar	11g

COLORFUL POSOLE

There are different types of posole that are all equally delicious. There is white, red, and green. The three colors vary depending on the type of chile used. The different versions typically include either pork or chicken and are normally served at special occasions.

2 tablespoons olive oil

1 large sweet onion, peeled and chopped

1 jalapeño, seeded and chopped (about 1 tablespoon)

2 teaspoons jarred minced garlic

4 cups gluten-free chicken broth, divided

2 (4-ounce) cans green chiles, drained

½ cup chopped fresh cilantro leaves

2 teaspoons ground cumin, divided

½ teaspoon dried oregano

½ teaspoon paprika

1 (15-ounce) can white hominy, rinsed and drained

1 (15-ounce) can pinto beans, rinsed and drained

2 cups shredded cooked pork

1 tablespoon lime juice

1 Heat olive oil in a large skillet over medium heat. Add onions and jalapeño and cook for 5 minutes or until onions are tender, stirring occasionally. Stir in garlic and cook for 30 seconds until fragrant. Spoon the onion mixture into a blender. Add ½ cup broth, chiles, and cilantro to the blender. Cover and blend until the mixture is smooth.

2 Cook the blended onion mixture and 1 teaspoon cumin in a large saucepan over medium heat for 5 minutes or until thickened, stirring often. Stir in the remaining broth, remaining cumin, oregano, paprika, hominy, and beans and heat to a boil. Reduce the heat to medium-low. Add pork and cook for 5 minutes, stirring occasionally. Stir in lime juice. Serve warm.

Stuffed Pepper Soup

This creative innovation brings the flavors of traditional stuffed peppers to a meaty, filling soup. Substitute ground turkey for beef for an equally delicious meat option.

1 teaspoon olive oil
1 pound 90/10 ground beef
½ teaspoon salt
⅛ teaspoon ground black pepper
1 large green bell pepper, seeded and diced
1 large red bell pepper, seeded and diced
1 cup peeled and diced sweet onion
2 teaspoons jarred minced garlic
1 (28-ounce) can diced tomatoes, undrained
1 (15-ounce) can tomato sauce
2 cups gluten-free beef broth
1 tablespoon light brown sugar, packed
1 teaspoon dried basil
1 teaspoon dried oregano
2 cups cooked long grain white rice

SERVES 6

Per Serving:

Calories	320
Fat	12g
Protein	20g
Sodium	825mg
Fiber	5g
Carbohydrates	33g
Sugar	11g

1. In a large pot, heat olive oil over medium heat. Add beef, salt, and black pepper. Cook for 7–8 minutes, stirring occasionally while breaking up beef, until browned. Drain beef of excess fat and add bell peppers, onions, and garlic. Cook for 2–3 minutes until onion is translucent.

2. Add tomatoes, tomato sauce, broth, brown sugar, basil, and oregano and stir to combine. Cover and simmer for 30 minutes until peppers are tender. Add cooked rice to soup, stir to combine, and cook for 10 minutes uncovered. Serve.

Maple Bacon Sweet Potato Soup

SERVES 4

Per Serving:

Calories	490
Fat	5g
Protein	12g
Sodium	575mg
Fiber	7g
Carbohydrates	100g
Sugar	47g

Savory bacon is the star of this show. This dish is a sweet and savory delight in every spoonful!

2 tablespoons dairy-free buttery spread
1 cup peeled and diced sweet onion
8 cups peeled and chopped sweet potato
2 cups gluten-free chicken broth
2 teaspoons ground cinnamon

½ teaspoon ground nutmeg
½ teaspoon salt
⅛ teaspoon ground black pepper
4 tablespoons pure maple syrup
6 strips cooked gluten-free bacon, crumbled

1   In a large pot, melt buttery spread over medium heat. Add in onions and sauté for 1–2 minutes until tender. Add in sweet potatoes, broth, and spices. Cover and bring to a boil. Let simmer for 15–20 minutes until potatoes have softened. Add maple syrup and stir.

2   Blend with an immersion blender or transfer to a blender and blend in batches until smooth and well combined. Serve topped with crumbled bacon.

Black Bean Soup

SERVES 4

Per Serving:

Calories	545
Fat	6g
Protein	33g
Sodium	1,300mg
Fiber	33g
Carbohydrates	89g
Sugar	11g

This easy Black Bean Soup is filled with an assortment of flavors that creates a multilayered product.

1 teaspoon olive oil
6 strips gluten-free bacon, finely chopped
1 medium sweet onion, peeled and chopped
2 tablespoons jarred minced garlic
1 cup gluten-free chicken broth
1½ cups canned chopped tomatoes, including liquid
2 tablespoons ketchup

2 teaspoons gluten-free Worcestershire sauce
¼ teaspoon salt
⅛ teaspoon ground black pepper
1 tablespoon chili powder
4 (15.5-ounce) cans black beans, drained and rinsed
2 tablespoons lime juice
½ cup chopped cilantro

1   Add olive oil in a large pot over medium heat. Add bacon and cook for 3–4 minutes. Stir in onions and cook for 3–4 minutes, stirring occasionally, until translucent. Stir in garlic and cook for 1 minute until fragrant.

2   Add broth, tomatoes, ketchup, Worcestershire sauce, salt, pepper, and chili powder. Stir in beans, turn the heat to high and bring to a low boil. Add lime juice and cook for 10 minutes. Serve with chopped cilantro.

Chicken Pot Pie Soup

If you liked chicken pot pie when you were a kid, then you will absolutely love this savory Chicken Pot Pie Soup. It tastes just like traditional chicken pot pie and is much easier to prepare—plus, you don't have to worry about the gluten-based crust if you make it in soup form!

2 tablespoons dairy-free buttery spread
1 cup peeled and diced russet potatoes
1 cup peeled and chopped sweet onion
½ cup chopped celery
1 cup peeled and chopped carrots
½ cup gluten-free all-purpose flour with xanthan gum
½ teaspoon salt
¼ teaspoon ground black pepper
2 cups gluten-free chicken broth
1 cup frozen corn
1 cup frozen peas
2 cups shredded cooked chicken

1 Heat buttery spread in a large pot over medium-high heat. Add potatoes, onions, celery, and carrots; cook and stir for 5–7 minutes until onions are tender.

2 Stir in flour, salt, and pepper until combined; whisk in broth. Bring to a boil over high heat, stirring occasionally.

3 Reduce heat; simmer uncovered for 10–15 minutes or until potatoes are fork-tender. Stir in corn, peas, and chicken and cook for 5–10 minutes until vegetables are heated through.

SERVES 6

Per Serving:

Calories	215
Fat	3g
Protein	18g
Sodium	360mg
Fiber	4g
Carbohydrates	29g
Sugar	6g

Egg Drop Soup

SERVES 4

Per Serving:

Calories	100
Fat	5g
Protein	9g
Sodium	150mg
Fiber	0g
Carbohydrates	5g
Sugar	1g

Stay at home tonight because this Egg Drop Soup is just as good as your best local Chinese restaurant! This light soup is a great starting course for many meal options.

3 cups gluten-free chicken broth
1 teaspoon ground ginger
¼ teaspoon garlic powder
½ teaspoon gluten-free soy sauce
½ teaspoon toasted sesame oil

1 tablespoon cornstarch
2 tablespoons cold water
3 large eggs, whisked
1 green onion, sliced

1 In a large saucepan, add broth, ginger, garlic powder, soy sauce, and sesame oil and bring to a boil over medium heat.

2 In a small bowl, whisk together cornstarch and water until cornstarch is dissolved. Slowly pour the mixture into broth and stir. Bring to a boil; cook and stir for 2 minutes or until thickened.

3 Reduce heat and simmer for 1–2 minutes. Slowly pour whisked eggs into hot broth, stirring constantly. The egg will spread and feather. Remove from the heat; stir in onions and serve immediately.

Tex-Mex Chicken Noodle Soup

SERVES 6

Per Serving:

Calories	430
Fat	7g
Protein	26g
Sodium	810mg
Fiber	3g
Carbohydrates	66g
Sugar	6g

Take your ordinary chicken noodle soup to the Southwest with this Tex-Mex twist! This immune-boosting soup tastes good and is good for you. The oregano, garlic, and chicken all have immune-boosting properties.

1 tablespoon olive oil
1 large sweet onion, peeled and diced
2 teaspoons jarred minced garlic
1 medium carrot, peeled and sliced into half-moons
1 (15-ounce) can corn, drained
1 tablespoon dried oregano
1 tablespoon ground cumin
2 teaspoons chili powder

½ teaspoon salt
1 (15-ounce) can diced tomatoes, including liquid
6 cups gluten-free chicken broth
1 (12-ounce) box gluten-free rotini pasta
2 cups shredded cooked chicken
2 tablespoons lime juice
¼ cup chopped fresh cilantro

1 Heat olive oil in a large pot over medium heat. Add onions and cook for 2 minutes until soft. Add garlic, carrots, and corn and stir until combined. Add oregano, cumin, chili powder, and salt and stir to combine.

2 Add tomatoes and chicken broth and simmer. Add pasta and cook to al dente according to the package directions. Add chicken and lime juice and stir to combine. Cook for 2 minutes. Serve topped with cilantro.

CHAPTER 10

Appetizers

Crispy Baked Buffalo Wings

SERVES 6

Per Serving:

Calories	620
Fat	42g
Protein	53g
Sodium	1,280mg
Fiber	0g
Carbohydrates	5g
Sugar	0g

SOME LIKE IT HOT

Many years ago, there were only a few choices of quality hot sauce. With the growing popularity of spicy flavors, you will now find lots of choices for hot sauces right in your local grocery store. Make sure to always check your labels to verify that a sauce is both gluten-free and dairy-free.

Prepare yourself for the best home-cooked buffalo wings that you've ever eaten! This incredibly simple recipe will give you irresistible wings every time. Serve with celery sticks and gluten-free and dairy-free ranch dressing.

4 pounds chicken wings, wingettes, and drumettes
½ cup gluten-free baking powder
1 teaspoon garlic powder
½ teaspoon salt
⅛ teaspoon ground black pepper
½ cup Frank's RedHot Sauce
4 tablespoons dairy-free buttery spread
1 tablespoon honey
1½ teaspoons cornstarch
1 tablespoon water

1. Adjust oven rack to the middle position. Preheat oven to 450°F. Line a rimmed baking sheet with aluminum foil, set a heatproof wire rack on the pan, and spray the rack with gluten-free nonstick cooking spray.

2. Pat wings dry with paper towels. Place wings in a large sealable plastic bag. Add baking powder, garlic powder, salt, and pepper and seal the bag. Shake and turn the bag to evenly coat wings.

3. Place wings skin-side up on the rack. Bake for 30 minutes, flip the wings over, and bake for an additional 20–30 minutes until wings are crispy and golden brown.

4. In a small saucepan, add hot sauce, buttery spread, and honey. Cook over medium heat for 1–2 minutes, stirring until ingredients are melted and combined. In a small bowl, combine cornstarch and water. Immediately add the cornstarch mixture to sauce and whisk to combine. Constantly whisk and cook sauce for 15–30 seconds until thickened.

5. Pour sauce into a large bowl. Immediately transfer hot wings to the large bowl and toss with sauce to coat.

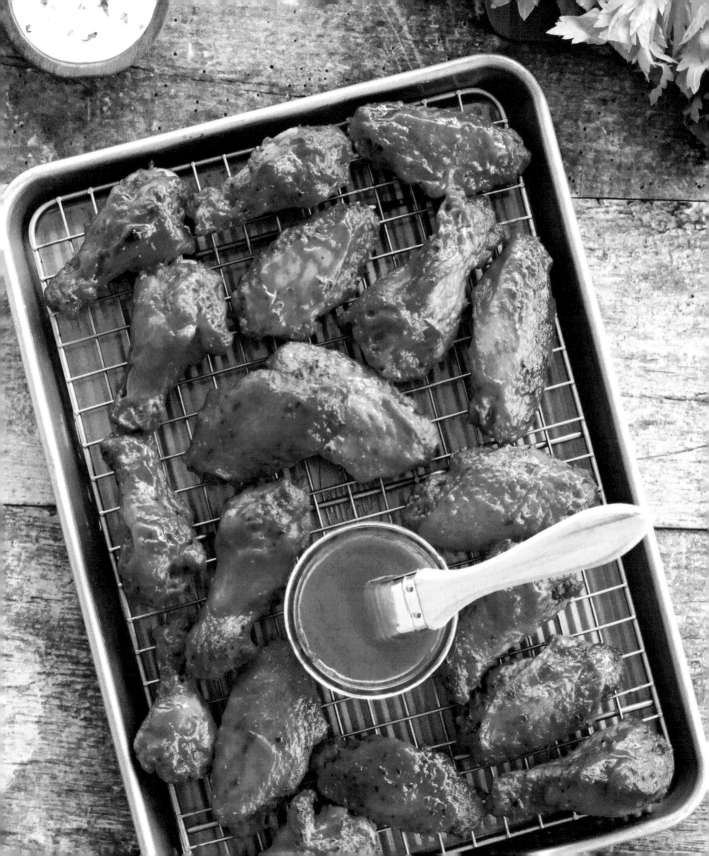

Fried Green Tomatoes

This is a traditional southern favorite that you can make to suit your dietary needs by using gluten-free cornmeal and gluten-free flour. This is a true taste of the South that nothing else can match!

SERVES 4

Per Serving:

Calories	820
Fat	67g
Protein	6g
Sodium	2,900mg
Fiber	3g
Carbohydrates	51g
Sugar	6g

GREEN TOMATOES

Green tomatoes are simply tomatoes that have not yet ripened. They have a tangy and almost sour flavor when uncooked, so they are not frequently eaten raw. However, when you bread and deep-fry them, the tanginess and sour flavor turn into a perfect combination of fresh, tangy, and savory flavors. Frying the tomatoes also softens them and makes them juicy.

TOMATOES

3 large firm green tomatoes
1 teaspoon salt
½ cup unsweetened almond milk
1½ teaspoons white vinegar
1½ cups vegetable oil
½ cup gluten-free all-purpose flour with xanthan gum
1 cup gluten-free cornmeal
½ cup cornstarch
1 tablespoon seasoned salt

REMOULADE SAUCE

1 cup mayonnaise
1 teaspoon horseradish sauce
½ teaspoon onion powder
½ teaspoon paprika
¼ teaspoon garlic powder
1 teaspoon lemon juice
¼ teaspoon salt

1 Slice tomatoes ¼" thick and place on a paper towel–lined plate. Salt tomatoes on both sides and let sit for 10 minutes. (Do not skip this step; it helps draw extra water out of tomatoes so they are crispier when fried.)

2 Add milk and vinegar into a pie pan or shallow dish and allow to sit for 1–2 minutes. Add tomatoes to the milk mixture.

3 Combine all the remoulade ingredients in a small bowl. Cover and refrigerate until serving.

4 Continue with tomatoes by heating oil in a large skillet over medium-high heat.

5 Combine flour, cornmeal, cornstarch, and seasoned salt to a pie pan or shallow dish. Mix until fully combined.

6 Dip milk-covered tomatoes into the flour mixture. Cover both sides of tomatoes with the mixture.

7 Place tomatoes into the skillet in batches of four or five. Do not crowd tomatoes; they should not touch each other. Cook 2 minutes on each side or until golden brown. Remove from pan and place on a paper towel–lined plate. Repeat with remaining tomatoes. Serve with remoulade sauce while tomatoes are still hot.

Avocado Spring Rolls with Cashew and Cilantro Dipping Sauce

These incredibly tasty avocado spring rolls taste just like the spring rolls at one of your favorite chain restaurants! Now you can make them at home with ingredients you can control.

DIPPING SAUCE

4 teaspoons white vinegar
1 teaspoon balsamic vinegar
½ cup honey
½ cup chopped cashews
1¼ cups chopped fresh cilantro
1 tablespoon jarred minced garlic
2 green onions, sliced
1 tablespoon granulated sugar
1 teaspoon ground cumin
½ teaspoon ground turmeric
¼ cup olive oil

FILLING

2 large avocados, peeled, pitted, and diced
½ cup chopped sun-dried tomatoes packed in oil
¼ teaspoon chopped fresh cilantro

WRAPPING

8 (8") round rice paper wrappers
2 cups vegetable oil

MAKES 8 ROLLS

Per Serving
(Serving Size: 2 rolls):

Calories	670
Fat	43g
Protein	8g
Sodium	72mg
Fiber	7g
Carbohydrates	67g
Sugar	37g

REFRIGERATING AVOCADOS

If you are not going to use both halves of an avocado, do not remove the pit from one of the halves. Sprinkle the unused portion with lime juice, wrap tightly with plastic wrap, and refrigerate to help it not turn brown right away. Make sure to remove the pit before eating.

1 In a medium microwave-safe bowl, stir together vinegars and honey and microwave for 1 minute.

2 In a food processor purée cashews, 1 cup cilantro, garlic, onions, sugar, cumin, and turmeric.

3 Add the cashew mixture to the vinegar mixture and stir to combine. Add olive oil and stir to fully combine. Cover and refrigerate.

4 In a medium bowl, stir together the filling ingredients.

5 Fill a 9" cake pan with warm water. Submerge a rice paper into the water for 2 seconds. Place the rice papers on a cutting board, smooth-side down.

6 Place 2 tablespoons filling in the center of a paper. Fold the left and right edges of the rice paper in, then starting from the bottom, roll up to cover the filling. Then keep rolling until you reach the end. The rice paper is sticky, so it will seal itself. Place on a plate and repeat with remaining rice paper wrappers.

7 Heat oil in a large work or skillet over medium-high heat. Fry spring rolls in batches of four at a time for 2 minutes on each side until lightly golden. Remove with a slotted spoon to a paper towel–lined plate to absorb excess oil. Serve with dipping sauce.

Smoked Salmon Dip

SERVES 8

Per Serving:

Calories	96
Fat	6g
Protein	6g
Sodium	410mg
Fiber	0g
Carbohydrates	3g
Sugar	0g

This recipe will impress your party guests and will be gone before you know it! The rich and smoky flavor of salmon and the rich dairy-free cream cheese make this a must-have for your next event.

8 ounces dairy-free cream cheese
½ teaspoon horseradish sauce
2 tablespoons dried dill
½ teaspoon jarred minced garlic
1 tablespoon lemon juice

¼ teaspoon salt
1 tablespoon capers, minced
1 green onion, sliced
8 ounces smoked salmon

1 Add all ingredients to the bowl of a food processor and pulse until salmon is chopped well and everything is combined. Do not overprocess.

2 Place dip in a small bowl, cover with plastic wrap, and refrigerator for at least 30 minutes before serving.

Easy Guacamole

SERVES 4

Per Serving:

Calories	195
Fat	16g
Protein	3g
Sodium	16mg
Fiber	8g
Carbohydrates	14g
Sugar	3g

This is the delicious, traditional homemade guacamole recipe that is a must-have for any authentic Mexican meal or your next potluck event. Buy the avocados that aren't super ripe yet one or two days before you need to use them. The most popular avocado to make guacamole is the Mexican Hass avocado.

3 large ripe avocados, peeled, pitted, and mashed
2 tablespoons lime juice
½ teaspoon salt
½ teaspoon ground cumin

½ medium sweet onion, peeled and diced
2 large Roma tomatoes, diced
½ cup chopped fresh cilantro
½ teaspoon jarred minced garlic

In a large bowl, stir together avocado and lime juice and toss to coat. Add salt and cumin and stir to combine. Fold in onions, tomatoes, cilantro, and garlic and stir to fully combine ingredients.

Deep-Dish Pizza Bites

These easy mini pizzas are perfect for lunch, an after-school snack, an appetizer, or a quick and easy dinner!

2 large eggs, whisked
½ teaspoon garlic powder
1 teaspoon dried basil
1 teaspoon dried oregano
1⅓ cups Bisquick Gluten Free Pancake & Baking Mix

½ cup water
⅓ cup olive oil
1½ cups shredded dairy-free mozzarella cheese, divided
¾ cup gluten-free pizza sauce

MAKES 12 BITES

Per Serving (Serving Size: 1 bite):

Calories	160
Fat	9g
Protein	5g
Sodium	300mg
Fiber	1g
Carbohydrates	14g
Sugar	5g

1　Preheat oven to 425°F. Spray a twelve-cup muffin tin with gluten-free nonstick cooking spray.

2　In a medium bowl, add eggs, garlic powder, basil, and oregano and stir until fully combined. Add Bisquick, water, and olive oil and mix well.

3　Fill each muffin well three-quarters full. Sprinkle 1 tablespoon dairy-free cheese over the top of batter. Spoon 1 tablespoon pizza sauce over cheese. Add another layer of cheese over sauce. Bake for 15 minutes. Allow to cool for 2 minutes before removing from pan.

Spinach, Sundried Tomatoes, and Artichoke Dip

This dip is served at many popular restaurants and is popular with good reason. It's rich and delicious! Serve with restaurant-quality gluten-free corn tortilla chips or your favorite gluten-free and dairy-free cracker.

1 (10-ounce) package frozen chopped spinach, defrosted and drained
2 (13.75-ounce) cans artichoke hearts, drained and chopped
1 cup chopped sun-dried tomatoes
½ cup mayonnaise

8 ounces dairy-free cream cheese
1 tablespoon lemon juice
½ teaspoon jarred minced garlic
½ teaspoon onion powder

SERVES 8

Per Serving:

Calories	215
Fat	15g
Protein	5g
Sodium	520mg
Fiber	3g
Carbohydrates	14g
Sugar	4g

1　Squeeze the excess liquid out of spinach. Add all ingredients to the bowl of a food processor and pulse until spinach and artichokes are chopped well and everything is combined. Do not overprocess.

2　Place dip in a small bowl, cover with plastic wrap, and refrigerator for at least 30 minutes before serving.

Sticky Asian Wings

These Sticky Asian Wings are a perfect balance of sweet and tangy. The flavors of the soy, apricot, and lime meld to turn ordinary wings into extraordinary!

Per Serving:

Calories	360
Fat	20g
Protein	27g
Sodium	470mg
Fiber	0g
Carbohydrates	18g
Sugar	12g

APRICOTS 101

Apricot is both the name for the tree and the fruit that grows on the tree. Apricots are incredibly healthy. They are loaded with vitamins K and A, potassium, copper, and phosphorus. They are believed to support heart health and have anti-inflammatory properties.

MARINADE

½ cup gluten-free soy sauce
½ cup lime juice
2 teaspoons jarred minced garlic
2 teaspoons jarred minced ginger
2 pounds chicken wingettes and drumettes

WING SAUCE

½ cup gluten-free apricot jam
½ teaspoon salt
⅛ teaspoon garlic powder
1 teaspoon jarred minced ginger
⅛ teaspoon onion powder
¼ cup lime juice

1 In a large sealable plastic bag, add the marinade ingredients, seal, and turn the bag a few times to coat wings. Refrigerate overnight, turning occasionally. Before cooking, drain and discard marinade.

2 Preheat oven to 375°F.

3 Line a 9" x 13" baking pan with aluminum foil. Spray a baking rack with gluten-free nonstick cooking spray and place into pan. Place wings on the rack and bake for 15 minutes.

4 In a medium saucepan, combine the wing sauce ingredients. Stir to fully combine. Cook over medium heat and bring to a low boil. Simmer for 2 minutes.

5 Remove wings from oven and baste with sauce.

6 Bake for an additional 40 minutes, turning and basting wings every 10 minutes.

7 Take wings out of the oven and turn the oven to broil. Broil wings for 2–5 minutes until lightly charred.

Loaded Mashed Potato Bites

Anyone who loves mashed potatoes will get a kick out of these tasty one-bite snacks.

3 cups cold mashed potatoes
4 strips gluten-free bacon, cooked and chopped
1 cup shredded dairy-free Cheddar cheese
1 green onion, sliced
2 large eggs, whisked
1½ cups gluten-free panko bread crumbs
2 cups vegetable oil

MAKES 24 BITES

Per Serving:

Calories	140
Fat	10g
Protein	1g
Sodium	200mg
Fiber	2g
Carbohydrates	12g
Sugar	1g

1 In a large bowl, mix together mashed potatoes, bacon, cheese, and green onion.

2 Using a small cookie scoop, scoop out the potato mixture and roll into 1½" balls. Dip balls into eggs and then dredge in panko, pressing to coat on all sides.

3 Heat oil in a large skillet over medium-high heat. Working in batches, add balls to hot oil and cook for 2–3 minutes on each side until golden and crispy. Transfer to a paper towel–lined plate. Allow to cool for 2–4 minutes before serving.

Party Meatballs

These meatballs are tender and full of bold, sweet flavor. Simmer them in a slow cooker and serve with toothpicks.

MEATBALLS
½ cup gluten-free bread crumbs
1 tablespoon Italian seasoning
½ tablespoon onion powder
½ teaspoon salt
1 tablespoon jarred minced garlic
6 tablespoons unsweetened almond milk
1 pound 90/10 ground beef
1 large egg, beaten

SAUCE
2 (12-ounce) bottles chili sauce
1 (32-ounce) jar gluten-free grape jelly

MAKES 24 MEATBALLS

**Per Serving
(Serving Size: 4 meatballs):**

Calories	570
Fat	10g
Protein	12g
Sodium	1,435mg
Fiber	1g
Carbohydrates	1g
Sugar	57g

1 Spray a slow cooker with gluten-free nonstick cooking spray.

2 Combine all the meatball ingredients in a large bowl. Use a cookie scoop or rounded tablespoon to form twenty-four meatballs. Place uncooked meatballs in the bottom of the slow cooker.

3 In a medium bowl, whisk together chili sauce and grape jelly. Pour over meatballs and cook on high for 3–4 hours until meatballs reach an internal temperature of 165°F.

Buffalo Chicken Dip

Sometimes you want the flavor of buffalo wings, but not the messy hands and face! This dip is a perfect solution. Scoop it up with restaurant-quality gluten-free tortilla chips, celery sticks, or your favorite gluten-free and dairy-free crackers.

2 (13-ounce) cans chicken breast, drained
½ cup mayonnaise
½ cup gluten-free and dairy-free ranch dressing
2 tablespoons gluten-free and dairy-free hot sauce

1 Preheat oven to 350°F and spray an 8" × 8" casserole dish with gluten-free nonstick cooking spray.

2 In a large bowl, add chicken, using a fork to shred it into small pieces. Add mayonnaise, ranch dressing, and hot sauce and stir to combine.

3 Transfer to prepared baking dish and bake for 20 minutes. Allow to cool for 5 minutes before serving.

Southwestern Queso Dip

This queso recipe is a creamy, dairy-free twist on the traditional party favorite that will satisfy your craving for traditional cheese. Add diced jalapeños for an extra blast of spice.

1 cup cashews
1 cup unsweetened cashew milk
¼ cup nutritional yeast
1 tablespoon olive oil
2 (15-ounce) cans black beans, drained and rinsed
1½ cups gluten-free chunky salsa
2 tablespoons gluten-free taco seasoning

1 Add water to a small saucepan and boil raw cashews in water for 5–10 minutes. Remove from heat and let cool in water, then drain. Blend in a food processor or blender with milk and yeast until smooth, scraping sides as needed.

2 Add the olive oil to a large skillet over medium heat. Add black beans, salsa, and taco seasoning and cook for 5–8 minutes, stirring until heated through. Stir in cashew sauce and stir to combine. Cook for 2–3 more minutes until thickened. Serve while hot.

Buffalo Chicken Bites

This recipe gives you the spicy, bold taste of game-day buffalo wings in easy-to-eat bites! They are also a great on-the-go snack for school or work.

1 (12.5-ounce) can chicken breast, drained
½ cup gluten-free and dairy-free buffalo wing sauce, divided
½ cup gluten-free and dairy-free ranch dressing, divided
2 cups shredded dairy-free Cheddar cheese
1½ cups Bisquick Gluten-Free Pancake & Baking Mix
¾ cup unsweetened almond milk

1 Preheat oven to 350°F degrees. Line a baking sheet with parchment paper.

2 In a large bowl, add chicken, ¼ cup buffalo wing sauce, and ¼ cup ranch dressing. Stir to fully coat chicken.

3 Add cheese and Bisquick to the chicken mixture. Mix until fully combined. Add milk and mix until fully combined.

4 Using a cookie scoop or a rounded tablespoon, make approximately thirty-six 1" balls from the mixture. Place balls on prepared baking sheet. Bake for 22–26 minutes until golden brown. Serve with remaining ¼ cup buffalo wing sauce and ¼ cup ranch dressing for dipping.

MAKES 36 BITES

**Per Serving
(Serving Size: 3 bites):**

Calories	180
Fat	10g
Protein	4g
Sodium	860mg
Fiber	0g
Carbohydrates	17g
Sugar	2g

APPETIZERS FOR DINNER

Appetizers are great for snacking on at dinner parties, but did you know that heavy appetizers also make great meals? Surprise your family and combine a couple of your favorite appetizers and serve them as the main course. You can also serve them with fresh gluten-free and dairy-free dinner rolls for a complete and enjoyable meal.

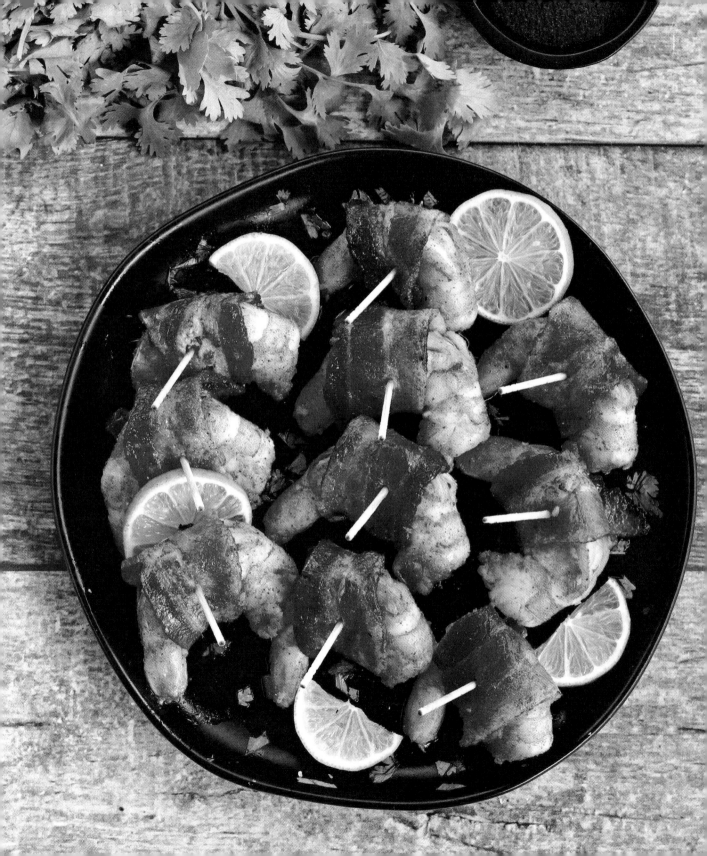

Chili Lime Bacon-Wrapped Shrimp

The sizzle of bacon wrapped around plump, fresh shrimp is an appetizer people will devour! This can easily be made into a healthier version by using turkey bacon. Sprinkle with freshly chopped cilantro, if desired.

¼ cup light brown sugar, packed
1 teaspoon onion powder
1 tablespoon jarred minced garlic
½ teaspoon chili powder
1 teaspoon paprika
¼ teaspoon kosher salt
2 tablespoons lime juice
2 tablespoons olive oil
20 large shrimp, peeled and deveined
10 strips gluten-free bacon, cut in half

SERVES 5

Per Serving:

Calories	340
Fat	27g
Protein	11g
Sodium	510mg
Fiber	0g
Carbohydrates	12g
Sugar	11g

1 Combine all of the ingredients except shrimp and bacon in a sealable plastic bag. Add shrimp, seal the bag, and turn over several times so marinade covers shrimp. Place in the refrigerator for 30 minutes.

2 Preheat oven to 450°F and line a jelly roll pan with aluminum foil and spray with gluten-free nonstick cooking spray.

3 Wrap each shrimp with half slice bacon, securing with a toothpick.

4 Bake for 10–15 minutes until bacon is crisp and shrimp turn pink.

Fried Pickles

SERVES 4

Per Serving:

Calories	250
Fat	15g
Protein	1g
Sodium	1,170mg
Fiber	1g
Carbohydrates	28g
Sugar	1g

HOW TO MAKE YOUR OWN PICKLES

Making your own pickles is easy! Slice small cucumbers the long way or slice them into rounds and combine them with apple cider vinegar, water, dill seed, garlic, and kosher salt in a Mason jar (look online for various recipes). With a little practice, and patience, you can have artful and delightful homemade pickles!

These sweet and crispy Fried Pickles will turn the ordinary hamburger into an extraordinary flavor celebration! You can also eat them as an appetizer with gluten-free and dairy-free ranch dressing for dipping.

½ cup unsweetened almond milk
1½ teaspoons white vinegar
2 cups sliced dill pickles, drained
½ cup gluten-free all-purpose flour with xanthan gum
½ cup gluten-free cornstarch
1 tablespoon seasoned salt
1½ cups vegetable oil

1 Add milk and vinegar to a pie pan or shallow dish and allow to sit for 1–2 minutes. Add pickles to the milk mixture.

2 Combine flour, cornstarch, and salt to a separate pie pan or shallow dish. Mix until fully combined.

3 Dip milk-covered pickles into the flour mixture. Cover both sides of pickles with the mixture. Place on a plate.

4 Heat oil in a large skillet over medium-high heat.

5 Place pickles into the skillet in batches and fry for 1–2 minutes until golden brown; remove with a slotted spoon and drain on a paper towel–lined plate. Repeat with remaining pickles.

Mexican Street Corn Dip

This recipe is a wonderful way to celebrate Cinco de Mayo, watch the big game, or just enjoy a quiet day on the front porch. It goes great with gluten-free blue corn tortilla chips.

8 ounces dairy-free cream cheese, softened

½ cup mayonnaise

1 teaspoon jarred minced garlic

½ teaspoon chili powder

½ teaspoon ground cumin

2 tablespoons lime juice

2 (15-ounce) cans corn, drained

2 tablespoons peeled and chopped red onion

½ cup chopped fresh cilantro

¼ teaspoon paprika

SERVES 6	
Per Serving:	
Calories	270
Fat	22g
Protein	4g
Sodium	430mg
Fiber	2g
Carbohydrates	16g
Sugar	4g

1 In a medium bowl, combine cream cheese, mayonnaise, garlic, chili powder, cumin, and lime juice and mix until fully combined and smooth.

2 Add corn, onions, and cilantro and stir to combine. Cover and refrigerate for at least 30 minutes before serving. Sprinkle with paprika before serving.

Easy Homemade Hummus

This hummus is creamy, full of flavor, and outrageously easy to make! You can add any number of gluten- and dairy-free ingredients to vary the flavor, like pine nuts or sun-dried tomatoes. Reserve the chickpea liquid in case you want to add any to thin out your hummus.

¼ cup tahini

¼ cup lemon juice

3 tablespoons olive oil, divided

2 teaspoons jarred minced garlic

1 teaspoon salt

½ teaspoon ground cumin

1 (15-ounce) can chickpeas, drained, divided

SERVES 6	
Per Serving:	
Calories	230
Fat	15g
Protein	7g
Sodium	560mg
Fiber	5g
Carbohydrates	19g
Sugar	3g

1 Add tahini and lemon juice to the bowl of a food processor and process for 1 minute.

2 Add 2 tablespoons olive oil, garlic, salt, and cumin to the mixture and process for 1 minute. Add half of chickpeas to the food processor and process for 1 minute. Scrape sides and bottom of the bowl, then add remaining chickpeas and process for 1–2 minutes until thick and smooth.

3 Transfer hummus to a small bowl and drizzle with remaining 1 tablespoon olive oil.

Seven-Layer Dip

WHAT TO USE FOR DIPS AND SPREADS

There are a variety of gluten-free and dairy-free crackers available. For example, gluten-free and dairy-free potato chips and tortilla chips are an easy and readily available option. Just make sure to always check your labels. Carrots or celery sticks are healthier options if you're counting calories or carbs.

Whether you are looking for an easy dip for the next party or just want something special for Saturday afternoon snacking, dive into the zesty flavor of this classic Seven-Layer Dip. The easy ingredient substitutions keep the flavors but ditch the dairy.

DAIRY-FREE SOUR CREAM

6 ounces dairy-free plain Greek yogurt

1 teaspoon lemon juice

DIP

2 tablespoons gluten-free taco seasoning

1 (16-ounce) can gluten-free refried beans

2 cups guacamole

1 cup gluten-free salsa

1 cup shredded lettuce

1 cup dairy-free Cheddar cheese shreds

¼ cup sliced black olives

½ cup diced green onion

½ cup chopped fresh cilantro

1 (11-ounce) bag gluten-free tortilla chips

1 Drain off any excess liquid from yogurt. Stir yogurt and lemon juice together in a small bowl. Cover and refrigerate at least 30 minutes before using.

2 In a small bowl, mix together sour cream and taco seasoning.

3 Spread beans onto the bottom of an 8" × 8" casserole dish sprayed with gluten-free nonstick cooking spray. Spread a layer of sour cream mixture over beans, then guacamole over the sour cream mixture, followed by a layer of salsa, then lettuce and cheese. Sprinkle olives, green onions, and cilantro over the top. Cover and refrigerate for 1 hour before serving. Serve with gluten-free tortilla chips.

Southwestern Spring Rolls

This recipe is an imaginative and delicious change from the traditional spring roll. You can always turn up the heat by adding diced jalapeños.

FILLING

½ cup chopped cooked chicken
1 large avocado, peeled, pitted, and diced
¼ cup canned corn, drained and rinsed
¼ cup canned black beans, drained and rinsed
¼ cup chopped fresh cilantro
1 teaspoon ground cumin
2 teaspoons lime juice

WRAPPING

8 (8") round rice paper wrappers
2 cups vegetable oil

1. In a medium bowl, stir together the filling ingredients.

2. Fill a 9" cake pan with warm water. Submerge a rice paper into the water for 2 seconds. Place the rice paper on a cutting board with smooth-side down.

3. Place 2 tablespoons filling in the center of the paper. Fold the left and right edges of the rice paper in, then starting from the bottom, roll up to cover the filling. Then keep rolling until you reach the end. The rice paper is sticky, so it will seal itself. Place on a plate and repeat with remaining rice paper wrappers.

4. Heat oil in a large work or skillet over medium-high heat. Fry spring rolls in batches of four at a time for 2 minutes on each side until lightly golden. Remove with a slotted spoon to a paper towel–lined plate to absorb excess oil and repeat with remaining rolls.

MAKES 8 ROLLS

Per Serving
(Serving Size: 2 rolls):

Calories	130
Fat	8g
Protein	5g
Sodium	40mg
Fiber	2g
Carbohydrates	10g
Sugar	0g

ALL TYPES OF SPRING ROLLS

Different varieties of spring rolls have been eaten in Asian countries for generations. The combinations of shrimp, beef, pork, vegetables, and fish are influenced by regional availability of ingredients and differing tastes from country to country. One of the newest versions to hit menus is the dessert spring roll, which can be filled with bananas, fruit, and chocolate.

Thai Chicken Skewers with Peanut Sauce

SERVES 4

Per Serving:

Calories	580
Fat	29g
Protein	59g
Sodium	76mg
Fiber	2g
Carbohydrates	15g
Sugar	8g

THE TASTE OF THAI FOOD

Thai food blends a mix of exotic flavors that is unlike any other food in the world. While it is true that many Thai dishes are very spicy, there are many perfectly mild dishes that are filled with fresh vegetables, healthy fruits, and flavor-packed sauces.

These perfectly marinated chicken skewers will take the trophy at any event, and the sauce is so good that you will never have enough! These marinated chicken skews are also perfect for a light dinner when paired with jasmine rice and Thai stir-fried vegetables. For extra peanut flavor, top with diced peanuts.

MARINADE

1 tablespoon gluten-free soy sauce
3 tablespoons lime juice
¼ teaspoon salt
⅛ teaspoon ground black pepper
1 tablespoon jarred minced garlic
1 tablespoon jarred minced ginger
½ teaspoon coriander
½ teaspoon ground cumin
½ teaspoon ground turmeric
2 tablespoons olive oil
2 pounds chicken tenders
¼ cup chopped fresh cilantro

DIPPING SAUCE

1 teaspoon jarred minced ginger
½ teaspoon jarred minced garlic
½ cup gluten-free peanut butter
2 teaspoons sesame oil
2 tablespoons gluten-free soy sauce
2 tablespoons lime juice
2 tablespoons light brown sugar, packed
¼ teaspoon sriracha
⅓ cup coconut milk beverage

1 In a medium bowl, whisk together soy sauce, lime juice, salt, pepper, garlic, ginger, coriander, cumin, turmeric, and olive oil. Add chicken and toss with marinade, cover, and refrigerate for 30 minutes.

2 Preheat grill. Skewer chicken tenders. Grill chicken for 4–5 minutes on each side until it is browned on both sides and cooked through. Sprinkle with cilantro.

3 Combine the dipping sauce ingredients in a small bowl until smooth and serve on the side.

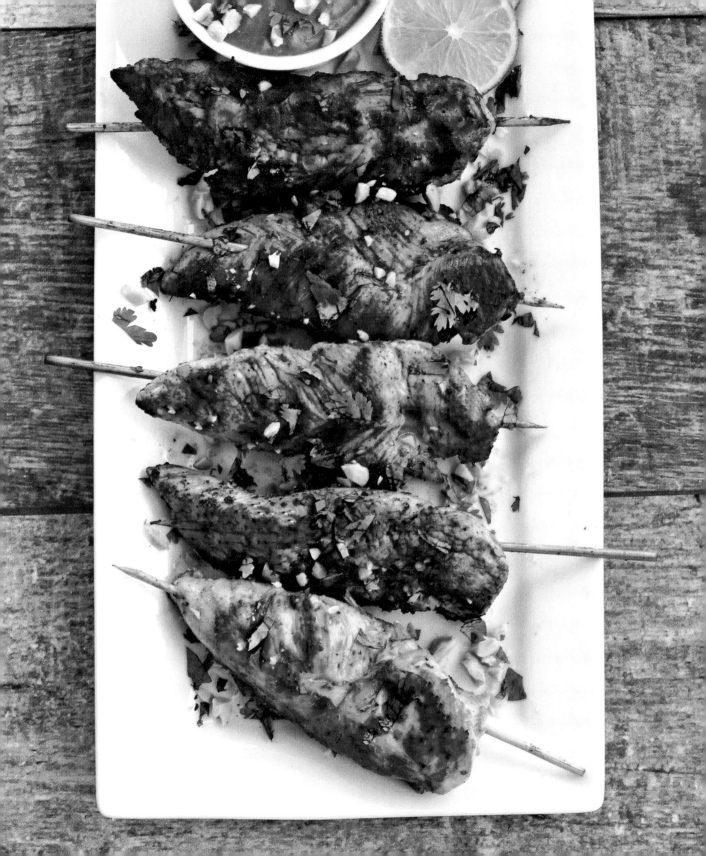

Italian Bruschetta

SERVES 4

Per Serving:

Calories	288
Fat	17g
Protein	4g
Sodium	410mg
Fiber	3g
Carbohydrates	25g
Sugar	7g

The taste of this traditional bruschetta recipe is straight out of Italy! Always use fresh and fully ripe Roma tomatoes for the best bruschetta.

8 large ripe Roma tomatoes, diced
6 fresh basil leaves, chopped
¼ teaspoon salt
⅛ teaspoon ground black pepper
2 tablespoons jarred minced garlic

4 tablespoons extra-virgin olive oil, divided
1 teaspoon balsamic vinegar
1 baguette gluten-free and dairy-free French bread

1 In a medium bowl, combine tomatoes, basil, salt, pepper, garlic, 1 tablespoon olive oil, and balsamic vinegar. Cover and refrigerate for 30 minutes.

2 Preheat oven to broil. Slice baguette, brush with remaining olive oil, and place on a baking sheet and broil for 1–2 minutes until bread is toasted. Top with the tomato mixture and serve.

Smoked Salmon with Cucumber and Dill

SERVES 6

Per Serving:

Calories	70
Fat	4g
Protein	5g
Sodium	220mg
Fiber	1g
Carbohydrates	3g
Sugar	1g

This sophisticated appetizer is one that you will be proud to take to even the most elegant events. This dip goes well with most varieties of gluten-free and dairy-free party crackers.

4 ounces dairy-free cream cheese, softened
2 tablespoons dried dill
2 tablespoons lemon juice

1 large English cucumber
4 ounces thinly sliced smoked salmon
½ teaspoon everything bagel seasoning

1 In a medium bowl, mix together cream cheese, dill, and lemon juice until smooth.

2 With a vegetable peeler, stripe cucumber, leaving a small strip of skin in between each peel. Slice cucumber into ¼" slices.

3 Place cucumber slices on a platter. Place ½ teaspoon cream cheese mixture on each cucumber. Fold strips of smoked salmon and place on top of the mixture. Sprinkle with everything bagel seasoning before serving.

Classic Deviled Eggs

No holiday meal would be complete without a chilled platter of fresh deviled eggs. If you're feeling adventurous, you can experiment with adding gluten-free bacon, seafood, or even green chiles.

6 large hard-boiled eggs, peeled and sliced in half, divided
2 tablespoons mayonnaise
½ teaspoon ground mustard
½ teaspoon white vinegar
¼ teaspoon salt
½ teaspoon dried dill

1 Remove yolks and place in a small bowl. Mash yolks with a fork and stir in mayonnaise, mustard, vinegar, and salt.

2 Fill egg whites evenly with the yolk mixture. Sprinkle with dill. Cover and chill in the refrigerator for at least 30 minutes before serving.

SERVES 6

Per Serving:

Calories	110
Fat	9g
Protein	6g
Sodium	190mg
Fiber	0g
Carbohydrates	1g
Sugar	1g

Pico de Gallo

After you try the authentic flavors of this classic fresh salsa, you will never buy premade salsa again! Use the freshest ingredients you can find.

12 large Roma tomatoes, chopped
1 cup peeled and chopped red onion
2 cups chopped fresh cilantro
1 small jalapeño pepper, veins and seeds removed, diced
3 tablespoons lime juice
½ teaspoon salt

Combine tomatoes, onions, cilantro, jalapeño, lime juice and salt in a small bowl. Cover and refrigerate for 30 minutes before serving.

SERVES 6

Per Serving:

Calories	18
Fat	0g
Protein	1g
Sodium	200mg
Fiber	1g
Carbohydrates	4g
Sugar	2g

Stuffed Mushrooms

SERVES 6

**Per Serving
(Serving Size:
5 mushrooms):**

Calories	320
Fat	23g
Protein	17g
Sodium	300mg
Fiber	2g
Carbohydrates	10g
Sugar	1g

MUSHROOM SHOPPING

To choose the best mushrooms, start by looking for the largest and firmest mushrooms at the supermarket. Avoid mushrooms that are slimy or look bruised and dented.

This recipe for classic Stuffed Mushrooms is full of flavor and beautifully browned, and it complements many dishes. You won't miss any of the dairy or gluten you usually find in traditional recipes!

1 tablespoon olive oil
¼ cup peeled and finely chopped sweet onion
½ teaspoon jarred minced garlic
1 pound gluten-free ground sausage
1 tablespoon dried sage
8 ounces dairy-free cream cheese
3 tablespoons nutritional yeast
⅓ cup gluten-free bread crumbs
3 teaspoons dried basil
1 teaspoon dried parsley
30 large fresh baby bella mushrooms, stems removed
3 tablespoons dairy-free buttery spread, melted

1 Preheat oven to 400°F. Spray a 9" × 13" baking dish with gluten-free nonstick cooking spray.

2 Heat olive oil in a large skillet over medium-high heat. Add onions and garlic and sauté for 30 seconds until garlic is fragrant. Add sausage and sage and cook for 6–8 minutes until sausage is no longer pink and onions are tender. Break up sausage into crumbles and drain. Add cream cheese and nutritional yeast; cook and stir until melted. Stir in bread crumbs, basil, and parsley.

3 Place mushroom caps in prepared baking pan, stem-side up. Brush with buttery spread. Spoon the sausage mixture into mushroom caps. Bake uncovered for 12–15 minutes until mushrooms are tender.

CHAPTER 11

Pressure Cooker and Slow Cooker

Pressure Cooker Mexican Rice

A pressure cooker makes this delicious rice recipe quickly and easily. This dish goes perfectly with homemade enchiladas or fajitas.

SERVES 6

Per Serving:

Calories	310
Fat	6g
Protein	7g
Sodium	235mg
Fiber	1g
Carbohydrates	56g
Sugar	5g

SPANISH RICE OR MEXICAN RICE?

There is some debate about what the difference between Spanish rice and Mexican rice is. While there is not a specific rice dish in Spain that fits the description, many areas of Mexico refer to this side dish as *Spanish rice*. To complicate matters, the combination of broth, tomato, onions, garlic, and spices varies from region to region in Latin America. Whatever name you give this dish, it is scrumptious!

2 tablespoons olive oil
¼ cup peeled and chopped sweet onion
1 teaspoon jarred minced garlic
2 cups long-grain white rice
2½ cups gluten-free chicken broth
¾ cup canned crushed tomatoes, including liquid
½ teaspoon ground cumin
½ teaspoon chili powder
½ teaspoon paprika
1 teaspoon salt
½ cup chopped fresh cilantro, divided

1 Set the pressure cooker to Sauté mode. When the display reads "Hot," add in olive oil, onions, and garlic. Sauté for 2–3 minutes or until garlic and onions are tender.

2 Add rice and stir until coated. Add in broth, tomatoes, cumin, chili powder, paprika, salt, and cilantro.

3 Press the Cancel button and place the lid on your pressure cooker and twist it so it locks in place and set the steam release knob to the Sealing position. Press the Manual button and set to 8 minutes. When the cooking cycle has finished, allow the pressure cooker to naturally release for 5 minutes. Once the pressure cooker reads "5 minutes," manually release by turning the knob to Venting. Hot steam will be released from the valve in venting mode. Once all steam has been released and the pressure valve lowers, remove the lid and serve. Take a fork and lightly fluff rice. Sprinkle with cilantro. Serve warm.

Pressure Cooker Collard Greens

This easy collard greens side dish is an age-old essential for Sunday lunch. The savory scent of slow-cooked collard greens will fill the house and keep everyone asking if lunch is ready yet! Serve it alongside Southern Chicken-Fried Steak (see recipe in Chapter 5).

1 tablespoon olive oil
8 strips thick-cut gluten-free bacon, sliced
½ cup peeled and diced sweet onion
2 teaspoons jarred minced garlic
2 cups gluten-free chicken broth
1 tablespoon apple cider vinegar
1 tablespoon light brown sugar, packed
2 teaspoons seasoned salt
1 (16-ounce) bag chopped collard greens

1 Set the pressure cooker to the Sauté setting. When the display reads "Hot," add olive oil. Add bacon, onions, and garlic and cook for 3–5 minutes, stirring occasionally, until tender.

2 Press the Cancel button. Add broth, vinegar, brown sugar, and salt; stir to combine. Add collard greens and put the lid on the pot and lock it into place. Set the steam release knob to the Sealing position. Press the Meat/Stew button and set to 35 minutes.

3 When the cooking cycle has finished, wait 10 minutes and then manually release the remaining steam by turning the knob to Venting. Hot steam will be released from the valve in venting mode. Once all steam has been released and the pressure valve lowers, remove the lid and serve. Serve warm.

SERVES 6

Per Serving:

Calories	234
Fat	18g
Protein	9g
Sodium	1,060mg
Fiber	3g
Carbohydrates	9g
Sugar	4g

NUTRITIONAL BENEFITS OF COLLARD GREENS

Collard greens are considered a superfood. They are a rich source of vitamins, minerals, and fiber. Collard greens are packed with vitamins K, B_6, C, A, and E. They are also low in calories and contain protein and fiber.

Slow Cooker Black Beans

SERVES 6

Per Serving:

Calories	290
Fat	2g
Protein	17g
Sodium	800mg
Fiber	12g
Carbohydrates	51g
Sugar	4g

Black beans are an easy and healthy side. Add a little cayenne pepper if you prefer things a little spicier.

1 pound dry black beans, picked over and rinsed
1 sweet onion, peeled and diced
2 teaspoons jarred minced garlic
1 bay leaf
2 teaspoons salt
6 cups water

1   Place black beans, onions, garlic, bay leaf and salt in a slow cooker. Add water. Cover and cook on high for about 3–4 hours until beans are soft, testing after 3 hours. If cooking on low, set it for 6–8 hours until beans are soft, testing after 6 hours.

2   Remove bay leaf and allow beans to cool for 10 minutes before serving.

Slow Cooker Apples and Cinnamon

SERVES 4

Per Serving:

Calories	250
Fat	2g
Protein	1g
Sodium	60mg
Fiber	7g
Carbohydrates	55g
Sugar	45g

This recipe for thick, sweet, and luscious slow-cooked apples and cinnamon tastes like a heaping helping of apple pie! Granny Smith apples are tart, but the brown sugar balances the flavor out well.

5 large Granny Smith apples, peeled and sliced into ½"-thick slices
2 tablespoons dairy-free buttery spread, melted
1 tablespoon fresh lemon juice
6 tablespoons light brown sugar, packed
1 teaspoon ground cinnamon
2 tablespoons apple cider

1   Spray a slow cooker with gluten-free nonstick cooking spray. Add apples, buttery spread, and lemon juice to the slow cooker and stir.

2   Sprinkle with brown sugar and cinnamon; toss to coat. Pour cider over apples. Cover and cook on low heat setting 3½ hours or until apples are tender.

Slow Cooker Pork Roast with Savory Gravy

This juicy cut of pork is the centerpiece for a cozy weekend dinner. Serve it alongside Roasted Garlic Potatoes and Honey-Glazed Carrots (see recipes in Chapter 7).

2 pounds pork loin roast

½ teaspoon salt

⅛ teaspoon ground black pepper

2 tablespoons olive oil

½ medium sweet onion, peeled and diced

2 tablespoons jarred minced garlic

½ cup gluten-free chicken broth

2 tablespoons gluten-free Worcestershire sauce

2 teaspoons dried thyme

1 teaspoon dried rosemary

1 tablespoon cornstarch

3 tablespoons water

1 Season pork with salt and pepper. Set the pressure cooker to the Sauté setting and add olive oil. Add pork and sear the sides a golden brown. Add onions and garlic and cook for 2 minutes until soft.

2 In a small bowl, stir together broth, Worcestershire sauce, thyme, and rosemary. Pour over pork. Press the Cancel button and put the lid on the pot and lock it into place. Set the steam release knob to the Sealing position. Press the Manual button and set to 30 minutes. When the cooking cycle has finished, manually release by turning the knob to Venting. Hot steam will be released from the valve in venting mode. Once all steam has been released and the pressure valve lowers, remove the lid and check that internal temperature of pork is 145°F.

3 Remove pork from the pressure cooker, place on a cutting board, cover with aluminum foil and allow to rest for 10 minutes.

4 Mix together cornstarch and water. Add to the pressure cooker with the juices. Turn pressure cooker on to Sauté and simmer until thickened. Slice pork, place on plates, and drizzle with gravy.

SERVES 8

Per Serving:

Calories	210
Fat	9g
Protein	26g
Sodium	270mg
Fiber	0g
Carbohydrates	4g
Sugar	2g

VARIOUS CUTS OF PORK

There are several cuts of pork, and with a little knowledge, you will become an expert at the meat counter. The cuts from the top of the pig are the loin, the pork chop, the sirloin, and baby back ribs. They tend to be more tender and leaner than other cuts. The cuts from the bottom of the pig are pork belly (bacon) and spare ribs. These cuts are best when smoked. And finally, the cut in the rear is the ham. It is best baked, cured, or smoked and sliced.

Pressure Cooker Baked Potatoes

SERVES 4

Per Serving:

Calories	110
Fat	0g
Protein	3g
Sodium	2mg
Fiber	2g
Carbohydrates	26g
Sugar	1g

These soft and creamy baked potatoes are rich in earthy flavor and cook in less than 30 minutes! Baked potatoes can be kept in the refrigerator in an airtight container for up to 3 days or frozen for up to 1 year.

1 cup water
4 medium russet potatoes

1 Place the metal trivet inside of the pressure cooker and add water.

2 Poke potatoes with a fork several times all over. Place potatoes on top of the wire rack. Place lid on pressure cooker and lock it into place. Set the steam release knob to the Sealing position. Press the Manual button and set to 14 minutes.

3 When the cooking cycle has finished, let it naturally release for 10 minutes, and then manually release by turning the knob to Venting. Hot steam will be released from the valve in venting mode. Once all steam has been released and the pressure valve lowers, remove the lid and serve.

Pressure Cooker Mashed Potatoes

SERVES 6

Per Serving:

Calories	155
Fat	3g
Protein	4g
Sodium	890mg
Fiber	2g
Carbohydrates	31g
Sugar	1g

Instant mashed potatoes are fast, but boxed options often contain gluten and milk-based ingredients. Cooking them in the oven can take an hour or more! Luckily, you can make them at home in a snap with your pressure cooker!

7 medium russet potatoes, peeled
4 cups water
⅓ cup dairy-free buttery spread
¼ cup unsweetened almond milk
2 teaspoons salt

1 Add potatoes to the cooker and pour water over them. Place lid on the pressure cooker and lock it into place. Set the steam release knob to the Sealing position. Press the Manual button and set to 12 minutes.

2 When the cooking cycle has finished, manually release pressure. Once all steam has been released and the pressure valve lowers, remove the lid and drain.

3 Transfer potatoes to a large bowl. Add buttery spread, milk, and salt and mash with a potato masher until you reach desired texture and smoothness.

Pressure Cooker New Orleans–Style Red Beans and Rice

This traditional recipe is bursting with Cajun flavors. If you soak the red beans ahead of time, you can savor the flavors of New Orleans in less than an hour.

2 tablespoons olive oil
1 pound gluten-free andouille sausage, sliced
1 cup peeled and chopped sweet onion
1 cup seeded and chopped green bell pepper
1 cup chopped celery
1 tablespoon jarred minced garlic
1 teaspoon dried thyme
2 teaspoons Cajun seasoning
4 cups gluten-free chicken broth
2 bay leaves
1 pound small red beans, soaked overnight or quick-soaked and drained
1 smoked ham hock
4 cups cooked white rice
2 green onions, sliced
¼ cup chopped fresh parsley

1. Set the pressure cooker to the Sauté mode and add olive oil. Add sausage and cook for 5 minutes until browned. Remove with a slotted spoon to plate and set aside.

2. Add onions, bell peppers, celery, and garlic. Cook for 5 minutes until onion is translucent. Stir in thyme and Cajun seasoning. Stir in broth, bay leaves, red beans, and ham hock.

3. Press the Cancel button and place the lid on pressure cooker and lock it into place. Set the steam release knob to the Sealing position. Press the Manual button and set to 30 minutes. Allow to completely release pressure naturally (15–30 minutes). Once all steam has been released and the pressure valve lowers, remove the lid and remove the ham hock, chop into bite-sized pieces, and return back to the pot. Remove bay leaves. Add the sausage back into the pot and stir. Select Sauté mode and allow beans to thicken for 5 minutes. Serve over rice and garnish with green onions and parsley.

SERVES 6

Per Serving:

Calories	660
Fat	18g
Protein	40g
Sodium	1,020mg
Fiber	24g
Carbohydrates	83g
Sugar	5g

THE TASTE OF CAJUN

The term *Cajun* refers to a group of French Canadians that relocated in the bayou lands of southern Louisiana in the eighteenth century. Their foods were heavily influenced by French cuisine and the local ingredients that were available. Cajun cuisine includes locally influenced pork, beef, seafood, and chicken dishes. Cajun foods are spiced with seasonings like paprika, cayenne pepper, garlic, and onion.

Pressure Cooker Whole Roasted Chicken

SERVES 6

Per Serving:

Calories	700
Fat	50g
Protein	52g
Sodium	600mg
Fiber	1g
Carbohydrates	3g
Sugar	0g

ORGANIC CHICKEN

Organic chicken is free from antibiotics and growth hormones sometimes used to make chickens larger. It might cost a little more, but try to stretch your budget to include it if possible—it's better for your health!

Sometimes the best things in life are simple, and this recipe for a whole roasted chicken is quick, easy, and oh so good! Serve alongside Italian Roasted Vegetables or Creamy Scalloped Potatoes (see recipes in Chapter 7).

1 teaspoon garlic powder
1 tablespoon onion powder
1 tablespoon dried oregano
1 tablespoon dried thyme
1 tablespoon dried sage
1 teaspoon salt
1 (4-pound) whole roasting chicken, innards removed
1 medium lemon, halved
2 tablespoons olive oil
1 cup gluten-free chicken broth

1. In a small bowl, combine seasonings. Dry chicken skin with paper towels. Rub the seasoning mixture all over chicken, including the cavity. Place lemons into the cavity.

2. Set the pressure cooker to the Sauté setting. Add olive oil and chicken, breast-side down, and cook for 4 minutes until golden brown. Using tongs, turn chicken over and cook for 4 minutes. Remove chicken and set aside.

3. Place a metal trivet into the pot and add broth. Place chicken on top of the trivet. Place lid on pressure cooker and lock it into place. Set the steam release knob to the Sealing position. Press the Manual button and set to 28 minutes. Allow to completely pressure release naturally (15–30 minutes). Once all steam has been released and pressure valve has lowered, remove the lid and let rest for 10–15 minutes. Serve immediately.

Pressure Cooker Hard-Boiled Eggs

Everyone can boil eggs, but not just everyone can boil the "perfect eggs"! You will get perfect and superfast boiled eggs with this technique.

1 cup water
6 large eggs

1 Place water in the pressure cooker. Add in an egg or steam rack and carefully set eggs as desired.

2 Place lid on pressure cooker and lock it into place. Set the steam release knob to the Sealing position. Press the Manual button and set to 5 minutes.

3 When the cooking cycle has finished, let pressure release naturally for 5 minutes, then manually release by turning the knob to Venting. Hot steam will be released from the valve in venting mode. Once all steam has been released and pressure valve has lowered, remove the lid. Carefully remove eggs from pressure cooker and place in a large bowl of ice water. Let eggs sit in water bath for 5 minutes. Remove eggs from water bath. Crack eggs and peel.

SERVES 6

Per Serving:

Calories	78
Fat	5g
Protein	6g
Sodium	62mg
Fiber	0g
Carbohydrates	1g
Sugar	1g

THE MANY USES OF HARD-BOILED EGGS

Keeping hard-boiled eggs in your refrigerator is a time-saver in the kitchen. Eggs are an excellent source of protein, vitamins, and minerals. Hard-boiled eggs are not only a great addition for salads but also for breakfast muffins like Bacon and Egg Muffins (see recipe in Chapter 2). Hard-boiled eggs are also an excellent topping for Asian and Indian dishes. Adding a hard-boiled egg to gluten-free ramen or curry chicken takes the texture, flavor, and nutritional value to another level.

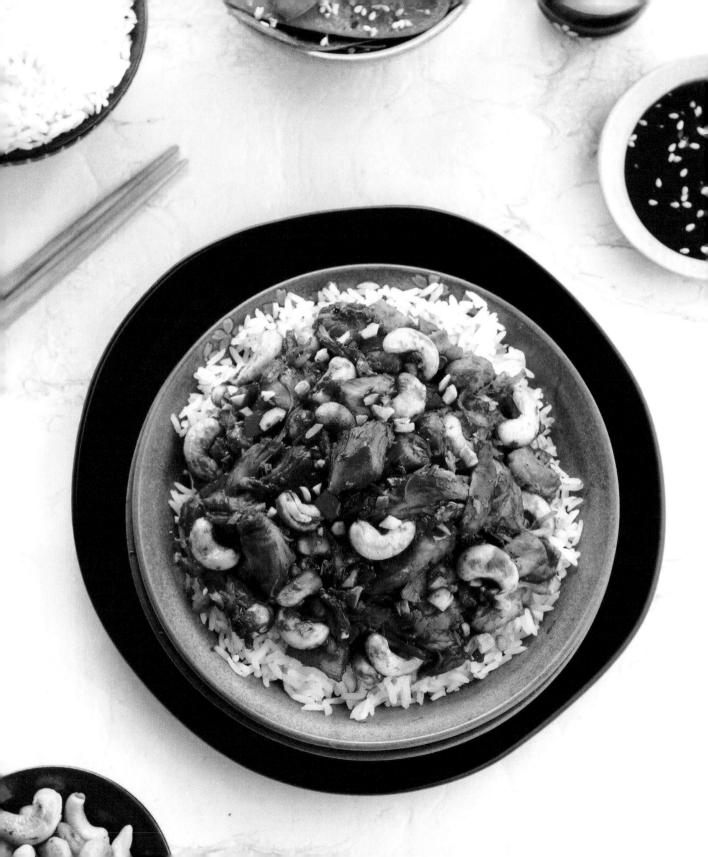

Pressure Cooker Cashew Chicken

Forget the fast-food option—with a pressure cooker, you have plenty of time to eat fresh, delectable cashew chicken made at home tonight! Serve alongside Sautéed Garlic Green Beans (see recipe in Chapter 7) and top with additional whole cashews, if desired.

SERVES 4

Per Serving:

Calories	700
Fat	27g
Protein	39g
Sodium	2,300mg
Fiber	2g
Carbohydrates	73g
Sugar	10g

2 tablespoons sesame oil, divided

½ cup gluten-free soy sauce

3 tablespoons rice wine vinegar

3 tablespoons ketchup

1 tablespoon honey

1 tablespoon jarred minced garlic

1 tablespoon jarred minced ginger

½ teaspoon Chinese five-spice powder

¼ teaspoon crushed red pepper flakes

1 pound boneless, skinless chicken breasts, cut into 1" pieces

3 tablespoons gluten-free cornstarch, divided

¼ teaspoon salt

¼ teaspoon ground black pepper

2 tablespoons water

1 cup chopped cashews

4 cups cooked rice

1 green onion, sliced

1 To make the sauce: in a medium bowl, whisk together 1 tablespoon oil, soy sauce, vinegar, ketchup, honey, garlic, ginger, five-spice powder, and red pepper flakes and set aside.

2 Add chicken to a sealable plastic bag. Pour in 2 tablespoons cornstarch, salt, and black pepper. Seal top and turn the bag several times to coat chicken.

3 Add remaining 1 tablespoon oil to the pressure cooker and turn it on to Sauté. Allow oil to heat up for 1 minute and then add coated chicken. Sear for 2 minutes.

4 Press the Cancel button and pour sauce into the pressure cooker. Stir to coat chicken with sauce. Place lid on pressure cooker and lock it into place. Set the steam release knob to the Sealing position. Press the Manual button and set to 10 minutes.

5 In a small bowl, stir to combine remaining 1 tablespoon cornstarch with water until cornstarch is dissolved.

6 When the cooking cycle has finished, manually release by turning the knob to Venting. Hot steam will be released from the valve in venting mode. Once all steam has been released and pressure valve has lowered, remove the lid. Press the Sauté button and pour the cornstarch mixture into the pressure cooker and whisk into sauce. Add cashews and continue stirring for 1–2 minutes until sauce has thickened. Serve over rice and sprinkle with green onions.

Pressure Cooker Steak Sandwich

SERVES 6

Per Serving:

Calories	390
Fat	20g
Protein	23g
Sodium	580mg
Fiber	3g
Carbohydrates	30g
Sugar	9g

TIPS FOR SLICING MEAT EASILY

A professional kitchen tip is to freeze beef before slicing it. Just 30 minutes in the freezer is enough to partially freeze thin cuts of meat, making it easier to slice the meat into thin strips. If your meat is totally frozen, do not completely defrost it entirely if you need to slice it. Defrost until it is partially frozen for an easier and neater slicing experience.

You can make the same steak sandwiches at home that you can find at popular delis, but this recipe can be made in just minutes and you can control the ingredients! Here, you'll serve it on dinner rolls to make steak sandwich sliders. Try it alongside Bacon and Tomato Macaroni Salad or Baked Sweet Potato Fries (see recipes in Chapter 7).

1 pound rib eye steak
½ teaspoon salt
½ teaspoon garlic powder
1 teaspoon dried thyme
½ teaspoon dried oregano
2 tablespoons olive oil
1 large green bell pepper, seeded and sliced
1 large red bell pepper, seeded and sliced
1 cup sliced mushrooms
1 large sweet onion, peeled and sliced
1 tablespoon gluten-free Worcestershire sauce
½ cup gluten-free beef broth
12 Soft Homemade Dinner Rolls (see recipe in Chapter 8)

1. Freeze steak for 30 minutes. Cut steak against the grain into very thin strips and set aside.

2. In a small bowl, add salt, garlic powder, thyme, and oregano. Stir to combine. Sprinkle on steak strips.

3. Set the pressure cooker to the Sauté setting and add olive oil. Sauté bell peppers, mushrooms, and onions for 5 minutes. Add the seasoned beef strips on top of sautéed vegetables.

4. In a small bowl, mix together Worcestershire sauce and beef broth. Pour the mixture over the meat and vegetables.

5. Place lid on the pressure cooker and lock it into place. Set the steam release knob to the Sealing position. Press the Manual button and set to 8 minutes.

6. When the cooking cycle has finished, let pressure release naturally for 12 minutes, then manually release by turning the knob to Venting. Hot steam will be released from the valve in venting mode. Once all steam has been released and pressure valve has lowered, remove the lid. Save broth to serve as au jus for dipping. Serve with the rolls.

Slow Cooker Southern-Style Pinto Beans

Pinto beans are a healthy source of protein and iron. They are low in fat and high in fiber. Adding them to your diet in creative and tasty ways allows you to take advantage of their many health benefits.

1 pound dry pinto beans, rinsed, picked over for tiny stones and soaked 6–8 hours or overnight
1 teaspoon chili powder
½ teaspoon dried oregano
1 tablespoon seasoned salt
1 teaspoon olive oil
3 slices pork fatback, chopped
4 cups water
1 small sweet onion, peeled and chopped

SERVES 12	
Per Serving:	
Calories	190
Fat	6g
Protein	9g
Sodium	20mg
Fiber	6g
Carbohydrates	26g
Sugar	2g

1   Add beans to a slow cooker and stir in chili powder, oregano, and salt.

2   Add olive oil to a large skillet and heat over medium-high heat. Add fat back to the skillet and cook for 2 minutes. Place meat and any rendered fat in the slow cooker with beans.

3   Pour water into slow cooker and add onions. Stir well to combine, place lid on and cook on high for 5 hours until beans are very tender.

Pressure Cooker Sweet Potatoes

This recipe for plump and fluffy sweet potatoes will cut your oven baking time in half and still give you perfect results! There are many herbs and spices that go well with sweet potatoes—try using chili pepper, garlic, ginger, nutmeg, rosemary, thyme, or cinnamon.

4 medium sweet potatoes
1½ cups water

SERVES 4	
Per Serving:	
Calories	110
Fat	0g
Protein	2g
Sodium	75mg
Fiber	4g
Carbohydrates	26g
Sugar	5g

1   Add a steaming trivet to the pressure cooker, place potatoes on top of the trivet, and pour in water.

2   Place lid on the pressure cooker and lock it into place. Set the steam release knob to the Sealing position. Press the Manual button and set to 18 minutes.

3   When the cooking cycle has finished, let pressure release naturally, about 15 minutes. Once all steam has been released and the pressure valve lowers, remove the lid and serve potatoes.

Texas-Style Slow Cooker Beef Chili

Per Serving:	
Calories	370
Fat	15g
Protein	24g
Sodium	1,220mg
Fiber	6g
Carbohydrates	36g
Sugar	11g

SANTA FE FRITO PIE

There is an unusual, but famous, chili treat—the Frito Pie—that is served at the classic Five and Dime General Store on the square in downtown Santa Fe, New Mexico, and you will see visitors walking around everywhere enjoying them. It is made by opening an individual bag of corn chips and ladling chili with pinto beans, chopped onions, and shredded Cheddar cheese. The good news is you can make a gluten-free and dairy-free version of Frito Pie using this Texas-Style Slow Cooker Beef Chili recipe and dairy-free shredded cheese; Fritos are both gluten- and dairy-free.

This amazing chili recipe will warm your heart and your body! Whether it's for game day or a meal on a cold day, you'll fill the bowls around your table with tasty goodness. Top your chili with cilantro and your favorite gluten-free corn chips.

1 tablespoon olive oil
1 teaspoon minced fresh garlic
1 large sweet onion, peeled and diced
2 large green bell peppers, seeded and diced
1 pound 90/10 ground beef
1 (4-ounce) can diced green chile peppers
1¾ cups gluten-free beef broth
1 (15-ounce) can pinto beans, drained and rinsed
1 (14-ounce) can diced tomatoes, including liquid
2 (8-ounce) cans tomato sauce
1 (6-ounce) can tomato paste
1 tablespoon ground cumin
2 tablespoons chili powder
1 teaspoon dried oregano
1 tablespoon light brown sugar, packed
1 teaspoon salt
¼ teaspoon ground black pepper

1 Heat olive oil in a large skillet over medium-high heat. Add garlic, onions, and green peppers and sauté for 2–5 minutes until vegetables are softened. Add beef and cook for 5–8 minutes until no longer pink; drain.

2 Add the beef mixture to a slow cooker. Add remaining ingredients and stir well to combine. Place top on the slow cooker and cook on low for 4–6 hours.

Rotisserie-Style Shredded Chicken

This recipe gives instructions on making shredded chicken in a pressure cooker or a slow cooker. Either way, you'll end up with juicy chicken you can use in tacos and on sandwiches. Serve with Baked Sweet Potato Fries (see recipe in Chapter 7).

CHICKEN
2 tablespoons olive oil

4 (6-ounce) boneless, skinless chicken breasts

ROTISSERIE SEASONING
1 tablespoon dried sage

1 tablespoon dried thyme

1 tablespoon onion powder

1 tablespoon dried oregano

1 teaspoon garlic powder

1 teaspoon salt

PRESSURE COOKER
1 cup gluten-free chicken broth

SLOW COOKER
2 cups gluten-free chicken broth

SERVES 6

Per Serving:

Calories	200
Fat	8g
Protein	27g
Sodium	455mg
Fiber	1g
Carbohydrates	3g
Sugar	0g

BUYING ROTISSERIE CHICKEN

Many grocery stores sell their own freshly made rotisserie chickens. Chicken is naturally gluten- and dairy-free, but unfortunately, the seasoning mixes the stores use may not be. It is always important to check the labels before buying a premade rotisserie chicken. There is also a chance of cross contamination when the chickens are not made in a dedicated gluten-free and dairy-free kitchen. One major retailer, Costco, labels its rotisserie chickens as gluten-free, and there is no dairy listed in the ingredients.

1. **For either appliance:** Add olive oil and chicken to the pot. Add all the rotisserie seasoning ingredients to a medium bowl and stir to combine. Pour broth into the bowl with the seasoning mix and stir. Pour seasoned chicken broth over chicken.

2. **For the pressure cooker:** Place lid on the pressure cooker and lock it into place. Set the steam release knob to the Sealing position. Press the Manual button and set to 12 minutes. When the cooking cycle has finished, let pressure release naturally for 10 minutes, then manually release by turning the knob to Venting. Hot steam will be released from the valve in venting mode. Once all steam has been released and pressure valve has lowered, remove the lid. Check that internal temperature of chicken is 165°F. Shred chicken with remaining liquid in the pot.

3. **For the slow cooker:** Cook on low 6–8 hours or on high 3–4 hours until the internal temperature reaches 165°F. Once the cook time is over, turn the slow cooker off. Pour half of the liquid out of the pot and shred chicken with remaining liquid in the pot. (The slow cooker version contains a bit more salt, 470mg, than the pressure cooker version.)

Pressure Cooker Barbecue Pulled Pork

This pulled pork recipe hits all the right barbecue notes—sweet but with some savory spices. Each bite is full of flavor, and it goes great on gluten-free and dairy-free homemade bread.

1 tablespoon light brown sugar, packed
1 tablespoon garlic powder
1 tablespoon onion powder
1 tablespoon chili powder
1 tablespoon salt
1 tablespoon paprika
1 tablespoon ground cumin
1 teaspoon mustard powder

1 (3-pound) boneless pork roast, cut into 2" cubes
1 tablespoon olive oil
1 cup gluten-free chicken broth
1 tablespoon apple cider vinegar
2 cups gluten-free barbecue sauce, divided

1. In a large bowl, combine brown sugar and all spices. Add in pork and toss to coat with the spice mixture.

2. Add olive oil to the pressure cooker and turn on to Sauté. Add pork pieces in a single layer. Brown on all sides, then transfer to a plate and set aside. Repeat with remaining pieces of pork. Press Cancel to turn the cooker off.

3. Add the broth, vinegar, and 1 cup barbecue sauce to cooker and stir to combine. Add in pork and stir to coat with the sauce mixture. Place lid on pressure cooker and lock it into place. Set the steam release knob to the Sealing position. Press the Manual button and set to 60 minutes.

4. When the cooking cycle has finished, let pressure naturally release. Once all steam has been released and pressure valve has lowered, remove the lid.

5. Transfer pork to a separate clean plate with a slotted spoon, leaving juices behind. Turn on to Sauté once more and let sauce simmer for 10 minutes until it has thickened and reduced by more than half. Shred pork with two forks.

6. Once sauce has reduced, skim the fat off the top with a spoon and discard. Add shredded pork and remaining 1 cup barbecue sauce into the cooker and toss to coat with sauce. Serve immediately.

Pressure Cooker Chicken Cacciatore

This remarkably simple but mouthwatering dish is a tried-and-true favorite. Serve it alongside gluten-free and dairy-free pasta, Italian Roasted Vegetables (see recipe in Chapter 7) or a Grilled Chicken Caesar Salad (see recipe in Chapter 3).

4 (4-ounce) bone-in, skin-on chicken thighs
1 teaspoon salt
⅛ teaspoon ground black pepper
2 tablespoons olive oil
1 tablespoon jarred minced garlic
1 small sweet onion, peeled and diced
1 large green bell pepper, seeded and diced
1 cup sliced mushrooms
1 cup diced celery
1 (14-ounce) can stewed tomatoes
3 tablespoons tomato paste
2 tablespoons Italian seasoning
¾ cup gluten-free chicken broth

SERVES 4	
Per Serving:	
Calories	270
Fat	13g
Protein	18g
Sodium	1,100mg
Fiber	4g
Carbohydrates	20g
Sugar	11g

1 Season chicken with salt and pepper. Set the pressure cooker to the Sauté setting and add olive oil. Add chicken and cook until browned, about 6 minutes per side. Transfer chicken to a plate.

2 Place garlic, onions, peppers, mushrooms, and celery in the pot; cook for 5 minutes until soft. Place chicken back in the pot; add tomatoes and tomato paste. Sprinkle with Italian seasoning and pour in chicken broth. Place lid on the pressure cooker and lock it into place. Set the steam release knob to the Sealing position. Press the Manual button and set to 11 minutes.

3 When the cooking cycle has finished, manually release pressure. Once all steam has been released and the pressure valve lowers, remove the lid and check chicken for doneness; an instant-read thermometer inserted near the bone should read 165°F. Serve.

Pressure Cooker Corned Beef and Cabbage

This recipe is more than just a St. Patrick's Day tradition. The tender corned beef and earthy cabbage will fill your stomach and heart on any cold day.

SERVES 6

Per Serving:

Calories	620
Fat	33g
Protein	57g
Sodium	3,400mg
Fiber	7g
Carbohydrates	29g
Sugar	6g

CORNED BEEF

Corned beef is readily available all year long. It comes prepackaged and will be in the meat department. Corned beef is naturally gluten- and dairy-free, but additives may not be. Corned beef is made from brisket and goes through a long curing process using large grains of rock salt and a brine. Make sure the corned beef you choose is labeled as gluten-free and there is no dairy listed in the ingredients. The pickling spice packet used in this recipe should come with the meat.

1 small yellow onion, peeled and sliced
2 teaspoons jarred minced garlic
Pickling spice packet from corned beef
3 cups water
1 (4-pound) corned beef brisket, rinsed
1 pound tiny potatoes
1 pound baby carrots
1 head cabbage, cut into 8 wedges

1 Place a metal trivet inside of the pressure cooker. Add onions, garlic, pickling spices, and water in the cooker. Place corned beef brisket, fat-side up, on a rack on top of onions. Place lid on pressure cooker and lock it into place. Set the steam release knob to the Sealing position. Press the Manual button and set to 85 minutes.

2 When the cooking cycle has finished, let pressure naturally release for 20 minutes, then manually release the remaining pressure. Once all steam has been released and pressure valve has lowered, remove the lid. Remove corned beef to a cutting board and cover with aluminum foil to keep warm.

3 Strain cooking liquid into a small bowl and discard solids. Return 1½ cups liquid to the cooker and reserve remaining liquid. Add potatoes, carrots, and cabbage to the cooker. Place lid on pressure cooker and lock it into place. Set the steam release knob to the Sealing position. Press the Manual button and set to 4 minutes. Manually release pressure. Once all steam has been released and pressure valve has lowered, remove the lid.

4 Slice corned beef against the grain. Spoon reserved cooking liquid over corned beef slices. Remove vegetables from the cooker with a slotted spoon and serve with corned beef.

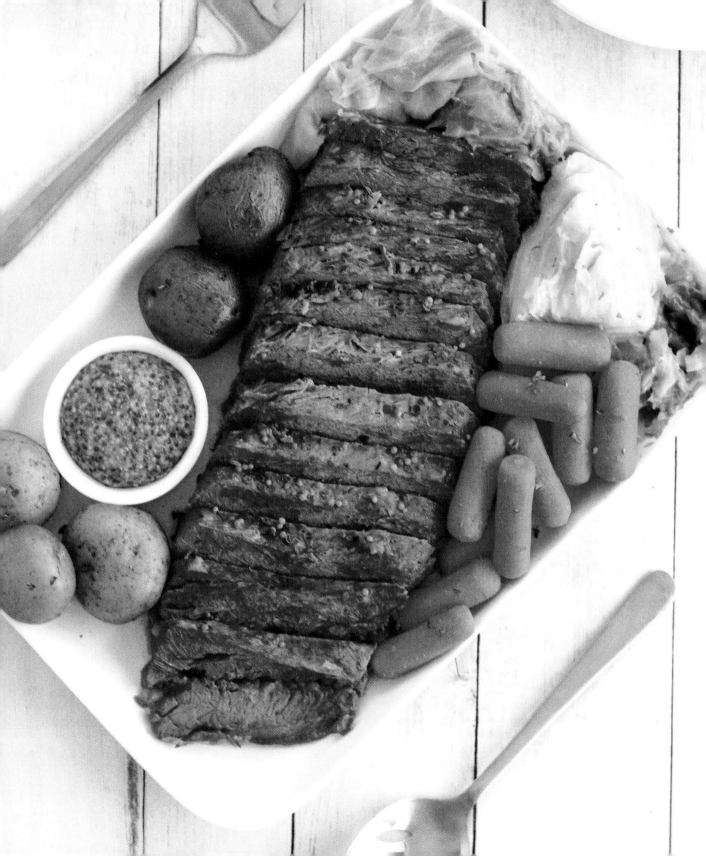

Slow Cooker Beef Tips and Gravy

SERVES 6

Per Serving:

Calories	400
Fat	17g
Protein	51g
Sodium	370mg
Fiber	0g
Carbohydrates	6g
Sugar	2g

A BEEF "TIP"

Beef labeled as *beef tips* is not necessarily the same as stew meat. While it is possible that your package of beef tips could be the least tender tips taken from steak or roasts, also called *stew meat*, beef tips could also be from better cuts. So double-check the label carefully to see which cut of meat was used in making your beef tips.

If you need a hands-off dish that still provides a hearty and delicious meal, try this recipe for Slow Cooker Beef Tips and Gravy. It goes perfectly with creamy Pressure Cooker Mashed Potatoes (see recipe in this chapter).

3 tablespoons olive oil, divided
3 pounds top sirloin, cubed
1 teaspoon seasoned salt
⅛ teaspoon fresh ground black pepper
1 cup peeled and diced sweet onion
2 tablespoons jarred minced garlic
1 cup sliced mushrooms
2 cups gluten-free beef broth
1 tablespoon gluten-free Worcestershire sauce
2 teaspoons Italian seasoning
1 teaspoon dried thyme
2 tablespoons cornstarch
3 tablespoons water

1 Heat 1 tablespoon olive oil in a large skillet over medium-high heat. Add beef, sprinkle with salt and pepper and cook for 2–4 minutes until seared on each side. Add 2 tablespoons of olive oil to the bottom of the slow cooker. Remove beef to slow cooker and top with onions, garlic, and mushrooms.

2 Add beef broth and Worcestershire sauce to the slow cooker and sprinkle beef with Italian seasoning and thyme.

3 Cover and cook on low for 6–7 hours or on high for 3–4 hours until beef is tender.

4 Whisk together cornstarch and water in a small bowl and add to slow cooker. Stir until sauce has thickened and cook on low for an additional 10 minutes before serving.

Pressure Cooker Indian Butter Chicken

This surprisingly easy-to-make chicken recipe is full of savory flavors and will give your dinner menu some flair. Butter Chicken is one of the most popular curries at any Indian restaurant around the world.

4 tablespoons dairy-free buttery spread

1 cup peeled and chopped sweet onion

3 tablespoons jarred minced garlic

2 tablespoons jarred minced ginger

1 tablespoon curry powder

2 teaspoons garam masala

1 teaspoon salt

¾ teaspoon smoked paprika

2 pounds boneless, skinless chicken thighs cut into 1" pieces

1 (15-ounce) can tomato sauce

1 cup full-fat unsweetened canned coconut milk

¼ cup chopped fresh cilantro

1 Add the buttery spread, onions, garlic, ginger, and all spices in the pressure cooker. Turn pressure cooker on to Sauté for 5 minutes, stirring occasionally. Press the Cancel button.

2 Add chicken and tomato sauce. Place lid on pressure cooker and lock it into place. Set the steam release knob to the Sealing position. Press the Manual button and set to 7 minutes.

3 When the cooking cycle has finished, manually release pressure by turning the knob to Venting. Hot steam will be released from the valve in venting mode. Once all steam has been released and pressure valve has lowered, remove the lid.

4 Stir in milk. Turn the pressure cooker on to Sauté again and simmer for 2 minutes to thicken sauce. Serve topped with cilantro.

SERVES 6

Per Serving:

Calories	260
Fat	9g
Protein	32g
Sodium	960mg
Fiber	2g
Carbohydrates	7g
Sugar	4g

WHAT IS GARAM MASALA?

Garam masala is a mixture of Indian spices that may differ from region to region. *Garam* means "hot" and *masala* means "spices," and while most garam masala spice mixtures are considerably hot, there are others that are mild. It typically includes cumin, coriander, cinnamon, nutmeg, turmeric, saffron, and cloves among others.

Slow Cooker Pot Roast with Savory Gravy

SERVES 6

Per Serving:

Calories	570
Fat	28g
Protein	42g
Sodium	600mg
Fiber	5g
Carbohydrates	36g
Sugar	5g

SLICE SOME *APIUM GRAVEOLENS*

Did you know that the scientific name for celery is *Apium graveolens*? Celery adds a great crunch when uncooked and a mellow flavor when cooked, and it is beneficial for arthritis pain, detoxifying the body, and weight loss.

When you need a plate of home-cooked comfort, this Slow Cooker Pot Roast with Savory Gravy recipe is always a good choice. It is tender, and the rich gravy goes perfectly with warm, buttery mashed potatoes as well.

1 tablespoon olive oil

1 teaspoon salt

1 (3-pound) chuck roast

2 cups baby carrots

1 cup sliced celery

1 cup halved baby potatoes

1 tablespoon onion powder

1 tablespoon dried sage

1 tablespoon dried thyme

1 teaspoon dried rosemary

1 teaspoon dried garlic powder

1 tablespoon apple cider vinegar

1 cup gluten-free beef broth

1 tablespoon cornstarch

1 tablespoon gluten-free all-purpose flour with xanthan gum

1 Add olive oil into a slow cooker. Salt beef roast and add to slow cooker. Add the carrots, celery, and potatoes.

2 In a small bowl, combine seasonings, vinegar, and broth and stir to combine. Pour the beef broth mixture over vegetables and beef.

3 Cook on high for 4–5 hours until vegetables and meat are tender. Using a slotted spoon, remove beef and vegetables to a platter and cover with aluminum foil to keep warm.

4 Pour liquid from the slow cooker into a small saucepan. Add cornstarch and flour and whisk over medium heat until fully combined. Bring to a slight boil, stirring until thickened. Remove the roast from the slow cooker and place on a cutting board to be sliced. Serve with gravy.

Pressure Cooker Chicken, Broccoli, and Rice

This recipe blends a symphony of savory flavors into a filling dish that will satisfy everyone at your dinner table. It's a one-dish wonder that's great for using up some leftover broccoli.

2 tablespoons olive oil

1 tablespoon jarred minced garlic

3 (6-ounce) boneless, skinless chicken breasts, cut into 1" cubes

1½ cups uncooked white rice

1⅓ cups gluten-free chicken broth

1 tablespoon gluten-free Worcestershire sauce

½ teaspoon salt

¼ teaspoon ground black pepper

1 teaspoon dried thyme

2 tablespoons onion powder

1 tablespoon lemon juice

3 cups unsweetened almond milk

3 tablespoons gluten-free all-purpose flour with xanthan gum

1 cup frozen broccoli florets

SERVES 4	
Per Serving:	
Calories	570
Fat	14g
Protein	37g
Sodium	570mg
Fiber	2g
Carbohydrates	67g
Sugar	1g

1 Add olive oil to pressure cooker and turn on to Sauté. Add garlic and chicken and cook for 1 minute, stirring occasionally so chicken gets browned on both sides.

2 Add rice, broth, Worcestershire sauce, salt, pepper, thyme, onion powder, lemon juice, and stir to combine. Place lid on cooker and lock it into place. Set the steam release knob to the Sealing position. Press the Manual button and set to 5 minutes.

3 In a small bowl, whisk together milk and flour and set aside.

4 When the cooking cycle has finished, manually release pressure by turning the knob to Venting. Hot steam will be released from the valve in venting mode. Once all steam has been released, remove the lid. Immediately add the milk mixture and mix until well combined.

5 Add the broccoli and place lid back on cooker and lock it in place. Set the steam release knob to the sealing position. Press the Manual button and set to 5 minutes. When the cooking cycle has finished, manually release pressure by turning the knob to Venting. Hot steam will be released from the valve in venting mode. Once all steam has been released, remove the lid, stir. and serve.

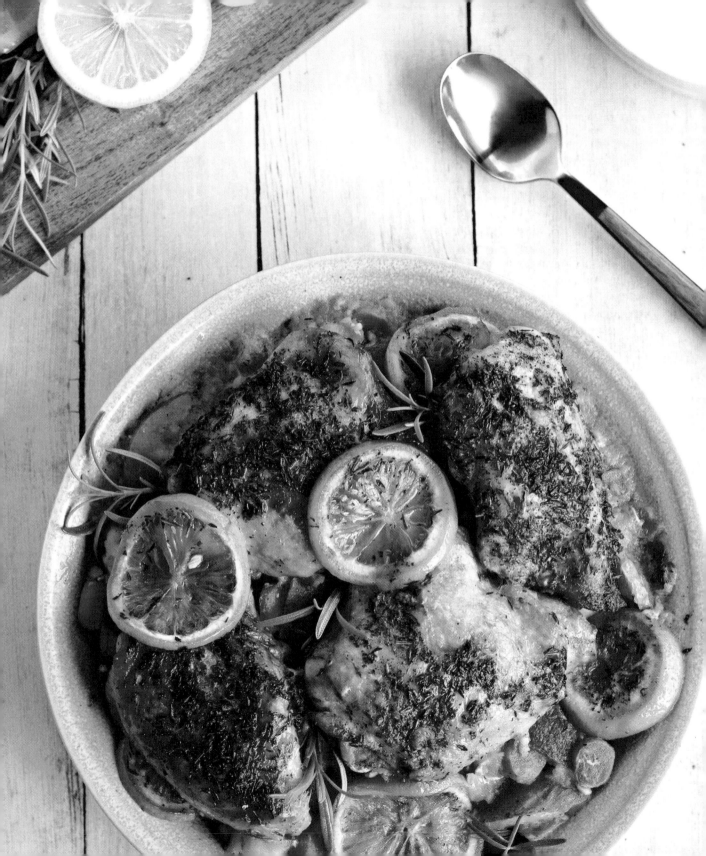

Slow Cooker Lemon Garlic Chicken

This quick and zesty Slow Cooker Lemon Garlic Chicken is your ticket to an easy weeknight dinner! The potatoes and vegetables make it a full meal.

4 cups quartered red potatoes

½ cup peeled and diced sweet yellow onion

1 cup peeled and sliced carrots

1 tablespoon jarred minced garlic

6 (4-ounce) bone-in, skin-on chicken thighs

½ teaspoon salt

¼ teaspoon ground black pepper

¼ cup olive oil

¼ cup lemon juice

½ teaspoon dried rosemary

1 teaspoon dried thyme

1 lemon, sliced

SERVES 6

Per Serving:

Calories	420
Fat	23g
Protein	24g
Sodium	300mg
Fiber	3g
Carbohydrates	27g
Sugar	4g

1. Place potatoes, onions, carrots, and garlic in the bottom of a slow cooker.

2. Sprinkle chicken thighs with salt and pepper and place in slow cooker. Pour olive oil evenly over top, followed by lemon juice, rosemary, and thyme. Place lemon slices over top.

3. Cook on high for 4 hours or on low for 8 hours. When chicken is finished cooking, remove and place on a baking sheet greased with gluten-free nonstick cooking spray. Preheat oven to broil and place baking sheet under the broiler for 3–4 minutes until chicken is browned and crisp. Remove lemon slices from the cooker and squeeze over chicken. Serve chicken with vegetables.

Slow Cooker Orange Chicken

SERVES 4

Per Serving:

Calories	490
Fat	19g
Protein	31g
Sodium	1,685mg
Fiber	1g
Carbohydrates	49g
Sugar	37g

STORE-BOUGHT MARMALADE

Marmalade is a fruit preserve made from the juice and peel of citrus fruits boiled with sugar and water. Jams and jellies are naturally gluten- and dairy-free, but always make sure to check your labels if you're buying them at the store.

This recipe makes the most flavorful, tender chicken covered in sweet, tangy sauce. Serve alongside steamed broccoli or Sautéed Garlic Green Beans (see recipe in Chapter 7).

¼ cup cornstarch
1 teaspoon salt
¼ teaspoon ground black pepper
3 (6-ounce) boneless, skinless chicken breasts, cut into 1" pieces
¼ cup vegetable oil
¾ cup orange marmalade
¼ cup gluten-free soy sauce
1 tablespoon rice vinegar
1 teaspoon sesame oil
1 teaspoon jarred minced garlic
1 teaspoon jarred minced ginger
1 tablespoon sesame seeds
2 tablespoons sliced green onion

1 Add cornstarch, salt, and pepper to a sealable plastic bag. Add chicken to the bag and seal. Turn bag over several times to coat chicken.

2 Heat vegetable oil in a large skillet over medium-high heat. Add chicken in a single layer and cook for 3–4 minutes on each side until browned, working in batches.

3 Coat a slow cooker with gluten-free nonstick cooking spray and add chicken.

4 In a small bowl, whisk together orange marmalade, soy sauce, vinegar, sesame oil, garlic, and ginger. Pour sauce over chicken and gently stir to coat. Cook on low for 2–3 hours. Sprinkle with sesame seeds and green onions, then serve.

CHAPTER 12

Desserts

Chocolate Chip Cookies

MAKES 48 COOKIES

Per Serving:

Calories	105
Fat	5g
Protein	1g
Sodium	80mg
Fiber	0g
Carbohydrates	13g
Sugar	7g

STORE-BOUGHT COOKIES

Finding store-bought gluten-free and dairy-free cookies is now easier than ever. There are more options now for a variety of cookie flavors from brands that make both gluten-free and dairy-free products, such as chocolate chip, sugar, and oatmeal, as well as graham crackers. They are shelf stable and can be found in the aisle with the other gluten-free products.

These traditional Chocolate Chip Cookies are just like the old favorites—but made in a gluten- and dairy-free way! They're melt-in-your-mouth soft and chewy, and they have just the perfect crispiness around the edges.

1 cup dairy-free buttery spread
¾ cup granulated sugar
¾ cup light brown sugar, packed
1 large egg
1 teaspoon molasses
1 teaspoon pure vanilla extract
2½ cups gluten-free all-purpose flour with xanthan gum
½ teaspoon baking soda
½ teaspoon gluten-free baking powder
½ teaspoon salt
2 cups gluten-free and dairy-free chocolate chips

1 Preheat oven to 375°F and line two baking sheets with parchment paper.

2 In a large bowl, beat buttery spread, granulated sugar, and brown sugar at medium speed until smooth and creamy.

3 Add egg, molasses, and vanilla extract and mix until fully combined.

4 In a medium bowl, stir together flour, baking soda, baking powder, and salt and stir to combine. Add the flour mixture to the buttery spread mixture and mix until fully combined. Add chocolate chips and mix on low until chips are fully combined.

5 Scoop batter with a greased 1½-tablespoons cookie scoop and place cookies 2" apart on prepared baking sheet.

6 Bake for 8–10 minutes until cookies start to turn golden brown. Allow to cool for 2–3 minutes before moving to a cooling rack. Store in an airtight container at room temperature for up to 3 days.

Fluffy Sugar Cookies

When you want the perfect cookie to take to the school party or the neighborhood get-together, try this recipe. These delicious sugar cookies are buttery and lightly sweet and can be topped with gluten-free sprinkles

¾ cup dairy-free buttery spread
¾ cup granulated sugar
1 large egg
1 tablespoon pure vanilla extract
⅛ teaspoon pure almond extract
1½ cups gluten-free all-purpose flour with xanthan gum
1 teaspoon gluten-free baking powder
⅛ teaspoon salt

MAKES 24 COOKIES

Per Serving:

Calories	67
Fat	2g
Protein	1g
Sodium	73mg
Fiber	0g
Carbohydrates	12g
Sugar	6g

1 Preheat oven to 375°F and line two baking sheets with parchment paper.

2 In a large bowl, beat buttery spread and sugar together on medium speed until smooth.

3 Beat in egg, vanilla extract, and almond extract.

4 In a small bowl, stir together flour, baking powder, and salt.

5 Slowly pour the flour mixture into batter and mix until fully combined.

6 Scoop batter with a greased 1½-tablespoons cookie scoop and place cookies 2" apart on a prepared baking sheet. Bake for 10–12 minutes or until the edges are very lightly browned. Allow cookies to cool for 2–3 minutes before moving to a cooling rack. Store in an airtight container at room temperature for up to 3 days.

The Perfect Pie Crust

SERVES 8

Per Serving:

Calories	150
Fat	8g
Protein	1g
Sodium	145mg
Fiber	0g
Carbohydrates	18g
Sugar	3g

PIE-MAKING MASTERY

Making homemade pie is very easy with canned pie fillings. Make a cherry, blueberry, peach, or lemon pie by using a 21-ounce can of pie filling. Make sure to always check labels for gluten and dairy ingredients.

You will be amazed at how tender, buttery, and flaky this easy-to-make pie crust is. It is ready for your favorite gluten- and dairy-free filling!

¼ cup dairy-free buttery spread, diced
¼ cup shortening
3 tablespoons ice-cold water
1¼ cups gluten-free all-purpose flour with xanthan gum
2 tablespoons granulated sugar
¼ teaspoon salt
1 large egg
¼ teaspoon apple cider vinegar

1. Put buttery spread, shortening, and water in separate small bowls. Put the bowls in the freezer for about 5 minutes.

2. Add remaining ingredients in the bowl of a stand-up mixer and mix with the paddle attachment until all ingredients are fully combined. (To make the pie crust if you do not have a mixer, cut buttery spread into flour, sugar and salt and then add the rest of the ingredients, mixing and forming into a ball.)

3. Shape dough into a ball, wrap in plastic wrap, and refrigerate at least 1 hour.

4. Remove from the refrigerator and let stand at room temperature for 15 minutes. Spay a 9" pie pan with gluten-free nonstick cooking spray.

5. Unwrap dough and place onto lightly floured parchment paper. Sprinkle dough with flour; top with plastic wrap or another sheet of parchment paper.

6. Use a rolling pin to roll dough out into a circle. Peel the plastic wrap or parchment paper off the top of dough circle.

7. Carefully place crust into prepared pie pan. Press dough into the bottom and sides (lift pie crust up and do not try to stretch it). Seal any cracks, if necessary. Fill and bake as directed in your pie recipe.

Butter Pound Cake

This Butter Pound Cake is a simple pound cake that is moist, buttery, and coated with a sweet buttery glaze that creates a perfect sweet, crunchy crust. Top it with fresh strawberries for a yummy addition and a lovely presentation!

CAKE
1 cup unsweetened almond milk
1 tablespoon white vinegar
1 cup dairy-free buttery spread
2 cups granulated sugar
4 large eggs
1 tablespoon pure vanilla extract
3 cups gluten-free all-purpose flour
    with xanthan gum
1 teaspoon gluten-free baking powder
½ teaspoon baking soda

GLAZE
⅓ cup dairy-free buttery spread, melted
¾ cup sugar
2 tablespoons water
2 teaspoons pure vanilla extract

1 Preheat oven to 325°F and spray a Bundt pan with gluten-free non-stick cooking spray.

2 In a small bowl, add milk and vinegar and allow to sit for 5 minutes to make buttermilk.

3 In a large bowl, beat buttery spread and sugar together on medium speed until smooth.

4 Add remaining cake ingredients to large bowl and mix until fully combined. The batter will be very thick. Pour batter into prepared Bundt pan and bake for 70 minutes or until a toothpick inserted in the center comes out clean.

5 Combine the glaze ingredients in a small saucepan over medium-low heat. Stir continuously until buttery spread is melted and sugar is dissolved, 2–3 minutes. Do not bring to a boil.

6 Poke holes all over warm cake with a knife and pour glaze evenly over cake while still in the pan. Allow cake to cool completely in the pan and then invert cake onto a serving plate. Store in an airtight container at room temperature for up to 3 days.

SERVES 16

Per Serving:

Calories	270
Fat	5g
Protein	2g
Sodium	225mg
Fiber	0g
Carbohydrates	52g
Sugar	35g

THE WONDERS OF BAKING SODA

Baking soda is used in cooking to help your baked goods rise and give them a crispier texture. But you will be interested to know that baking soda is also a great stove-top cleaner, a trash can deodorizer, a dishwasher cleaner, a shower grout cleaner, and a powerful stain remover.

Fudgy Brownies

SERVES 9

Per Serving:

Calories	210
Fat	5g
Protein	3g
Sodium	320mg
Fiber	2g
Carbohydrates	39g
Sugar	29g

SCHOOL BAKE SALE BASICS

When you cook for a bake sale, be sure to wrap each item either individually or in the way the group requests. Also be sure to label gluten- and dairy-free options as such, and display them in their own container to avoid cross contamination. Chances are, other people at the event will have dietary restrictions and will be happy to see your offering!

These will be the hit of the school bake sale! They have a rich flavor and excellent texture.

½ cup dairy-free buttery spread, melted
1 tablespoon pure vanilla extract
¾ cup granulated sugar
½ cup light brown sugar, packed
2 large eggs, room temperature
¾ cup gluten-free all-purpose flour with xanthan gum
½ cup cocoa powder
½ teaspoon baking soda
½ teaspoon salt

1. Preheat oven to 350°F and line an 8" × 8" baking pan with parchment paper and coat the bottom and sides with gluten-free nonstick cooking spray or buttery spread.

2. In a large bowl, add buttery spread, vanilla extract, granulated sugar, and brown sugar and mix until fully combined.

3. Add in eggs one at a time and mix until fully combined.

4. In a medium bowl, stir together flour, cocoa powder, baking soda, and salt.

5. Slowly add the flour mixture to the buttery spread mixture and mix until fully combined and smooth.

6. Pour brownie batter into prepared baking pan. Bake for 30–35 minutes or until a toothpick inserted in the center comes out just barely clean and the sides of brownies start to pull away from the pan. Let brownies cool completely, about 30 minutes, in the pan before slicing. Store in an airtight container at room temperature for up to 3 days.

Classic Vanilla Cake with Chocolate Buttercream

This moist and fluffy vanilla cake is ideal for stacking in layers for a dramatic presentation. The cake has just the right crumb texture, and the frosting is creamy and delicious! Many grocery stores now carry gluten-free and dairy-free ice cream, so you can now have ice cream with your slice of vanilla cake.

CAKE

⅔ cup dairy-free buttery spread

1½ cups granulated sugar

3 large eggs

1 tablespoon pure vanilla extract

2¼ cups gluten-free all-purpose flour with xanthan gum

3½ teaspoons gluten-free baking powder

½ teaspoon salt

1½ cups unsweetened almond milk

CHOCOLATE BUTTERCREAM FROSTING

1 cup dairy-free buttery spread

2 teaspoons pure vanilla extract

¼ teaspoon pure almond extract

1 cup cocoa powder

⅛ teaspoon salt

4 cups confectioners' sugar

3 tablespoons milk

SERVES 16

Per Serving:

Calories	340
Fat	7g
Protein	3g
Sodium	315mg
Fiber	2g
Carbohydrates	65g
Sugar	49g

1. Preheat oven to 350°F and spray two 9" round cake pans with gluten-free nonstick cooking spray.

2. In a large bowl, cream together buttery spread and sugar until smooth. Add eggs and vanilla extract and mix until fully combined.

3. Add flour, baking powder, and salt and mix until combined. Pour in milk and mix for 2 minutes on medium until batter is smooth.

4. Pour batter into prepared cake pans. Bake for 30–35 minutes or until a toothpick inserted in the center comes out clean. Cool in pans for 10 minutes and then remove from the pans and transfer to a wire rack to finish cooling, about 10–15 minutes. Allow cake to completely cool before frosting.

5. In a large bowl, cream buttery spread until smooth. Add vanilla and almond extracts and mix until fully combined. Add cocoa powder and salt and mix until fully combined. Add the confectioners' sugar 1 cup at a time and mix until fully combined. Add milk and beat until smooth and spreadable. Spread frosting between layers of cake and cover the top and sides. Store in an airtight container at room temperature for up to 3 days.

Cinnamon Roll Cake

This special treat has both the texture and taste of a gooey cinnamon roll, but you can make it in a fraction of the time! Bring it to a brunch gathering for people of all ages.

SERVES 16

Per Serving:

Calories	300
Fat	5g
Protein	2g
Sodium	240mg
Fiber	0g
Carbohydrates	60g
Sugar	41g

CAKE
3 cups gluten-free all-purpose flour with xanthan gum
¼ teaspoon salt
1 cup granulated sugar
4 teaspoons gluten-free baking powder
1½ cups unsweetened almond milk
2 large eggs
2 teaspoons pure vanilla extract
½ cup dairy-free buttery spread, melted

TOPPING
1 cup dairy-free buttery spread, softened
1 cup light brown sugar, packed
2 tablespoons gluten-free all-purpose flour with xanthan gum
1 tablespoon ground cinnamon

GLAZE
2 cups confectioners' sugar
5 tablespoons unsweetened almond milk
1 teaspoon pure vanilla extract

1. Preheat oven to 350°F and spray a 9" × 13" glass baking pan with gluten-free nonstick cooking spray.

2. In a large bowl, add flour, salt, sugar, baking powder, milk, eggs, and vanilla and mix until fully combined. Add buttery spread and mix until fully combined. The cake batter will be very thick and sticky. Pour into prepared baking pan.

3. In a medium bowl, beat together the topping ingredients until smooth.

4. Drop tablespoons of topping into cake batter and use a knife to swirl it around.

5. Bake at 350°F for 35–40 minutes or until a toothpick inserted in the center comes out clean.

6. In a separate medium bowl, mix together the glaze ingredients until smooth. Pour over warm cake and serve. Store in an airtight container at room temperature for up to 3 days.

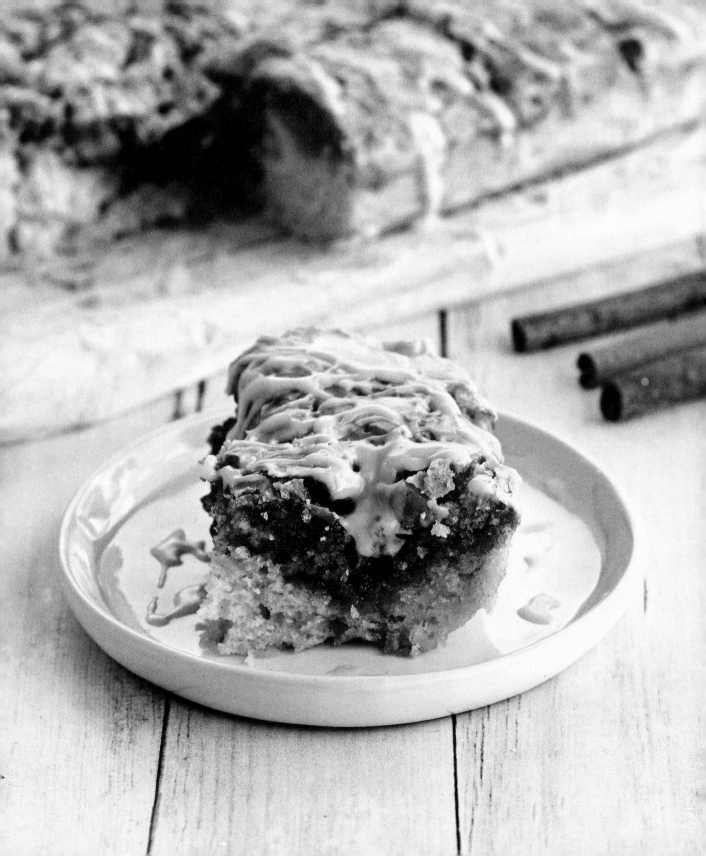

Pumpkin Bread Cookies

Per Serving:

Calories	105
Fat	1g
Protein	1g
Sodium	125mg
Fiber	0g
Carbohydrates	22g
Sugar	13g

PUMPKIN PIE SPICE IT

Pumpkin pie spice has a distinctive flavor and smell. It contains ground cinnamon, ground ginger, ground allspice, ground nutmeg, and ground cloves. It adds a warm and deep flavor profile to these cookies.

These super moist Pumpkin Bread Cookies taste just like pumpkin bread! They are a light and fluffy snack treat perfect for autumn events.

COOKIES

1 teaspoon baking soda
1 cup canned pumpkin
½ cup dairy-free buttery spread
1 cup sugar
1 large egg, room temperature
1 teaspoon pure vanilla extract
2 cups gluten-free all-purpose flour with xanthan gum
¼ teaspoon salt
1 tablespoon pumpkin pie spice
1 teaspoon ground cinnamon

GLAZE

½ cup confectioners' sugar
1 teaspoon pure vanilla extract
¼ teaspoon pumpkin pie spice
4 tablespoons pure maple syrup
1 teaspoon unsweetened almond milk

1 Preheat oven to 350°F and line two baking sheets with parchment paper.

2 In a small bowl, stir together baking soda and canned pumpkin and set aside for 2 minutes.

3 In a large bowl, beat buttery spread and sugar together on medium speed until smooth. Add egg and beat until the mixture is light and fluffy. Add the pumpkin mixture and vanilla extract into the buttery spread mixture and mix until fully combined.

4 In a medium bowl, stir together flour, salt, and spices. Pour the flour mixture into the pumpkin mixture and mix until fully combined. The cookie batter will be thick.

5 Scoop batter with a greased 1½-tablespoons cookie scoop and place cookies 2" apart on prepared baking sheets.

6 Bake for 15–20 minutes or until bottoms of cookies are lightly golden brown.

7 Combine the glaze ingredients in a small bowl and stir until smooth. Drizzle over warm cookies. Store cookies in an airtight container at room temperature for up to 3 days.

Apple Bundt Cake

This gluten-free Apple Bundt Cake is a super moist cake that is loaded with fresh apples and crunchy pecans and covered in a buttery brown sugar glaze. You can use freshly picked apples or a store-bought variety.

CAKE

1 cup unsweetened almond milk

1 tablespoon white vinegar

1 cup dairy-free buttery spread

2 cups granulated sugar

4 large eggs

1 tablespoon pure vanilla extract

3 cups gluten-free all-purpose flour
with xanthan gum

1 teaspoon gluten-free baking powder

½ teaspoon baking soda

1 tablespoon ground cinnamon

3 cups peeled and chopped Gala apples

1 cup chopped pecans

GLAZE

⅓ cup dairy-free buttery spread, melted

¾ cup light brown sugar, packed

2 tablespoons water

2 teaspoons pure vanilla extract

¼ teaspoon ground cinnamon

1. Preheat oven to 325°F. Spray a Bundt pan with gluten-free nonstick cooking spray.

2. Add milk and vinegar to a small bowl and allow to sit for 5 minutes to make buttermilk.

3. In a large bowl, beat buttery spread and sugar together on medium speed until smooth. Add eggs and vanilla extract and mix until combined. Add flour, baking powder, baking soda, and cinnamon and mix until fully combined. Add the milk mixture and stir until fully combined. The batter will be very thick. Stir in apples and pecans.

4. Pour batter into prepared Bundt pan and bake for 70 minutes or until a toothpick inserted in the center comes out clean.

5. Combine the glaze ingredients in a small saucepan over medium-low heat. Stir continuously until buttery spread is melted and brown sugar is dissolved, 2–3 minutes. Do not bring to a boil.

6. Poke holes all over warm cake with a knife and pour glaze evenly over cake while still in the pan.

7. Allow cake to cool completely in the pan and then invert cake onto a serving plate. Store in an airtight container at room temperature for up to 3 days.

SERVES 16

Per Serving:

Calories	285
Fat	5g
Protein	3g
Sodium	225mg
Fiber	1g
Carbohydrates	56g
Sugar	37g

HAVE FUN WITH BUNDT PANS

Creative manufacturers are now making Bundt pans in every shape and size under the sun, such as a mini Bundt, a square Bundt, a gingerbread house–shaped Bundt, and swirling design Bundt. Look for different options to make your dessert into a piece of art!

Peanut Butter Cookies

MAKES 36 COOKIES

Per Serving:

Calories	70
Fat	3g
Protein	1g
Sodium	65mg
Fiber	0g
Carbohydrates	10g
Sugar	6g

OTHER TYPES OF BUTTERS

If you or a loved one also has a peanut allergy, you can try other butters that might work better, such as almond butter, cashew butter, soy butter, sunflower seed butter, hazelnut butter, or combinations of peas, flax, and pumpkin. Most of these options can be substituted 1:1 for peanut butter, but look on the product brand's website to double-check substitution ratios before using.

These Peanut Butter Cookies are perfectly soft, chewy, and a little crisp around the edges. This is a classic cookie made with just a few simple ingredients in less than an hour.

½ cup plus 1 tablespoon granulated sugar, divided
½ cup light brown sugar, packed
½ cup dairy-free buttery spread, softened
½ cup gluten-free peanut butter
1 large egg
1 teaspoon molasses
1¼ cups plus 1 tablespoon gluten-free all-purpose flour with xanthan gum, divided
¾ teaspoon baking soda
½ teaspoon gluten-free baking powder

1 Add ½ cup granulated sugar, brown sugar, buttery spread, and peanut butter in a large bowl and mix with a mixer at medium speed until fully combined and creamy.

2 Mix in egg and molasses until fully combined.

3 In a medium bowl, stir together flour, baking soda, and baking powder.

4 Slowly pour the flour mixture into the peanut butter mixture and mix until fully combined. The cookie dough will be like soft Play-Doh.

5 Cover cookie dough and refrigerate for 30 minutes.

6 Preheat oven to 375°F. Line two baking sheets with parchment paper.

7 Scoop 1 tablespoon of dough and roll into a ball. Place onto prepared baking sheets 2" apart.

8 Add remaining tablespoon flour into a small bowl. Dip the bottom of a fork into the flour and then press down on the tops of cookies to make a crisscross "x" shape. Sprinkle the tops of cookies with remaining sugar.

9 Bake for 10–12 minutes or until light brown on the edges. Allow cookies to cool for 3–5 minutes before moving to a cooling rack. Store in an airtight container at room temperature for up to 3 days.

Pineapple Upside Down Cake

This recipe for sweet and sticky Pineapple Upside Down Cake is incredibly moist and full of pineapple flavor. It features a caramelized pineapple topping and an incredibly buttery cake.

SERVES 9

Per Serving:

Calories	300
Fat	4g
Protein	3g
Sodium	275mg
Fiber	1g
Carbohydrates	64g
Sugar	47g

TOPPING

¼ cup dairy-free buttery spread, melted

⅔ cup light brown sugar, packed

1 (20-ounce) can sliced pineapple, drained

9 maraschino cherries, stems removed

CAKE

⅓ cup dairy-free buttery spread

1 cup sugar

1 teaspoon pure vanilla extract

1 large egg

1⅓ cups gluten-free all-purpose flour with xanthan gum

1½ teaspoons gluten-free baking powder

½ teaspoon salt

1 cup unsweetened almond milk

1   Preheat oven to 350°F and spray a 9" × 9" pan with gluten-free nonstick cooking spray.

2   Pour melted buttery spread into the bottom of the pan. Sprinkle brown sugar over buttery spread. Place pineapple slices on top of brown sugar and then place a cherry in the center of each pineapple slice.

3   Cream buttery spread and sugar together. Add vanilla extract and egg and mix until fully combined.

4   Add flour, baking powder, and salt to the mixture and mix until fully combined. Pour in milk and mix for 2 minutes on medium speed until batter is smooth.

5   Pour cake batter over fruit in the cake pan. Bake for 50–55 minutes or until a toothpick inserted in the center comes out clean. Cool cake for 10 minutes, then invert cake onto a serving plate and serve warm. Store in an airtight container at room temperature for up to 3 days.

Carrot Cake with Cream Cheese Frosting

This carrot cake is super moist and deliciously spiced, and it has the perfect balance of sweet carrots and raisins, chopped pecans, juicy pineapple, and the light and delicate flavor of coconut.

SERVES 16

Per Serving:

Calories	375
Fat	8g
Protein	5g
Sodium	305mg
Fiber	2g
Carbohydrates	74g
Sugar	60g

HEALTH BENEFITS OF CARROTS

Carrots are good for you in so many ways. They are one of the highest sources of vitamin A and also contain a whole list of vital nutrients, including vitamin K, potassium, copper, vitamin B_6, and fiber.

CAKE

1½ cups applesauce

2 cups granulated sugar

3 large eggs

2 cups gluten-free all-purpose flour with xanthan gum

1 teaspoon baking soda

½ teaspoon gluten-free baking powder

2 teaspoons ground cinnamon

¼ teaspoon ground nutmeg

⅛ teaspoon ground cloves

¼ teaspoon ground allspice

½ teaspoon salt

2 cups peeled and grated carrots

1 cup shredded sweetened coconut

1 cup crushed pineapple in juice (not syrup), do not drain

½ cup raisins

½ cup chopped pecans

1 teaspoon pure vanilla extract

CREAM CHEESE FROSTING

1 cup dairy-free buttery spread, softened

2 (8-ounce) packages dairy-free cream cheese, softened

3 cups confectioners' sugar

2 tablespoons lemon juice

1 teaspoon pure vanilla extract

1. Preheat oven to 350°F. Cut parchment paper for the bottom of two 8" cake pans and spray with gluten-free nonstick cooking spray.

2. In a large bowl, mix applesauce, sugar, and eggs until fully combined.

3. In a medium bowl, stir together flour, baking soda, baking powder, cinnamon, nutmeg, cloves, allspice, and salt. Stir in carrots, coconut, pineapple, raisins, pecans, and vanilla extract into the applesauce mixture. Add the flour mixture to batter and mix until fully combined. Divide batter equally between prepared cake pans.

4. Bake on the middle rack for 35–40 minutes or until a toothpick inserted in the center comes out clean and the sides of cakes are pulling away from the pans.

5. In a large bowl, beat buttery spread and cream cheese together on medium speed until smooth and creamy. Beat in confectioners' sugar 1 cup at a time. Beat in lemon juice and vanilla extract.

6. Cool cakes in the pans for about 10–15 minutes. Then use a knife to loosen cakes around the edges of the pans and invert cakes onto a cooling rack to completely cool before frosting. Spread frosting between layers of cake and cover top and sides. Store in an airtight container in the refrigerator for up to 3 days.

Better Than Banana Bread Cookies

These cookies are as tasty as banana bread and very versatile! They are super moist, yet light and fluffy, and can be made with or without gluten-free and dairy-free chocolate chips. This is a simple recipe that your whole family will love!

3 large ripe bananas, peeled and mashed
1 teaspoon baking soda
½ cup dairy-free buttery spread
1 cup sugar
1 large egg
1 teaspoon pure vanilla extract
2 cups gluten-free all-purpose flour with xanthan gum
⅛ teaspoon salt
½ teaspoon ground cinnamon
¼ teaspoon ground nutmeg

1 Preheat oven to 350°F and line two baking sheets with parchment paper.

2 In a medium bowl, mix together bananas and baking soda and let sit for 2 minutes.

3 In a large bowl, beat buttery spread and sugar together on medium speed until smooth. Add egg and vanilla extract and mix until the mixture is light and fluffy.

4 Add the banana mixture to the buttery spread mixture.

5 In a medium bowl, stir together flour, salt, and spices.

6 Pour the flour mixture into the banana mixture and mix until fully combined.

7 Scoop batter with a greased 1½-tablespoons cookie scoop and place cookies 2" apart on prepared baking sheets.

8 Bake for 11–13 minutes or until golden brown. Allow cookies to cool for 2–3 minutes before moving to cooling rack. Store in an airtight container at room temperature for up to 3 days.

MAKES 24 COOKIES

Per Serving:

Calories	80
Fat	1g
Protein	1g
Sodium	110mg
Fiber	0g
Carbohydrates	17g
Sugar	9g

PICK YOUR BEST BANANAS

The best bananas for this recipe will have some brown spots on the peel. When the sugar content has increased in the ripening process, the brown spots will begin appearing. It normally takes 3 to 4 days for green bananas to fully ripen.

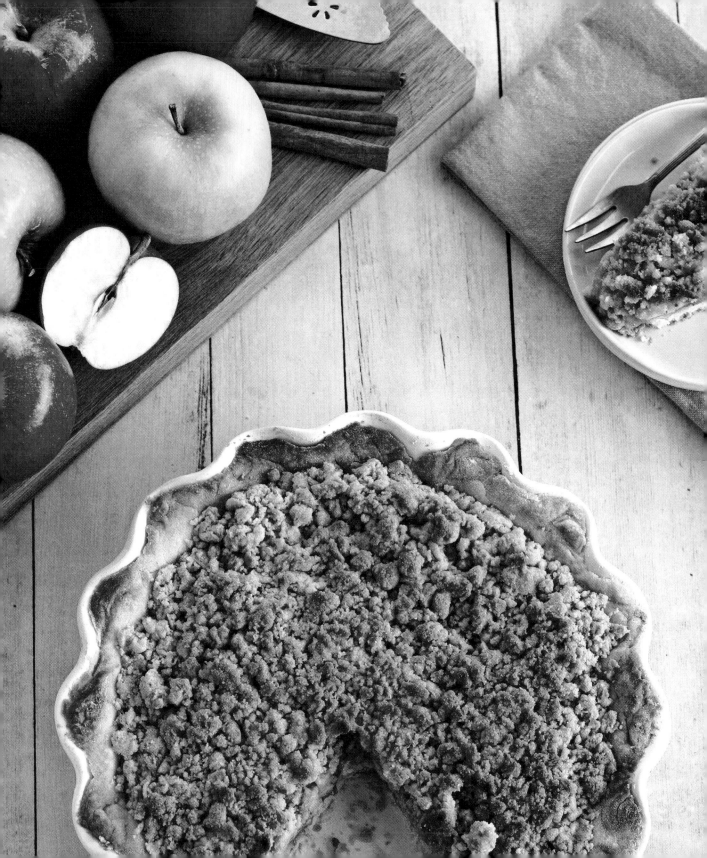

Dutch Apple Pie

This traditional Dutch Apple Pie will make you a believer in gluten-free and dairy-free baking! It's easy to make, and it is a great dessert for any holiday or special occasion.

FILLING

6 cups thinly sliced apples, such as Jazz apples

1 tablespoon lemon juice

⅔ cup granulated sugar

¼ cup gluten-free all-purpose flour with xanthan gum

1 tablespoon ground cinnamon

½ teaspoon ground nutmeg

⅛ teaspoon salt

PIE CRUST

1 (9") gluten-free and dairy-free pie crust (see The Perfect Pie Crust recipe in this chapter)

TOPPING

1 cup gluten-free all-purpose flour with xanthan gum

½ cup light brown sugar, packed

½ cup dairy-free buttery spread

SERVES 8

Per Serving:

Calories	410
Fat	11g
Protein	2g
Sodium	260mg
Fiber	2g
Carbohydrates	74g
Sugar	42g

1 Preheat oven to 425°F.

2 Add apples to a large bowl and sprinkle with lemon juice and toss to coat apples.

3 In a small bowl, stir together sugar, flour, cinnamon, nutmeg, and salt. Sprinkle mixture over apples and toss until apple slices are evenly coated. Transfer apple mixture into pie crust.

4 In a medium bowl, combine the topping ingredients with a fork or pastry blender until the mixture resembles small crumbs. Sprinkle apple mixture with topping.

5 Place pie pan on a baking sheet. Cover the pie crust edge with a 3" aluminum foil strip, to prevent overbrowning. Bake on the middle rack for 40 minutes. Remove the foil from the crust and then cover the top of the pie loosely with aluminum foil and bake for an additional 10 minutes until pie crust and crumb topping are deep golden brown and filling begins to bubble. Transfer to a cooling rack and allow pie to cool for 2–3 hours at room temperature before serving. Cover leftovers and keep at room temperature for 24 hours or refrigerated for up to 4 days.

Cowboy Cookies

MAKES 48 COOKIES

Per Serving:

Calories	100
Fat	6g
Protein	1g
Sodium	105mg
Fiber	0g
Carbohydrates	9g
Sugar	4g

These Cowboy Cookies are so named because this recipe originated in Texas. They're a combination of oatmeal cookies and chocolate chip cookies in one package!

1½ cups gluten-free all-purpose flour with xanthan gum
1½ teaspoons gluten-free baking powder
1½ teaspoons baking soda
2 tablespoons ground cinnamon
½ teaspoon salt
¾ cup dairy-free buttery spread
¾ cup sugar
¾ cup light brown sugar, packed
2 large eggs
2 teaspoons pure vanilla extract
1½ cups gluten-free and dairy-free chocolate chips
1½ cups gluten-free quick oats
1 cup sweetened coconut shreds
1 cup chopped pecans

1 Preheat oven to 350°F and line three baking sheets with parchment paper.

2 In a small bowl, mix together flour, baking powder, baking soda, cinnamon, and salt.

3 Add buttery spread to a large bowl and beat with a mixer at medium speed until smooth and creamy. Beat in sugars until combined. Add eggs, one at a time, and vanilla extract and beat until smooth.

4 Add the flour mixture and mix until fully combined. Add chocolate chips, oats, coconut, and pecans and mix until combined.

5 Using a greased 1½-tablespoons cookie scoop, place cookies 2" apart on prepared baking sheets.

6 Bake for 15–17 minutes until edges are lightly browned. Allow cookies to cool for 5 minutes before transferring to wire racks to cool further. Store in an airtight container at room temperature for up to 3 days.

Cinnamon Apple Fries

If you have never had Cinnamon Apple Fries, then you are in for a life-changing experience! These special treats are sweet and crisp apples lightly fried and covered in cinnamon and sugar. To add another layer of deliciousness, try dipping them in gluten-free and dairy-free whipped cream, caramel sauce, melted chocolate sauce, or strawberry sauce.

4 Granny Smith apples, peeled and cut into sticks
1 tablespoon lemon juice
3 cups vegetable oil
1 cup cornstarch
½ teaspoon salt
1 teaspoon ground cinnamon
1 cup sugar

1 In a large bowl, toss apples with lemon juice.

2 Heat oil in a large skillet over high heat.

3 Add cornstarch and salt to a large sealable plastic bag. Add apples to the bag, seal, and turn over and shake to coat apple slices.

4 Fry apple slices in oil for 2–3 minutes until golden brown.

5 Remove the fried apples from the skillet with a slotted spoon and place on a paper towel–lined plate to drain. Repeat with remaining apple slices.

6 In a large bowl, combine cinnamon and sugar. Toss apples in the mixture and serve warm.

SERVES 4

Per Serving:

Calories	560
Fat	17g
Protein	1g
Sodium	300mg
Fiber	5g
Carbohydrates	103g
Sugar	66g

White Cake with Almond Vanilla Buttercream

This super moist cake is tender and beautiful. Its simple flavors make it a perfect birthday or other special event cake.

MAKE YOUR CAKES LOOK FABULOUS

Successfully applying frosting to cake is a work of art, and there are some tricks that can make everyone a frosting artist. Before you start, make sure your cake is fully cooled. Always carefully trim off the uneven sections of the cake. Add a thin layer of frosting called the "crumb coat" to seal in stray crumbs before you apply a second frosting layer. Use an offset spatula to spread and a pastry bag for the finishing touches. Practice makes perfect!

CAKE

⅔ cup dairy-free buttery spread

1⅔ cups granulated sugar

1 teaspoon pure almond extract

2¼ cups gluten-free all-purpose flour with xanthan gum

3½ teaspoons gluten-free baking powder

½ teaspoon salt

1½ cups unsweetened almond milk

5 large egg whites

ALMOND VANILLA BUTTERCREAM

1 cup dairy-free buttery spread

1½ teaspoons pure vanilla extract

¼ teaspoon pure almond extract

4 cups confectioners' sugar

1. Preheat oven to 350°F. Cut parchment paper for the bottom of two 8" cake pans and spray with gluten-free nonstick cooking spray.

2. In a large bowl, beat together buttery spread and sugar on medium speed until smooth. Add almond extract and mix to combine. Add flour, baking powder, and salt and mix until fully combined. Add milk and mix until fully combined.

3. Beat in egg whites and mix on high for 2 minutes.

4. Divide the batter evenly between prepared cake pans.

5. Bake on the middle rack for 23–28 minutes or until a toothpick inserted in the center comes out clean and the sides of cakes are pulling away from the pans.

6. In a large bowl, beat buttery spread at medium speed until smooth. Add vanilla and almond extracts. Mix until fully combined.

7. Add confectioners' sugar 1 cup at a time and mix until combined.

8. Cool cakes in the pans for about 10–15 minutes. Then use a knife to loosen cakes around the edges of the pans and invert cakes onto a cooling rack to completely cool before frosting. Spread frosting between layers of cake and cover top and sides. Store in an airtight container for up to 3 days.

Strawberry Cupcakes with Strawberry Buttercream Frosting

These fresh strawberry cupcakes are moist and tender, have no artificial colors or flavors, and are full of fresh strawberries in every bite.

CUPCAKES

½ cup unsweetened almond milk
2 teaspoons white vinegar
¼ cup dairy-free buttery spread
1½ cups granulated sugar
½ teaspoon pure vanilla extract
3 large eggs
1½ cups gluten-free all-purpose flour with xanthan gum
1½ teaspoons gluten-free baking powder
½ teaspoon salt
1 cup strawberry purée

STRAWBERRY BUTTERCREAM FROSTING

1 cup dairy-free buttery spread, softened
½ cup strawberry purée
¼ teaspoon lemon juice
¼ teaspoon pure vanilla extract
3 cups confectioners' sugar

1. Preheat oven to 350°F and line two twelve-cup cupcake tins with baking cup liners.

2. In a small bowl, combine milk and vinegar and allow to sit for 5 minutes to make buttermilk.

3. In a large bowl, beat buttery spread and sugar. Add vanilla. Add eggs one at a time to the mixture and mix until fully combined.

4. In a medium bowl, stir together flour, baking powder, and salt. Add the flour mixture to the buttery spread mixture. Mix until combined. Add strawberry purée and the milk mixture to batter. Mix until combined.

5. Scoop batter into prepared cupcake tins. Bake for 20 minutes or until a toothpick inserted in the center of a cupcake comes out clean. Remove cupcakes to a rack to cool. Allow to completely cool before frosting, about 30 minutes.

6. In a large bowl, beat buttery spread until smooth. Use a spatula to scrape down the sides of the bowl before adding the next ingredients.

7. Add strawberry purée, lemon juice, and vanilla extract and mix until fully combined. Use a spatula to scrape down the sides of the bowl before adding powdered sugar.

8. Add confectioners' sugar 1 cup at a time. Mix until frosting is firm. Refrigerate frosting for 5 minutes before either piping or spreading on top of cupcakes.

MAKES 24 CUPCAKES

Per Serving:

Calories	170
Fat	3g
Protein	1g
Sodium	160mg
Fiber	0g
Carbohydrates	35g
Sugar	28g

MAKING STRAWBERRY PURÉE

You can easily make your own strawberry purée at home using fresh strawberries. First wash, dry, and stem berries. Place the berries in a food processor or blender and process until liquidy with slight pulp. One pint of strawberries will yield about 1½ cups purée. You can also use frozen strawberries, but thaw them first for about 15 minutes before processing. A 1-pound package of frozen strawberries will yield about 2 cups purée.

Lemon Crinkle Cookies

MAKES 24 COOKIES

Per Serving:

Calories	90
Fat	2g
Protein	1g
Sodium	125mg
Fiber	0g
Carbohydrates	18g
Sugar	11g

These soft, zesty lemon cookies are a lemon lover's dream come true! They are bursting with bright flavor and are super easy to whip together.

¾ cup dairy-free buttery spread
1 cup sugar
1 teaspoon pure vanilla extract
1 large egg
1½ tablespoons lemon juice
1 teaspoon dried lemon peel
1¾ cups gluten-free all-purpose flour with xanthan gum
¼ teaspoon baking soda
½ teaspoon gluten-free baking powder
½ teaspoon salt
½ cup confectioners' sugar

1   In a large bowl, beat buttery spread and sugar together on medium speed until smooth. Add vanilla extract, egg, lemon juice, and lemon peel and mix until fully combined.

2   Add flour, baking soda, baking powder, and salt and mix until fully combined.

3   Cover and refrigerate dough for 1 hour. Preheat oven to 350°F and line two baking sheets with parchment paper.

4   Add the confectioners' sugar to a small bowl. Scoop dough with a greased 1½-tablespoons cookie scoop and roll cookies in confectioners' sugar. Roll to cover all sides and place sugared dough balls 2" apart on prepared baking sheets.

5   Bake for 12–13 minutes until cookies start to turn golden brown. Allow cookies to cool for 5 minutes before moving to a cooling rack. Store in an airtight container in the room temperature for up to 3 days.

Double Chocolate Chip Cookies

These Double Chocolate Chip Cookies are rich and decadent. You can also substitute the regular chocolate chips for white chocolate chips for an easy variation on this recipe.

½ cup dairy-free buttery spread

¼ cup granulated sugar

¾ cup light brown sugar, packed

1 large egg, room temperature

1 tablespoon unsweetened almond milk

2 teaspoons pure vanilla extract

1½ cups gluten-free all-purpose flour with xanthan gum

¼ teaspoon salt

½ cup cocoa powder

1 teaspoon baking soda

1 cup gluten-free and dairy-free chocolate chips

MAKES 24 COOKIES

Per Serving:

Calories	130
Fat	5g
Protein	2g
Sodium	125mg
Fiber	1g
Carbohydrates	17g
Sugar	9g

1　Preheat oven to 350°F degrees and line two baking sheets with parchment paper.

2　In a large bowl, beat buttery spread, granulated sugar, and brown sugar on medium speed until creamy.

3　Beat in egg, milk, and vanilla and mix until fully combined.

4　In a medium bowl, stir together flour, salt, cocoa powder, and baking soda.

5　Add the flour mixture to the buttery spread mixture and mix until fully combined. Add in chocolate chips and mix until fully combined.

6　Scoop cookie dough using a greased 1½-tablespoons cookie scoop and place cookies onto prepared baking sheets 2" apart. Bake for 11–12 minutes.

7　Allow cookies to cool on the baking sheet for at least 5 minutes before transferring to a wire rack to cool completely. Store in an airtight container at room temperature for 3 days.

Mini "Cheesecakes"

If you are a big fan of traditional cheesecakes, then you will truly love these cute, Mini "Cheesecakes" made with gluten- and dairy-free cashew cream and pecan crust! They are an easy no-bake dessert and make a very elegant addition to any dessert table.

MAKES 12 "CHEESECAKES"

Per Serving:

Calories	300
Fat	21g
Protein	4g
Sodium	30mg
Fiber	3g
Carbohydrates	24g
Sugar	14g

FILLING

1½ cups cashews

⅔ cup full-fat unsweetened canned coconut milk, refrigerated

⅓ cup lemon juice

⅓ cup coconut oil, melted

⅓ cup pure maple syrup

1 teaspoon pure vanilla extract

CRUST

1 cup pecans

1 cup soft pitted dates, packed

¼ teaspoon pure vanilla extract

½ teaspoon ground cinnamon

⅛ teaspoon sea salt

1 To prepare cashews for filling, add cashews to a medium heatproof bowl, cover with boiling water, and let them soak for 1 hour. Then drain.

2 Line two twelve-cup muffin tins with baking cup liners.

3 In a food processor, add the crust ingredients and process until the mixture resembles a loose dough. Press 1 tablespoon into the bottom of each muffin cup.

4 Scoop ⅔ cup off the top of the cold (and hardened) milk from the top of the can (leaving the clear liquid underneath) and add to a blender. Add soaked and drained cashews, lemon juice, coconut oil, maple syrup, and vanilla extract and blend together until very smooth.

5 Pour the cashew mixture over the crusts in the muffin tin. Cover with aluminum foil and place in the freezer for 2–3 hours to allow the mixture to set. When ready to serve, allow to thaw for 5 minutes at room temperature. Store leftovers in an airtight container in the refrigerator for up to 3 days.

Old-Fashioned Oatmeal Raisin Cookies

Your family will cherish the comforting scent of oatmeal cookies baking in your kitchen when you make this simple and quick cookie recipe! It's easy to whip up, and you probably already have the ingredients on hand.

½ cup dairy-free buttery spread

½ cup granulated sugar

½ cup light brown sugar, packed

½ teaspoon pure vanilla extract

1 large egg

1 cup gluten-free all-purpose flour with xanthan gum

½ teaspoon baking soda

½ teaspoon gluten-free baking powder

¼ teaspoon salt

1 teaspoon ground cinnamon

1½ cups gluten-free quick oats

1 cup raisins

1 Preheat oven to 375°F. Line two baking sheets with parchment paper.

2 In a large bowl, beat together buttery spread, granulated sugar, and brown sugar on medium speed until smooth. Add vanilla extract and egg and mix until fully combined.

3 Add flour, baking soda, baking powder, salt, cinnamon, oats to the mixture and mix until fully combined. Mix in raisins until fully combined.

4 Scoop dough with a greased 1½-tablespoons cookie scoop and place cookies 2" apart on a parchment-lined baking sheet.

5 Bake for 10–12 minutes until cookies start to turn golden brown. Allow cookies to cool for 2–3 minutes before moving to a cooling rack. Store in an airtight container at room temperature for up to 3 days.

MAKES 24 COOKIES

Per Serving:

Calories	105
Fat	2g
Protein	1g
Sodium	94mg
Fiber	1g
Carbohydrates	21g
Sugar	14g

Apple Crisp

SERVES 6

Per Serving:

Calories	410
Fat	5g
Protein	4g
Sodium	275mg
Fiber	4g
Carbohydrates	86g
Sugar	34g

This recipe combines the sweet and tender flavor of baked apples with fresh oats and rich brown sugar. Top it with gluten-free and dairy-free vanilla ice cream for a fabulous treat!

TOPPING

½ cup gluten-free all-purpose flour with xanthan gum

½ cup gluten-free quick oats

½ cup light brown sugar, packed

½ teaspoon gluten-free baking powder

¼ teaspoon ground cinnamon

⅛ teaspoon salt

⅓ cup dairy-free buttery spread

FILLING

4 cups peeled and chopped Granny Smith apples

3 tablespoons dairy-free buttery spread, melted

2 tablespoons gluten-free all-purpose flour with xanthan gum

1 tablespoon lemon juice

3 tablespoons unsweetened almond milk

1 teaspoon pure vanilla extract

¼ cup light brown sugar, packed

½ teaspoon ground cinnamon

⅛ teaspoon salt

1 Preheat oven to 375°F and spray an 8" × 8" baking pan with gluten-free nonstick cooking spray.

2 In a medium bowl, combine the topping ingredients with a fork or pastry blender until it resembles small crumbs. Refrigerate while you prepare the filling.

3 Add apples to a large bowl.

4 In a small bowl, stir together buttery spread and flour until well blended. Add lemon juice, milk, and vanilla extract and stir to combine. Add brown sugar, cinnamon, and salt and stir until fully combined.

5 Pour the mixture over apples and toss to coat. Pour the apple mixture into prepared baking pan and spread into an even layer. Sprinkle topping evenly over apples. Bake for 30–35 minutes or until golden brown. Remove from the oven and cool for 10 minutes before serving.

Pistachio Cookies

If you love pistachio ice cream, you are going to love these cookies! They are lightly crunchy on the outside and chewy in the middle.

½ cup dairy-free buttery spread, softened
¾ cup light brown sugar, packed
¼ cup granulated sugar
1 box (3.5-ounce) gluten-free pistachio instant pudding
1 large egg
2 tablespoons unsweetened almond milk
½ teaspoon pure almond extract
½ teaspoon gluten-free green food coloring
1½ cups gluten-free all-purpose flour with xanthan gum
¼ teaspoon salt
1 teaspoon baking soda
½ cup finely chopped pistachios

1 Preheat oven to 350°F degrees and line three baking sheets with parchment paper.

2 In a large bowl, beat buttery spread until creamy. Add brown sugar and granulated sugar and beat until creamy.

3 Beat in pudding mix, egg, milk, and almond extract until fully combined. Add green food coloring and mix until fully combined.

4 In a medium bowl, mix together flour, salt, and baking soda. Add the flour mixture to the buttery spread mixture and mix until fully combined. Add nuts and mix until fully combined.

5 Scoop cookie dough using a 1½-tablespoons cookie scoop, place cookies onto prepared baking sheets 2" apart, and bake for 10–12 minutes. Allow cookies to cool on the baking sheet for at least 5 minutes before transferring to a wire rack to cool completely. Store cookies in an airtight container at room temperature for up to 3 days.

MAKES 36 COOKIES

Per Serving:

Calories	70
Fat	2g
Protein	1g
Sodium	120mg
Fiber	0g
Carbohydrates	13g
Sugar	8g

THE POWER OF PISTACHIOS

Not only are pistachios delicious in baking, but they are also a tasty and healthy snack on their own. They are a great source of vitamins B_2, B_3, and B_5 and are full of copper, zinc, and calcium. They are also are proven to promote healthy cholesterol and reduce blood pressure.

Coconut Cream Pie

SERVES 8

Per Serving:

Calories	670
Fat	38g
Protein	5g
Sodium	200mg
Fiber	2g
Carbohydrates	83g
Sugar	72g

This sweet and creamy Coconut Cream Pie is great for entertaining or special occasions. The coconut crust and vanilla custard filling covered with whipped coconut cream is sure to please your guests!

CRUST

2 large egg whites

2⅔ cups shredded sweetened coconut

3 tablespoons dairy-free buttery spread, melted

FILLING

⅓ cup gluten-free all-purpose flour with xanthan gum

⅔ cup sugar

2 cups coconut milk beverage (carton)

2 large egg yolks

1 cup shredded sweetened coconut

1 tablespoon pure vanilla extract

1 teaspoon dairy-free buttery spread

TOPPING

1 (14-ounce can) coconut cream, refrigerated overnight

1 teaspoon pure vanilla extract

¾ cup confectioners' sugar

2 tablespoons cornstarch

1 Preheat oven to 350°F and grease a 9" pie pan with gluten-free non-stick cooking spray.

2 In a large bowl, stir together egg whites, shredded coconut, and buttery spread. Pat the mixture into prepared pie pan to make crust. Bake crust for 20–25 minutes or until golden brown.

3 In a medium saucepan, mix together flour, sugar, milk, and egg yolks. Cook and stir over medium-high heat until mixture comes to a boil. Boil for only 1 minute. Remove from heat and add coconut, vanilla extract, and buttery spread. Pour custard filling into crust. Cover and refrigerate for 3 hours.

4 Chill a large bowl and whisk attachments of a mixer in the freezer for 10 minutes.

5 Scrape out the top of the chilled and thickened coconut cream (leaving the liquid behind) and place hardened coconut cream in chilled bowl. Beat for 30 seconds with mixer until creamy. Then add vanilla extract, confectioners' sugar, and cornstarch and mix for 1 minute until creamy and smooth. Use immediately or cover and refrigerate. Before serving pie, spread coconut whip on top of pie or on each individual slice. Store leftovers covered in the refrigerator for up to 3 days.

Hummingbird Cake with Cream Cheese Frosting

This moist cake is a southern classic flavored with bananas, pineapple, and cinnamon and covered in a rich cream cheese frosting topped with toasted pecans. Some say the cake was named after the hummingbird because it is sweet enough to attract hummingbirds.

CAKE

⅓ cup unsweetened almond milk

1 teaspoon white vinegar

1 cup dairy-free buttery spread

2 cups granulated sugar

4 large eggs

1 tablespoon pure vanilla extract

3 cups gluten-free all-purpose flour with xanthan gum

½ teaspoon gluten-free baking powder

1 teaspoon baking soda

1 teaspoon ground cinnamon

1 teaspoon salt

3 large ripe bananas, peeled and mashed

1 (8-ounce) can crushed pineapple, including liquid

1 cup chopped pecans

FROSTING

1 cup dairy-free buttery spread

2 (8-ounce) packages dairy-free cream cheese

2 tablespoons lemon juice

1 tablespoon pure vanilla extract

3 cups confectioners' sugar

½ cup chopped pecans

SERVES 16

Per Serving:

Calories	440
Fat	17g
Protein	4g
Sodium	540mg
Fiber	2g
Carbohydrates	69g
Sugar	48g

1. Preheat oven to 350°F and spray two 9" round cake pans with gluten-free nonstick cooking spray.

2. In a small bowl, add milk and vinegar and allow to sit for 2–3 minutes to make buttermilk.

3. In a large bowl, cream together buttery spread and sugar until smooth. Add eggs one at a time and vanilla extract and mix until fully combined.

4. Add flour, baking powder, baking soda, cinnamon, and salt and mix until fully combined. Pour in the milk mixture and mix for 2 minutes on medium until batter is smooth. Add bananas, pineapple, and 1 cup pecans and mix until fully combined.

5. Divide batter evenly between the two cake pans. Bake for 30–35 minutes or until a toothpick inserted in the center comes out clean. Cool in pans for 10 minutes and then transfer to a wire rack to finish cooling, about 10–15 minutes.

6. In a large bowl, cream buttery spread and cream cheese together until smooth. Add lemon juice and vanilla extract and mix until fully combined. Add confectioners' sugar 1 cup at a time and beat until smooth and spreadable.

7. Allow cake to completely cool before frosting. Spread frosting between layers of cake and cover top and sides. Sprinkle the top of frosted cake with ½ cup chopped pecans.

Red Velvet Cookies

These delicious cookies are soft, chewy, and chocolaty! Pour a tall glass of ice-cold dairy-free milk to drink with them.

MAKES 24 COOKIES

Per Serving:

Calories	125
Fat	5g
Protein	2g
Sodium	230mg
Fiber	0g
Carbohydrates	17g
Sugar	9g

½ cup dairy-free buttery spread, softened
¾ cup light brown sugar, packed
¼ cup granulated sugar
1 large egg
1 tablespoon unsweetened almond milk
2 teaspoons pure vanilla extract
1 tablespoon gluten-free red food coloring
1½ cups gluten-free all-purpose flour with xanthan gum
¼ teaspoon salt
¼ cup cocoa powder
1 teaspoon baking soda
1 cup gluten-free and dairy-free chocolate chips

1. In a large bowl, beat buttery spread until creamy. Add brown sugar and granulated sugar and beat until creamy.

2. Beat in egg, milk, and vanilla extract and mix until fully combined. Add red food coloring and mix until fully combined.

3. In a medium bowl, mix together flour, salt, cocoa powder, and baking soda and whisk together until fully combined.

4. Add the flour mixture to the buttery spread mixture and mix until fully combined. Mix in chocolate chips until fully combined. Cover cookie dough and refrigerate for at least 1 hour.

5. Preheat oven to 350°F degrees and line two baking sheets with parchment paper.

6. Scoop cookie dough using a 1½-tablespoons cookie scoop and roll into twenty-four balls. Place cookie balls onto prepared baking sheets 2" apart and bake for 11–12 minutes. (The cookies will not spread too much while baking but you will flatten them next.)

7. Take cookies out of the oven and press down on warm cookies to slightly flatten. Allow cookies to cool on baking sheets for at least 5 minutes before transferring to a wire rack to cool completely. Store in an airtight container at room temperature for 3 days.

Chocolate-Covered Coconut Macaroons

The combination of melted chocolate and sweet, crunchy toasted coconut makes these macaroons extraordinary. They're good enough to be featured in a fancy bakery!

3 large egg whites
¼ teaspoon cream of tartar
⅛ teaspoon salt
¼ teaspoon pure almond extract
½ cup granulated sugar
⅔ cup gluten-free all-purpose flour with xanthan gum
4 cups sweetened shredded coconut
1½ cups gluten-free and dairy-free chocolate chips
2 teaspoons coconut oil melted

MAKES 21 MACAROONS

Per Serving:

Calories	210
Fat	13g
Protein	3g
Sodium	75mg
Fiber	1g
Carbohydrates	20g
Sugar	13g

1 Preheat oven to 350°F degrees and line two baking sheets with parchment paper.

2 In a large bowl, use a mixer to beat egg whites, cream of tartar, and salt until foamy. Add almond extract. Add sugar 1 tablespoon at a time and continue to beat. Add flour 1 tablespoon at a time and continue to beat until stiff. Stir in shredded coconut.

3 Scoop out dough using a 1½-tablespoons cookie scoop and place on prepared baking sheets.

4 Bake for 18–20 minutes until the cookie edges start to turn golden brown. Remove from the oven and allow cookies to cool completely before dipping them in chocolate.

5 In a microwave-safe dish, melt chocolate chips for 1–2 minutes, then stir and continue microwaving 30 seconds at a time until chips melt and are smooth. Once chocolate chips are fully melted, add coconut oil and stir. Dip the top of each cookie into the melted chocolate. Allow chocolate to cool for 1–2 minutes before serving cookies. Store in an airtight container at room temperature for up to 3 days.

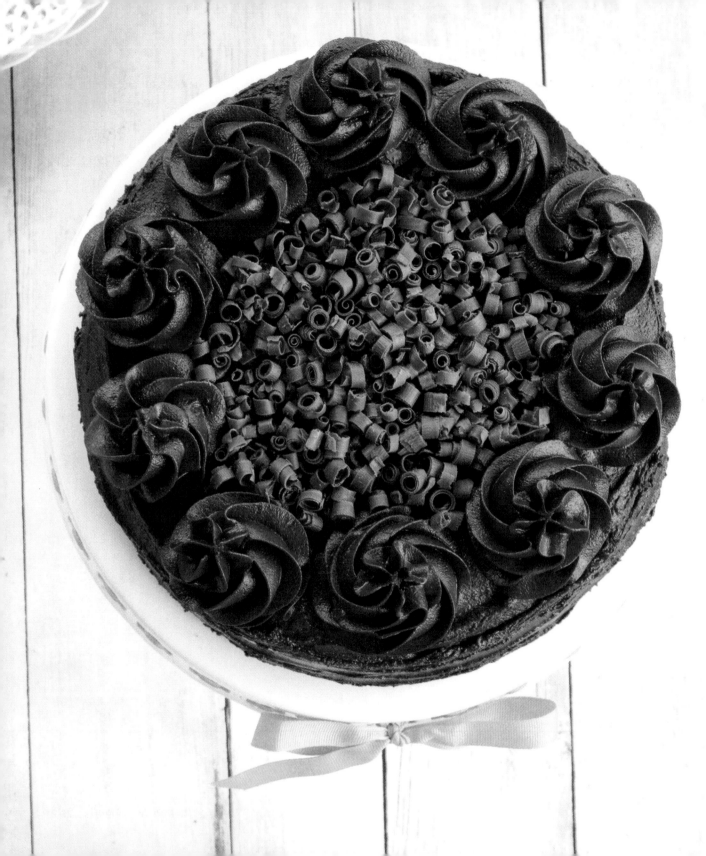

Easy Gluten-Free Chocolate Cake with Chocolate Buttercream Frosting

This delicious Easy Gluten-Free Chocolate Cake with Chocolate Buttercream Frosting is the perfect birthday cake (or graduation cake or anniversary cake or any other celebration cake). The person you're celebrating will love being able to enjoy an old favorite. You can spread the frosting on top of the cake in a basic way, or get creative with swirls and gluten-free toppings.

SERVES 16

Per Serving:

Calories	360
Fat	7g
Protein	3g
Sodium	445mg
Fiber	3g
Carbohydrates	71g
Sugar	55g

CAKE

1 cup unsweetened almond milk

1 tablespoon white vinegar

2 cups gluten-free all-purpose flour with xanthan gum

1 teaspoon salt

1 teaspoon baking soda

½ teaspoon gluten-free baking powder

½ teaspoon ground cinnamon

½ cup plus 1 tablespoon dairy-free buttery spread, softened

2 cups granulated sugar

2 large eggs

1 teaspoon pure vanilla extract

¾ cup cocoa powder

¾ cup boiling water

CHOCOLATE BUTTERCREAM FROSTING

1 cup dairy-free buttery spread

2 teaspoons pure vanilla extract

¼ teaspoon pure almond extract

1 cup cocoa powder

⅛ teaspoon salt

4 cups confectioners' sugar

3 tablespoons unsweetened almond milk

1 Preheat oven to 350°F degrees. Cut parchment paper for the bottom of two 8" cake pans and spray with gluten-free nonstick cooking spray.

2 In a small bowl, combine milk and vinegar and allow to sit for 5 minutes to make buttermilk.

3 In a medium bowl, stir together flour, salt, baking soda, baking powder, and cinnamon.

4 In a large bowl, beat buttery spread and sugar together on medium speed until smooth.

5 Add eggs and vanilla extract to the buttery spread mixture and mix until fully combined.

6 Add the flour mixture to the buttery spread mixture and mix until fully combined.

7 Add the milk mixture to the buttery spread mixture and mix until fully combined.

continued on next page

continued

8　Add cocoa powder to batter and mix until fully combined.

9　Add boiling water to batter and mix until fully combined.

10　Divide batter evenly between prepared cake pans.

11　Bake on the middle rack for 30–35 minutes or until a toothpick inserted in the center comes out clean and the side of cake is pulling away from the side of the pan.

12　Cool cakes in the pans for about 10–15 minutes. Then use a knife to loosen cakes around the edges of the pans and invert cakes onto a cooling rack to completely cool before frosting.

13　In a large bowl, beat buttery spread at medium speed until smooth. Add vanilla and almond extracts and mix until fully combined.

14　Add the cocoa powder and salt and mix until fully combined.

15　Add confectioners' sugar 1 cup at a time and mix until fully combined.

16　Add milk and beat until smooth and spreadable. Spread frosting between layers of cake and cover top and sides. Store leftovers in an airtight container for up to 3 days.

Chocolate Peanut Butter Brownies

The combination of chocolate and peanut butter is always a crowd-pleaser. If you need a change from traditional brownies, try this recipe.

½ cup dairy-free buttery spread, melted
1 tablespoon pure vanilla extract
¾ cup granulated sugar
½ cup light brown sugar, packed
2 large eggs, room temperature
¾ cup gluten-free all-purpose flour with xanthan gum
½ cup cocoa powder
½ teaspoon baking soda
½ teaspoon salt
¼ cup gluten-free peanut butter

SERVES 9

Per Serving:

Calories	255
Fat	8g
Protein	4g
Sodium	345mg
Fiber	2g
Carbohydrates	40g
Sugar	29g

1 Preheat oven to 350°F and line an 8" × 8" baking pan with parchment paper and coat the bottom and sides with gluten-free nonstick cooking spray or buttery spread.

2 In a large bowl, add buttery spread, vanilla extract, granulated sugar, and brown sugar and mix until fully combined.

3 Add in eggs one at a time and mix until fully combined.

4 In a medium bowl, stir together flour, cocoa powder, baking soda, and salt.

5 Slowly add the flour mixture to the buttery spread mixture and mix until fully combined and smooth.

6 Pour the brownie batter into prepared baking pan. Drop 6 tablespoons of peanut butter on top of brownie batter in two rows of three. Take a knife and drag it through peanut butter and brownie batter to make a swirl pattern.

7 Bake for 30–35 minutes or until a toothpick inserted in the center comes out just barely clean and the sides of brownies start to pull away from the pan. Let brownies cool completely, about 30 minutes, in the pan before slicing. Store in an airtight at room temperature container for up to 3 days.

Frosted Coconut Cake

SERVES 16

Per Serving:

Calories	400
Fat	12g
Protein	2g
Sodium	340mg
Fiber	1g
Carbohydrates	73g
Sugar	58g

Nothing looks as elegant as a beautiful, snow-white coconut cake on an elaborate cake stand. This coconut cake recipe will impress everyone, even at weddings and other important events!

CAKE

⅔ cup dairy-free buttery spread

1⅔ cups granulated sugar

1 teaspoon pure almond extract

2¼ cups gluten-free all-purpose flour with xanthan gum

3½ teaspoons gluten-free baking powder

½ teaspoon salt

1½ cups unsweetened coconut milk beverage (carton)

2 cups sweetened shredded coconut

5 large egg whites

FROSTING

1 cup dairy-free buttery spread, softened

1½ teaspoons pure vanilla extract

¼ teaspoon pure almond extract

4 cups confectioners' sugar

1 cup sweetened shredded coconut

1. Preheat oven to 350°F. Cut parchment paper for the bottom of two 8" cake pans and spray with gluten-free nonstick cooking spray.

2. In a large bowl, beat together buttery spread and sugar on medium speed until smooth. Add almond extract and mix to combine. Add flour, baking powder, and salt and mix until fully combined. Add the coconut milk and shredded coconut and mix until fully combined.

3. Beat in egg whites and mix on high for 2 minutes.

4. Divide batter evenly between prepared cake pans.

5. Bake on the middle rack for 23–28 minutes or until a toothpick inserted in the center comes out clean and the sides of the cake are pulling away from the sides of the pan.

6. In a large bowl, beat buttery spread at medium speed until smooth. Add vanilla and almond extracts. Mix until fully combined.

7. Add confectioners' sugar 1 cup at a time to the buttery spread mixture and mix until fully combined.

8. Add coconut and mix until fully combined.

9. Cool cakes in the pans for about 10–15 minutes. Then use a knife to loosen cakes around the edges of the pans and invert cakes onto a cooling rack to completely cool before frosting. Spread frosting between layers of cake and cover top and sides. Store in an airtight container for up to 3 days.

Cinnamon Roll Cookies

These Cinnamon Roll Cookies are an unexpected treat at a dessert buffet. Each one is like eating a tiny cinnamon roll!

COOKIES

½ cup dairy-free buttery spread
½ cup light brown sugar, packed
¼ cup sugar
2 large eggs
2 teaspoons pure vanilla extract
2½ cups plus 1 tablespoon gluten-free all-purpose flour with xanthan gum, divided
1 teaspoon gluten-free baking powder
½ teaspoon baking soda
¼ teaspoon salt

FILLING

¼ cup light brown sugar, packed
1 tablespoon ground cinnamon

GLAZE

¼ cup light brown sugar, packed
3 tablespoons dairy-free buttery spread, melted
1 cup confectioners' sugar
1 tablespoon unsweetened almond milk

MAKES 24 COOKIES

Per Serving:

Calories	75
Fat	2g
Protein	1g
Sodium	110mg
Fiber	0g
Carbohydrates	14g
Sugar	14g

1 In a large bowl, beat together buttery spread, brown sugar, and granulated sugar at medium speed until smooth.

2 Add eggs and vanilla extract and mix until fully combined. In a medium bowl, stir together 2½ cups flour, baking powder, baking soda, and salt. Pour the flour mixture into the buttery spread mixture and mix until fully combined.

3 Sprinkle remaining 1 tablespoon flour on a piece on parchment paper. Remove cookie dough from the bowl and shape it into a ball.

4 Form dough round about 7" in diameter and 1" thick.

5 Mix brown sugar and cinnamon together in a small bowl. Pour the mixture over cookie dough and pat down lightly.

6 Roll dough into a log shape. Wrap log in parchment paper, place on a baking sheet, and refrigerate for 1 hour.

7 Preheat oven to 375°F and line two baking sheets with parchment paper.

8 Using a knife or a pastry scraper, cut dough into ½" slices. Carefully put cookie slices on prepared baking sheets about 2" apart. Bake cookies for 10–12 minutes until golden around the edges.

9 In a small bowl, stir together brown sugar and buttery spread. Add confectioners' sugar and stir until it starts to thicken. Add milk to thin out glaze. Drizzle glaze all over the cookies, just like a cinnamon roll. Allow cookies to cool for 2–3 minutes before moving to cooling rack.

Apple Pie Blondies

MAKES 9 BLONDIES

Per Serving:

Calories	450
Fat	5g
Protein	4g
Sodium	460mg
Fiber	2g
Carbohydrates	101g
Sugar	86g

This soft, blonde brownie is topped with delicious cinnamon apples and maple vanilla glaze. It includes all of your favorite apple pie flavors atop buttery cake blondies.

FILLING

1 tablespoon dairy-free buttery spread

2 cups peeled and diced Red Delicious apples

2 tablespoons light brown sugar, packed

1 teaspoon ground cinnamon

1 teaspoon pure vanilla extract

BLONDIE

½ cup dairy-free buttery spread, softened

¾ cup light brown sugar, packed

2 large eggs

1 tablespoon pure vanilla extract

1½ cups gluten-free all-purpose flour with xanthan gum

1 teaspoon gluten-free baking powder

1 teaspoon ground cinnamon

⅛ teaspoon ground nutmeg

½ teaspoon salt

GLAZE

1 cup confectioners' sugar

3 tablespoons pure maple syrup

1 teaspoon pure vanilla extract

1. Preheat oven to 350°F and line an 8" × 8" baking pan with parchment paper and coat with gluten-free nonstick cooking spray.

2. In a small saucepan, add buttery spread, apples, brown sugar, cinnamon, and vanilla extract. Cook over medium heat for 1–2 minutes until buttery spread is melted. Stir diced apples to fully coat. Allow the mixture to come to a slight boil. Cook for 2–3 minutes until apples are soft and remove from the heat.

3. In a large bowl, beat buttery spread and brown sugar together on medium speed until smooth. Add eggs and vanilla extract and mix until fully combined.

4. Add flour, baking powder, cinnamon, nutmeg, and salt and mix until ingredients are fully combined. The blondie batter will be sticky.

5. Pour batter into prepared pan. Pour apple filling on top of blondie batter and spread to cover evenly.

6. Bake for 35–45 minutes until golden brown. The sides on the blondies will start to pull away from the sides of the pan.

7. Allow blondies to cool for 1 hour before adding glaze.

8. In a small bowl, stir together the glaze ingredients until smooth. Drizzle glaze on top of warm blondies.

9. Remove blondies from the pan by carefully lifting them up with the parchment paper. Refrigerate in an airtight container up to 3 days.

Peanut Butter Blossoms

These classic cookies got a gluten- and dairy-free makeover so you won't miss out on them! Although the traditional Hershey's Kisses are gluten-free, they are not dairy-free. Don't worry, because this recipe has a homemade chocolate filling that has all the flavor of the traditional cookie.

MAKES 36 COOKIES

Per Serving:

Calories	125
Fat	5g
Protein	2g
Sodium	85mg
Fiber	1g
Carbohydrates	15g
Sugar	10g

COOKIES

½ cup granulated sugar

½ cup light brown sugar, packed

½ cup dairy-free buttery spread

½ cup gluten-free peanut butter

1 large egg

1 teaspoon molasses

1¼ cups gluten-free all-purpose flour with xanthan gum

¾ teaspoon baking soda

½ teaspoon gluten-free baking powder

¼ cup granulated sugar for rolling

DAIRY-FREE CHOCOLATE PEANUT BUTTER FILLING

¾ cup gluten-free peanut butter

4 tablespoons cocoa powder

1 tablespoon pure vanilla extract

¾ cup confectioners' sugar

5 tablespoons unsweetened almond milk

1 In a large bowl, beat together granulated sugar, brown sugar, buttery spread, and peanut butter at medium speed until fully combined and creamy. Mix in egg and molasses until combined.

2 In a medium bowl, stir together flour, baking soda, and baking powder.

3 Slowly pour the flour mixture into batter and mix until fully combined. The cookie dough will be like soft Play-Doh.

4 Cover cookie dough and refrigerate for 30 minutes.

5 Preheat oven to 375°F and line two baking sheets with parchment paper. Add ¼ cup granulated sugar to a small bowl. Scoop tablespoonfuls of dough and roll into balls with your hands. Roll balls in granulated sugar and place onto prepared baking sheets.

6 Bake for 10–12 minutes or until light brown on the edges.

7 As soon as you bring cookies out of the oven, use the back of a rounded teaspoon to make an indent in the center of the cookie. Allow cookies to cool for 2–3 minutes before moving to a cooling rack. Cool completely before adding filling.

8 In a large bowl, mix together the peanut butter, cocoa powder, and vanilla extract until fully combined. Add confectioners' sugar and mix until combined. Add milk and mix until smooth. Either pipe or spoon filling into the centers of cookies. Store in an airtight container at room temperature for up to 3 days.

Weekly Meal Plans

	M	T	W	T	F	S	S
Week 1							
Breakfast	Easy Blueberry Banana Muffins (Chapter 2)	Breakfast Burritos (Chapter 2)	Banana Chocolate Peanut Butter Overnight Oats (Chapter 2)	Southern Buttermilk Biscuits (Chapter 8)	Fluffy Homemade Pancakes (Chapter 2)	Double Chocolate Muffins (Chapter 2)	Homestyle Waffles (Chapter 2)
Lunch	Asian Chicken Lettuce Wraps (Chapter 3)	Grilled Chicken Caesar Salad (Chapter 3)	Southwest Tricolored Quinoa Salad (Chapter 3)	Egg Roll Bowl (Chapter 3)	Loaded Burger Bowls (Chapter 3)	Grilled Chicken Chimichurri Salad (Chapter 3)	Greek Chicken Wraps (Chapter 3) with Flatbread (Chapter 8)
Dinner	Crispy Salmon Cakes (Chapter 6) with Baked Sweet Potato Fries (Chapter 7)	Mongolian Beef (Chapter 5) with Sautéed Garlic Green Beans (Chapter 7)	Crispy Baked Chicken Thighs (Chapter 4) with Italian Roasted Vegetables (Chapter 7)	Fish Tacos (Chapter 6) with Southwestern Black Bean and Corn Salad (Chapter 7)	Asian Apricot Chicken (Chapter 4) with Easy Rice Pilaf (Chapter 7)	Oven-Baked St. Louis–Style Ribs (Chapter 5) with Loaded Bacon Ranch Potato Salad (Chapter 7)	Prime Rib (Chapter 5) with Balsamic-Roasted Brussels Sprouts (Chapter 7)
Dessert	Chocolate Chip Cookies (Chapter 12)	Apple Crisp (Chapter 12)	Fudgy Brownies (Chapter 12)	Butter Pound Cake (Chapter 12)	Cinnamon Roll Cake (Chapter 12)	Coconut Cream Pie (Chapter 12)	Easy Gluten-Free Chocolate Cake with Chocolate Buttercream Frosting (Chapter 12)

Week 2

	M	T	W	T	F	S	S
Breakfast	Easy Apple Cinnamon Crumb Muffins (Chapter 2)	Western Frittata (Chapter 2)	Chocolate Cake Donuts (Chapter 2)	Tater Tot Breakfast Casserole (Chapter 2)	Breakfast Cookies (Chapter 2)	Cinnamon Roll French Toast Casserole (Chapter 2)	Crepes (Chapter 2)
Lunch	Creamy Italian Pasta Salad (Chapter 3)	Southern Chicken Salad (Chapter 3)	Crispy Southwest Wraps (Chapter 3)	Soy Ginger Vegetable Stir-Fry (Chapter 3)	Tuna Salad Avocado Bowls (Chapter 3)	Deep-Dish Pizza Bites (Chapter 10)	Taco Salad (Chapter 3)
Dinner	Pecan-Crusted Honey Mustard Salmon (Chapter 6) with Roasted Garlic Potatoes (Chapter 7)	Pork Tenderloin (Chapter 5) with Savory Stuffing (Chapter 7)	Swedish Meatballs (Chapter 5) with Honey-Glazed Carrots (Chapter 7)	Taco Soup (Chapter 9) with Southern Sweet Corn Bread (Chapter 8)	Chicken Piccata (Chapter 4) with Garlic Breadsticks (Chapter 8)	Pressure Cooker Corned Beef and Cabbage (Chapter 11)	Chicken and Dumplings (Chapter 5) with Pressure Cooker Mashed Potatoes (Chapter 11)
Dessert	Fluffy Sugar Cookies (Chapter 12)	Apple Bundt Cake (Chapter 12)	Hummingbird Cake with Cream Cheese Frosting (Chapter 12)	Cowboy Cookies (Chapter 12)	Pineapple Upside Down Cake (Chapter 12)	Dutch Apple Pie (Chapter 12)	White Cake with Almond Vanilla Buttercream (Chapter 12)

STANDARD **US/METRIC** MEASUREMENT CONVERSIONS

VOLUME CONVERSIONS

US Volume Measure	Metric Equivalent
⅛ teaspoon	0.5 milliliter
¼ teaspoon	1 milliliter
½ teaspoon	2 milliliters
1 teaspoon	5 milliliters
½ tablespoon	7 milliliters
1 tablespoon (3 teaspoons)	15 milliliters
2 tablespoons (1 fluid ounce)	30 milliliters
¼ cup (4 tablespoons)	60 milliliters
⅓ cup	90 milliliters
½ cup (4 fluid ounces)	125 milliliters
⅔ cup	160 milliliters
¾ cup (6 fluid ounces)	180 milliliters
1 cup (16 tablespoons)	250 milliliters
1 pint (2 cups)	500 milliliters
1 quart (4 cups)	1 liter (about)

WEIGHT CONVERSIONS

US Weight Measure	Metric Equivalent
½ ounce	15 grams
1 ounce	30 grams
2 ounces	60 grams
3 ounces	85 grams
¼ pound (4 ounces)	115 grams
½ pound (8 ounces)	225 grams
¾ pound (12 ounces)	340 grams
1 pound (16 ounces)	454 grams

OVEN TEMPERATURE CONVERSIONS

Degrees Fahrenheit	Degrees Celsius
200 degrees F	95 degrees C
250 degrees F	120 degrees C
275 degrees F	135 degrees C
300 degrees F	150 degrees C
325 degrees F	160 degrees C
350 degrees F	180 degrees C
375 degrees F	190 degrees C
400 degrees F	205 degrees C
425 degrees F	220 degrees C
450 degrees F	230 degrees C

BAKING PAN SIZES

American	Metric
8 × 1½ inch round baking pan	20 × 4 cm cake tin
9 × 1½ inch round baking pan	23 × 3.5 cm cake tin
11 × 7 × 1½ inch baking pan	28 × 18 × 4 cm baking tin
13 × 9 × 2 inch baking pan	30 × 20 × 5 cm baking tin
2 quart rectangular baking dish	30 × 20 × 3 cm baking tin
15 × 10 × 2 inch baking pan	30 × 25 × 2 cm baking tin (Swiss roll tin)
9 inch pie plate	22 × 4 or 23 × 4 cm pie plate
7 or 8 inch springform pan	18 or 20 cm springform or loose bottom cake tin
9 × 5 × 3 inch loaf pan	23 × 13 × 7 cm or 2 lb narrow loaf or pate tin
1½ quart casserole	1.5 liter casserole
2 quart casserole	2 liter casserole

Index